Oral health of Australian children

This book is available as a free fully-searchable ebook from

www.adelaide.edu.au/press

Oral health of Australian children

The National Child Oral Health Study 2012–14

Edited by

Loc G. Do and A. John Spencer

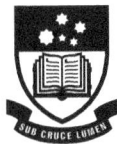

THE UNIVERSITY
of ADELAIDE

UNIVERSITY OF
ADELAIDE PRESS

Published in Adelaide by

University of Adelaide Press
Barr Smith Library
The University of Adelaide
South Australia 5005
press@adelaide.edu.au
www.adelaide.edu.au/press

The University of Adelaide Press publishes externally refereed scholarly
books by staff of the University of Adelaide. It aims to maximise access to
the University's best research by publishing works through the internet as
free downloads and for sale as high quality printed volumes.

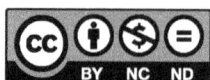

For the full Cataloguing-in-Publication data please contact the National
Library of Australia: cip@nla.gov.au

ISBN (paperback) 978-1-925261-40-0
ISBN (ebook: PDF): 978-1-925261-41-7
DOI: http://dx.doi.org/10.20851/ncohs

Editors: Ali White and Julia Keller
Cover design: Emma Spoehr
Cover image: © iStockphoto
Paperback printed by Griffin Press, South Australia

Contributors

Authors

Najith Amarasena, Australian Research Centre for Population Oral Health, The University of Adelaide, SA, Australia

Jason Armfield, Australian Research Centre for Population Oral Health, The University of Adelaide, SA, Australia

Peter Arrow, Australian Research Centre for Population Oral Health, The University of Adelaide, SA, Australia & Dental Health Services, Department of Health, Western Australia

David Brennan, Australian Research Centre for Population Oral Health, The University of Adelaide, SA, Australia

Sergio Chrisopoulos, Australian Research Centre for Population Oral Health, The University of Adelaide, SA, Australia

Loc Do, Australian Research Centre for Population Oral Health, The University of Adelaide, SA, Australia

Martin Dooland, Australian Research Centre for Population Oral Health, The University of Adelaide, SA, Australia

Anne Ellershaw, Australian Research Centre for Population Oral Health, The University of Adelaide, SA, Australia

Diep Ha, Australian Research Centre for Population Oral Health, The University of Adelaide, SA, Australia

Jane Harford, Australian Research Centre for Population Oral Health, The University of Adelaide, SA, Australia

Lisa Jamieson, Australian Research Centre for Population Oral Health, The University of Adelaide, SA, Australia

Xiangqun Ju, Australian Research Centre for Population Oral Health, The University of Adelaide, SA, Australia

Kostas Kapellas, Australian Research Centre for Population Oral Health, The University of Adelaide, SA, Australia

Carmen Koster, Australian Research Centre for Population Oral Health, The University of Adelaide, SA, Australia

Liana Luzzi, Australian Research Centre for Population Oral Health, The University of Adelaide, SA, Australia

Gloria Mejia, formerly Australian Research Centre for Population Oral Health, The University of Adelaide, SA, Australia

Karen Peres, Australian Research Centre for Population Oral Health, The University of Adelaide, SA, Australia

Marco Peres, Australian Research Centre for Population Oral Health, The University of Adelaide, SA, Australia

Kaye Roberts-Thomson, Australian Research Centre for Population Oral Health, The University of Adelaide, SA, Australia

A John Spencer, Australian Research Centre for Population Oral Health, The University of Adelaide, SA, Australia

Administrative personnel

Rose Thomas, Australian Research Centre for Population Oral Health, The University of Adelaide, SA, Australia

Ali White, Australian Research Centre for Population Oral Health, The University of Adelaide, SA, Australia

Acknowledgements

Collaborating state and territory health departments

New South Wales Health, Centre for Oral Health Strategy

Victorian Department of Human Services, Dental Health Unit

Queensland Health, Oral Health Unit

South Australian Dental Service

Western Australian Dental Health Services

Tasmanian Health Services, Oral Health Services

Australian Capital Territory, Community Health Dental Program

Northern Territory Health, Health Development and Oral Health Section

Funding sources for the 2012–14 National Child Oral Health Study

National Health and Medical Research Council, Partnership Grant # APP1016326.

State and Territory Health Departments.

Colgate Palmolive

The Australian Dental Association

Steering Committee

Emeritus Professor A John Spencer (co-chair)

Associate Professor Loc G Do (co-chair)

Professor Kaye Roberts-Thomson

Professor David Brennan

Dr Gloria Mejia

Dr Martin Dooland

Professor Fredrick Wright

Mr Andrew McAuliffe

Preface

Dental caries (tooth decay) is the most common oral disease and among the most prevalent health conditions in Australian children. It is therefore not surprising that child oral health is never out of sight of those concerned with health and health care delivery in Australia. Fortunately, research continues to shed light on the biological mechanisms of tooth decay and reveal more opportunities to intervene to improve oral health.

Improvement in children's oral health is needed for two simple reasons. First, oral diseases, mainly tooth decay, cause infection, discomfort, pain and suffering for the child and affect the family through those distressing symptoms and the burden of costly and sometimes difficult treatment. Second, poor oral health early in life is the strongest predictor of further oral disease in adult life. Effective treatments are sometimes scarce and can be expensive, affecting patient access.

For more than 60 years Australia has pursued measures to reduce or prevent tooth decay in children. The National Health and Medical Research Council (NHMRC), with its core membership that includes the leading public health officials from all States and Territories, has provided advice in support of public water fluoridation since 1952. Australia first introduced water fluoridation in 1953 and since then has achieved one of the highest population coverage rates when compared to similar countries. An internationally recognised Australian study in the 1960s reported on the effectiveness of fluoridated toothpaste in preventing and minimising caries. The combination of water fluoridation as a public health intervention and the use of fluoridated toothpaste as an individual action (used so widely as to mimic a population health initiative) has transformed child oral health. Compared to the 1950s, the prevalence of caries in children has more than halved and the number of teeth with caries has decreased by about 90%.

Access to dental services, prompt diagnosis and early treatment are key to limiting the impact of children's poor oral health. Those dental services can also help prevent oral disease. Australia has seen decades of mixed public and private delivery of childhood dental services, and this varies considerably across States and Territories. Access to dental services is still a challenging issue and developing evidence-based policy is now both vital and timely.

Most of what we currently know about child oral health has come from surveys of school dental services. In order to get a better picture to inform improvements in policy, it became increasingly important to document oral health in the wider population and to explore which children experience poorer oral health.

NHMRC's work focuses on fostering the creation of knowledge and improving standards of individual and public health throughout Australia. NHMRC funding is directed to the highest quality health and medical research which then contributes to the evidence base for sound policy and practices, in oral health and other fields, through its translation into health advice or guidelines.

NHMRC's research funding mechanisms have supported this extensive population-based study of child oral health and the use of dental services in Australia. The study was conducted as a Partnership Project, with researchers at The University of Adelaide and in every state and territory health authority.

The Partnerships Projects Scheme is a highly effective NHMRC funding scheme that reflects the real world by guaranteeing true connections between researchers and health practitioners or policy makers. These partnerships ensure that important issues identified by those delivering services or drafting Australian health policy are jointly examined by researchers and their partners. In this particular study, the state and territory health authorities brought their connections and opportunities to the table in their partnership with The University of Adelaide researchers.

The outcome of this partnership is a study where considerable effort has been made to ensure the quality and depth of data collected. Trends in child oral health, especially tooth decay and dental fluorosis, as well as preventive dental behaviours and the use of dental services, are presented. The resulting dataset will support extensive further investigation, including special analyses of Aboriginal and Torres Strait Islander child oral health and preventive dental behaviours.

The contributors to this book are research academics who are interested in oral health at both the individual and population level and the collected materials reflect their multidisciplinary approach. The book provides valuable perspectives on child oral health and how to improve it, including the role of dental services. I imagine that it will be appreciated by health authorities, academics, and dental practitioners.

Importantly, this book presents a national resource and seeks to maximise the opportunity to explore and learn about child oral health. Since 2013, NHMRC has been an active advocate of improving access to research and health data for the purpose of improving the quality of research and its translation, and, in so doing, improve health outcomes for all Australians. The range and quality of data within this resource will contribute to that goal.

The complexities of childhood oral disease and adult oral health described in this book provide some context for NHMRC's long history in recommending public water fluoridation. At the time of publishing, NHMRC is revising the evidence that underpins our 60-year history of recommending this public health intervention to prevent or minimise tooth decay.

On behalf of NHMRC, I congratulate the research partners in the nationally significant study that underpins *Oral health of Australian children: The National Child Oral Health Study 2012–14*. I welcome this publication and all that it offers those working to improve the oral health of Australian children, adolescents and adults.

Professor Anne Kelso AO

Chief Executive Officer

National Health and Medical Research Council

December 2016

Executive Summary

LG Do and AJ Spencer

The key challenges in child oral health in Australia are the ongoing population burden of childhood oral diseases for society and the affected individuals and the substantial proportion of children with an unfavourable pattern of use of dental services. There is a need to respond by improving population and individual-level prevention of oral diseases, the organisation and delivery of dental services that put children with better oral health and a favourable pattern of dental care.

The ultimate purpose of this collaborative work is to describe and interpret the findings on oral health and dental behaviours and practices of Australian children so as to stimulate discussion about how to meet the abovementioned challenges. This work is the first national project in Australia since the late 1980s investigating child oral health as well as its associated factors.

The 2012–14 National Child Oral Health Study (NCOHS) was a cross-sectional study of the child population aged 5–14 years in Australia. A total of 24,664 children aged 5 to 14 years from 841 participating schools completed the study. The study sample was selected in a complex multistage, stratified sampling design. Sophisticated weighting procedure was employed to take into account potential variations in probabilities of selection and response rates. Therefore, this report presents estimates as representative of child oral health in Australia.

This collaborative work provides a detailed 'snapshot' of child oral health in Australia. In doing so, it describes the levels of dental caries and its components, dental fluorosis and other oral health conditions. It also describes the other protective factors such as toothbrushing and the use of fluoridated toothpastes. The use of dental services by children so as to manage existing oral disease and to contribute to the prevention of dental caries are detailed. Important information of the patterns of dietary intake that might impact on child oral health are presented. The report describes patterns of oral health status and behaviours of a nationally representative sample of Indigenous children. Further, socioeconomic inequalities in child oral health and behaviours are examined. Finally, the report presents information on child oral health using frameworks that emphasise variation by the socioeconomic characteristics of children's households and their reported pattern of dental service use across Australian states and territories.

Child oral health

Dental caries

Dental caries is the most prevalent and important oral disease in Australian children.

- There has been small improvement in dental caries experience in the primary dentition since the 1987–88 National Oral Health Survey. During the same period, dental caries experience in the permanent dentition has been substantially improved.

- Just over 40% of children aged 5–10 years had experienced caries in their primary teeth. On average, children had 1.5 primary teeth with caries experience. However, over one-quarter of children aged 5–10 years had untreated dental caries in their primary dentition.

- Just under one-quarter of children aged 6–14 years had experienced caries in their permanent teeth with an average of 0.5 teeth per child. Over one in ten children aged 6–14 years had untreated dental caries in their permanent teeth.

- Dental caries experience in both primary and permanent dentitions clustered among a small proportion of the population. Some 20% of 5–10-year-old children and 17% of 11–14-year-old children had over 80% of the total population burden of dental caries in the primary dentition and permanent dentition respectively.

Childhood caries experience showed reasonably consistent social patterning.

- Caries experience and its components were consistently higher among children from households where parents had less education and low income. There were also variations by Indigenous identity and residential location.

- The social patterning by the abovementioned factors was particularly strong for indicators of untreated dental caries and tooth loss because of dental caries.

Social patterning in dental caries experience

Individual and area-level socioeconomic factors have strong and consistent association with indicators of caries experience in Australian children. Such patterning points to the role of social factors as determinants of dental caries and use of dental services in the population.

Caries experience of Australian children was examined across all states and territories.

- There were significant variations in the prevalence and severity of dental caries across states and territories.

- Northern Territory and Queensland had consistently higher indicators of caries experience than the national average. Children in those two jurisdictions were more likely to have dental caries as well as greater severity of the disease.

Dental fluorosis

Australia's guidelines on the use of fluorides have given primacy to the continued fluoridation of water supplies between 0.6 and 1.1 mg/L water depending on climate. The actual population exposure is set to achieve a near maximal reduction in dental caries without an unacceptable level of dental fluorosis. Fluoridated toothpaste is recommended for use by young children from the age of 18 months. Both water fluoridation and toothpaste use are associated with an increase in the prevalence of any fluorosis.

This is the first ever national snapshot of the prevalence and severity of dental fluorosis in Australian children.

- Any fluorosis (a TF score of 1+) was found to have a prevalence of 16.8% (95%CI: 15.5–18.1).
- A small percentage (0.9% (95%CI: 0.7–1.1)) of children had more definitive dental fluorosis (having a TF 3+ score). Very few children were observed with moderate to severe dental fluorosis (TF scores of 4 or 5).

Dental care

Access to dental care is a major policy issue in Australia. This report has focussed on Australian children's first visit to a dental provider and their current visiting behaviour.

There is variation among dental authorities on the recommended age at which a child should make their first dental visit. Some dental professional groups have recommended that a child should make their first visit soon after the eruption of their first teeth. Public health groups have recommended that a child make a dental visit before 2 years of age. However, previous research has shown that many children do not make a dental visit before the commencement of school. It is for this reason that this report has documented the proportion of children who have made their first visit at 5 years of age or younger.

- Just over 57% of children have made a visit before the age of 5 years.
- This percentage was higher for children in households where the parents had higher education and income and lower among Indigenous children and children who made their last dental visit for a dental problem.
- This percentage also varied across states and territories.
- One in ten children aged 5–14 years had never made a dental visit. This percentage was one in four among children aged 5–6 years.
- There were significant gradients in the percentage of children never having a dental visit by parental education and income.
- This percentage was lower in states and territories where school dental service had greater coverage.

It is recommended to have regular dental visits. However, a proportion of the population still reported irregular dental visiting patterns.

- Just over one-fifth of the children had an irregular visiting pattern.
- This proportion was higher among those children from households where parents had less education or low income. It was also higher among those children whose reason for their last dental visit was a dental problem.

Place of dental visit was dependent on availability and affordability of dental services which vary across jurisdictions.

- Over 56% of Australian children who had ever made a dental visit last attended private dental services. The remaining proportion made their last dental visit at public dental services, which was dominated by school dental services.
- The use of private dental services was socially patterned with a lower percentage of parents with less education and low income reporting that their child last visited a private practice.
- The percentage of children visiting a private dental practice varied greatly across states and territories. This percentage was highest in NSW and Victoria and lowest in Northern Territory and Tasmania.

Dental service use

- A high proportion of children who had never visited a dental provider by the age of 5–6 years highlighted the substantial change required in dental visiting early in a child's life.

- Although the proportion of children with irregular dental visiting was not high, this is a difficult group to access and to modify their behaviour. This creates a policy challenge in that these children are not readily identified and targeted.

- Regardless of whether parents seek care for their child through the school dental services or private practices, there needs to be an active management of each child's frequency of visiting. This is required to reduce or eliminate that percentage of children who have unacceptable periods of no visiting and who exist largely outside the dental system. There needs to be stronger recognition of the desirability of varying the frequency of visits according to risk of disease.

Several clinical preventive services have well-established efficacy. These include fissure sealants. The efficacy of dental sealants is high if they are applied to a tooth soon after its eruption into the mouth.

- Only 27% of children aged 6–14 years had one or more sealants and, on average, only 1.0 permanent molars had a sealant placed among all Australian children.

- The use of fissure sealants was an in-office preventive measure which varied substantially across states and territories.

Dental health behaviours

- Approximately one-third of children reportedly commenced toothbrushing with fluoridated toothpaste before 18 months of age.

- Over one-quarter of children reportedly commenced toothbrushing with fluoridated toothpaste after the age of 30 months.

It is recommended that children's teeth be cleaned (wiped or brushed) from the time of the eruption of teeth, but that toothpaste be introduced at 18 months of age. Late commencement of toothpaste use (after age 30 months) is not recommended.

- Children in families whose parents have higher educational attainment and income have a higher likelihood of early use of toothpaste. Indigenous children and children whose parents were born overseas and children who made their last dental visit for a problem have a higher likelihood of delayed use of toothpaste.

Regular toothbrushing daily is important in maintaining oral health.

- Nearly half of the children were reported to brush their teeth the recommended twice a day.
- Brushing twice a day was more common among those children in households where the parents had higher levels of education or income and living in major cities, but lower among Indigenous children or children whose last dental visit was for a dental problem.

Dental health behaviours

- The issue of the balance of prevention of caries and dental fluorosis is an important matter in Australia. Consideration might be given to a campaign to inform parents about the Australian guidelines for the use of fluorides, including toothpaste.

- There is a compelling argument for giving priority to actions to improve child oral health that are more universal, i.e. reach large numbers of children, are more passive, i.e. require little individual effort, and are more proportionate, i.e. benefit mostly those with the greatest burden of oral disease. While this might start with water fluoridation, it needs to be combined with actions at other levels which are consistent with the criteria for improving child oral health.

General health behaviours

General health behaviours are not only important for overall health but also for dental health. These behaviours include consumption of tap water and sugar-containing foods and beverages. Consumption of the former provides necessary exposure to fluoride while consumption of the latter increases risk for dental caries and other general health conditions.

- While most children consumed tap water, over one-quarter of children consumed some bottled water. This was higher among children whose parents had lower education or lower income.
- Almost one-fifth of Australian children drank four or more glasses of sugar-sweetened beverages in a usual day. Almost half of Australian children had four or more serves of sugar-containing snacks in a usual day. Inverse socioeconomic gradients in this level of sugary consumption were substantial.

General health behaviours

A sizeable proportion of Australian children were likely to exceed the recommended daily sugar intake from foods and drinks. Some children also consumed bottled water which does not contain fluoride. The social patterning in these health behaviours was a further concern.

Overall

Despite some improvement, child oral health has remained a significant population health issue in Australia in the 21st Century. The evidence documented in this book has pointed to substantial inverse social patterning of oral health status, dental service use, dental and general behaviours among Australian children.

The identification of the numerous factors and the relation between them at an individual child, family, school and community level poses both difficulties and opportunities for programs to improve child oral health and reduce social inequalities in child oral health.

1 Children's oral health — assessing and improving oral health

AJ Spencer and LG Do

Being orally healthy means that people can eat, speak and socialise without discomfort or embarrassment and without active disease in their mouth which affects their overall wellbeing (UK Department of Health 1994). Australians of all ages have an expectation of being orally healthy, but this is particularly relevant to children. Children constitute a special population group requiring attention and consideration because of the importance of maximising the opportunities of childhood as a key developmental stage and the foreshadowing of later adult oral health and wellbeing.

There are two highly prevalent oral diseases and disorders affecting the teeth and their supporting tissues: dental caries (decay) and periodontal diseases (gum disease). There are a number of less frequently occurring but nonetheless important oral diseases of the oral mucosa as well as disorders such as developmental defects, dental impactions, malocclusions, tooth wear, jaw joint dysfunction and dental and oral trauma (AHMAC, Steering Committee for National Planning for Oral Health 2001). Among children, dental caries, early stage periodontal disease (gingivitis), and developmental defects like dental fluorosis, oral mucosal lesions and trauma, are the most frequent and impacting oral diseases and disorders. These conditions severally and collectively cause pain and discomfort, eating difficulties, speech and cognition dysfunction, embarrassment and social marginalisation. These impacts are no different to the impacts of many other diseases and ill-health. Just as the mouth is an integral part of the body, oral health is an essential component of overall child health and quality of life.

1.1 Risks and prevention of dental caries

Among children, dental caries is the leading oral disease. It has high prevalence and associated high impact on children and their families. Its presence dominates the need for dental services and the cost of them both to families and society.

Historically, Australian children have experienced a high level of oral disease. In the immediate post-WW2 period, Australian children had one of the highest levels of dental caries among comparable developed countries (Barnard 1956). By the 1990 decade Australia's child oral health surveillance had reported a marked improvement in experience of dental caries. However, in the last two decades, the improvement in oral health of Australian children has ceased or even reversed (Armfield et al. 2010).

Whilst dental caries is mostly preventable, it remains the most common form of childhood infection, resulting in costly treatment and having an adverse impact on quality of life (Casamassimo et al. 2009). Dental caries among Australian children remains a significant health issue which creates burdens on the individual, the family and the community (NACOH 2004).

The underlying risk behaviours for dental caries have remained largely unchanged: Australians have a high per capita consumption of sugars (Australian Bureau of Statistics 2016). The form in which those sugars are consumed has changed but free sugar consumption remains high, well in excess of the recently announced recommendations by the World Health Organization (World Health Organization 2015). Toothbrushing practices are varied (Armfield & Spencer 2012) and the resulting removal of dental plaque is incomplete. Little improvement in the mechanics of toothbrushing has occurred, leaving the outcome one of plaque control rather than plaque removal. As a result, the fundamental aetiological factors for dental caries, sugars and dental plaques remain commonplace in the population.

What has changed is the possibility of counter-balancing the risk behaviours associated with dental caries with effective population preventive programs. Some 60 years of research has led to the development and implementation of two key population preventive programs: water fluoridation and the widespread and regular use of fluoridated toothpaste. Water fluoridation is a safe and effective public health program (National Health and Medical Research Council 2007). First introduced in Australia in 1953, its population coverage grew over the next few decades to reach two-thirds of the Australian population (Spencer 1984). More recently in the 2000 decade onwards, population coverage gain increased and has re-stabilised at around 90% coverage (NSW 2013). Fluoridated toothpaste was introduced into the Australian oral care product market in the early 1970s. Its penetration into homes grew rapidly and fluoridated toothpaste is used by most people. While fluoridated toothpaste is strictly an individual behaviour its widespread use mimics a population measure. Its efficacy is well established and has changed little over time. Although various aspects of its formulation have changed, this has generally not been in the key caries prevention component, fluoride.

The gains made in child dental caries in Australia are generally accepted to be largely as a result of the extensive water fluoridation programs and use of fluoridated toothpaste. However, such programs have been reasonably stable for many years. Where certain circumstances exist, continued risk behaviours can dominate, overwhelming preventive activities that may be present in varying degrees, resulting in experience of caries. So despite improvements, dental caries remains one of the most prevalent chronic diseases in children. For example, the prevalence of dental caries in permanent teeth in 6–15-year-old Australian children in 2004 was 36.3% (Armfield et al. 2007) whereas the prevalence of the most frequent general health condition, asthma, was 15.7% in 2001 (Australian Institute of Health and Welfare 2005).

Children's experience of dental caries is strongly age-related. At the beginning of school, at age 5–6 years, a little more than half of the children have had experience of caries in their primary/deciduous (baby) teeth with an average of two teeth with decay experience. At the end of primary school, at age 12 years, most primary teeth have exfoliated and the successor and additional posterior permanent (adult) teeth have erupted.

A little less than half of all children have had some experience of caries in their permanent teeth, but on average they have experienced only one tooth with decay. However, the distribution of decay experience at both ages is uneven. Many children have no or very low experience of decay, while a small minority have experienced much higher levels of decay.

The circumstances where risk can overwhelm prevention tend to be socially patterned. Caries prevalence and severity is unevenly distributed across social groups formed by educational level of parents or household income. Therefore, socioeconomic inequality in child oral health exists. Worryingly there is evidence that inequality in caries in children has widened in the decade between 1992/93 and 2002/03 (Do et al. 2010).

Numerous challenges exist in further reducing dental caries among Australian children. The two longstanding preventive approaches require further attention. About 10% of the Australian population live in areas without water fluoridation. Those reticulated water supplies currently not fluoridated should be the target of policy to assist them in fluoridating. Families without access to fluoridated water supplies need guidance on how to provide fluoride via other mechanisms. Both sugars in the diet and toothbrushing are individual behaviours shaped in the family and by the context in which those families live, work, and play. Not only is guidance needed for families on sugar consumption and toothbrushing practices, appropriate behaviour needs to be promoted. Successful promotion of healthy behaviours requires a mix of incentives and disincentives operating at the individual, family and community levels. While the oral care products industry has played a vital role thus far in shaping toothbrushing behaviours, more nuanced messages need to be promulgated in order for more Australian children to comply with current guidelines. Altering Australians consumption of sugars, especially to meet WHO recommendations about the percentage of energy derived from the consumption of free sugars, is only in its infancy as a health target. Those with an interest in oral health must work together with other health groups to develop and implement policy that will bring about such a change.

1.2 Describing and understanding child oral health

Several levels of activity have been involved in describing and understanding child oral health in Australia. Surveillance on child oral health that is ongoing collection of core indicators of child oral health has been conducted in Australia since 1977 through the state and territory school or community dental services. This time-series information has provided a robust picture of the trends in child oral health. Its ongoing collection also provides an early warning of any change in child oral health. However, there has been a decrease in the reach of the state and territory school or community dental services and information derived from these services is presented with the caveat that it represents only the users of those dental services. The picture of child oral health from those data is likely to be socially biased, but the extent of that bias is difficult to assess as Australia has rather little population survey data on child oral health with which to compare.

So another level of activity needed is periodic population surveys. The Australian National Oral Health Plans call for periodic population oral health surveys of child and adult oral health, alternating between a focus on children and adults (NACOH2004; OHMG 2016). The National Survey of Adult Oral Health (NSAOH) was conducted across 2004–06 by the Australian Research Centre for Population Oral Health (ARCPOH) at The University of Adelaide and the state and territory public dental services (Slade et al. 2007). The National Oral Health Plans call for a national survey of child oral health some five years later. Unlike surveillance activity such national surveys are built around population samples and the collection of extensive information on the social circumstances of participants, preventive and risk behaviours, and dental visiting. Nowadays such national surveys include a combination of oral epidemiologic (clinical) and self-reported oral health indicators.

A further level of activity is observational research on child oral health. Such research is distinguished from surveys per se by the presence of specific hypotheses that drive aspects of the information collected and the analyses performed. However, research hypotheses can also be embedded into survey procedures, greatly increasing the usefulness of the survey information. A complete description of child oral health and the continued development of our understanding of risk and protective factors require all three activities: surveillance, population surveys and observational research.

1.3   The role of dental services in child oral health

Dental services have an increasing potency in eliminating pain and discomfort, resolving infection, and restoring form and function for those with oral disease (Spencer 2012). Dental services have never been more able to provide high quality dental care. Therefore, it is natural to extrapolate from the sophistication and observed benefits of individual dental care to a presumed efficacy in the prevention of oral diseases including caries for the population. The repeated recurrence of caries across most individuals' life while regularly using dental services is the starkest evidence of the difficulty dental services have in 'curing' people from caries. If the evidence of individual cure is scant, then attribution of achievement in reducing a substantial proportion of caries in populations is misplaced.

In general, dental services are attributable for only modest variation in caries at a population level because:

- clinical preventive dental services have only a moderate strength of association with caries prevention; and,
- population exposure to clinical preventive dental services is far from universal.

Limited coverage shrinks the population preventive benefit that can be attributed to clinical services (Tugwell et al. 1984; Fletcher et al. 1988; Rockhill, Kawachi & Colditz 2000; Rockhill 2005; Rockhill, Newman & Weinberg 2008). There is a need to refocus attention on how to achieve improvements in population coverage with a favourable pattern of use of dental services, provision of appropriate clinical preventive services and the efficacy of those clinical preventive services to prevent caries, especially in children.

Clinical preventive services cannot be brought to bear on a child's caries risk unless there is a sustained favourable pattern of use of dental services. Use of dental services is an individual decision; however, the structural and procedural features of the dental services system shape the likelihood of favourable use of dental services (Arnljot et al. 1987). Further, favourable use begets future decisions to continue in such a pattern of use. Therefore, the features of the dental services system are vitally important to optimising the provision of clinical preventive services.

A substantial level of resources, approximately one billion dollars annually, is being directed to dental services for children (aged 0–17 years) in Australia. Of the $6.1 billion spent on dental care in Australia in 2007–08, it is estimated that 22% was for dental services for children aged 5–17 years (Australian Institute of Health and Welfare 2007).

Australia in the early 1970s implemented the Australian School Dental Scheme. This Scheme was to be a universal, free, school-based and largely provided by dental therapists. The Scheme expanded rapidly until 1981 when it reverted to being the responsibility of states and territories (Biggs 2008). The following years have seen spasmodic and varied policy around children's use of dental services. Federal policy on private health insurance, including dental insurance, and specific subsidies like the Teen Dental Plan, a voucher scheme predominantly for private dentistry, then more recently the Child Dental Benefits Scheme with its Medicare Australia administered payment to private and public providers of dental services to children, have characterised the varied national context for use of dental services.

The proportion of children reporting making a dental visit in a year grew rapidly in the 1970s under the Australian School Dental Scheme (ASDS) (Spencer & Brown 1986). Early growth of the infrastructure for the school dental services saw services directed to areas and schools at greater disadvantage in accessing dental services. Visiting was institutionalised and on set rosters. Groups with previously limited access to dental services were drawn into a favourable pattern of use. However, the ASDS tied grants for capital and operating expenses for the state and territory school dental services quickly began to diminish and ceased in 1981. Thereafter federal funding for the school dental services was no longer identified within Commonwealth health grants to the states/territories (Spencer 1983).

States and territories made independent decisions on what level of support they could provide school- or community-based dental services for children. In the early 1990s some 66% of children aged 5–11 years and 47% of children aged 12–17 years indicated their last dental visit was to a SDS or public dental service (PDS). Since the mid-1990s coverage by the SDS has rapidly decreased among 5–11-year-olds and somewhat less rapidly among 12–17-year-olds. By 2008, only 40% of 5–11-year-olds and 35% of 12–17-year-olds had their last visit to the SDS/PDS (Ellershaw & Spencer 2009). The dental health system has become increasingly pluralistic with markedly different percentages of children using SDS/PDS across states and territories.

The features of the dental services system that may be associated with use of those services have been studied. Two WHO-coordinated International Collaborative Studies of Oral Health Care Systems: ICS I (Arnljot et al. 1987) and ICS II (Chen et al. 1997) were multinational studies which compared different dental service systems in order to discover the approaches that were effective in improving population oral health. The ICS I tested the hypothesis that availability, accessibility and acceptability of dental care impacted on oral health status. The ICS II broadened its aim to investigate how factors in the dental care system, the socio-environmental characteristics and individual characteristics, affected oral health behaviours and status and oral health-related quality of life. Despite a limitation in lack of comparable data quality between countries, these two studies had an effect on the oral health policy of some participating countries.

The underlying concept of the ICS is highly applicable to current Australia because such a multi-system situation resembles the situation between and within Australian state/territories. Yet this natural laboratory on the dental system effects on child oral health has been little studied.

One of the few studies to compare effectiveness of private and public settings for dental services in Australia revealed rather unexpected results (Gaughwin et al. 1999). After controlling for other factors children who visited both private and public services and who visited public services only, had better oral health status compared with those who made private sector visits only. The Gaughwin study was conducted only in South Australia and prior to the implementation of policies such as school dental service co-payments, private insurance rebates, Teen Dental Schemes and the like. Contemporary and larger-scale evidence is needed to further explore the effect of different system settings and policies.

State and territory dental policy has focussed on what has become for most a residual program through their school, community or public dental services. The result is considerable variation in the actual arrangements for child dental services between states and territories. Individual states and territories make decisions about allocation of general health funds to dentistry and child dental services. States and territories have been and continue to be in quite different positions in the extent of dental service infrastructure and proportions of the child population who use some form of public dental service. As a result, the organisation of dental services for children can be grouped in three broad groups by percentage of the child population who use public dental services: Low coverage in NSW and Victoria; Moderate coverage in Qld, SA, ACT and Tasmania; and, high coverage in WA and the NT. The higher the coverage the greater the involvement of more traditional school dental services. The lower the coverage the more services are provided through community or public dental services.

Increasingly, parents have had to make alternative arrangements to visit private dentists and specialists. This is something the majority of parents have successfully negotiated, with or without private health insurance.

Most children still report visiting a dental provider in the last 12 months and many have a pattern of visiting that fits well with a recommended favourable visiting pattern: visiting a known provider for a check-up at least every two years with the interval determined by individual needs (Ellershaw & Spencer 2011). However, there is a minority who do not visit at an acceptable regularity, for a check-up, or the same provider. This minority of children includes some children with no or minimal disease experience, but also some with high levels of experience of caries. The overlap of the high disease experience group and those with an unfavourable visiting pattern is only partial. Further, while membership of these groups is associated with socioeconomic circumstance, it is not tightly clustered among those of lower socioeconomic circumstances. A minority of low socioeconomic background children are members of these groups. Instead membership is spread unevenly from low through to high socioeconomic circumstance children.

A further issue in improvements in oral health through dental services is the appropriateness of the provision of clinical preventive services to individual children and the efficacy of those clinical preventive services. The push for dental services to be more focussed on 'cure' for a child with dental caries is seen within what in Australia is called 'the minimum intervention approach' to clinical services (Mount 2003; 2007), and in the worldwide interest in caries classification and management systems like ICDAS (Pitts 2004) or the Nyvad system (Nyvad et al. 1999) and risk assessment and tailored individual interventions. In terms of counselling and education we are seeing renewed enthusiasm for individual behavioural change through techniques such as motivational interviewing (Weinstein et al. 2006) and efforts to increase oral health literacy (Horowitz & Kleinman 2008).

While potentially of value to the individual, there is still questioning about whether these approaches will have any substantial influence on population oral health. What goes on in the provision of clinical dental services is the result of a negotiation between providers and individuals, influenced by a complex set of social, economic and political factors, operating at a population level. This includes the structure and processes of the dental services system. However, the 'push' in these directions supports the notion that clinical dental services can be part of the solution to prevention of caries in children and justifies a desire to learn what works and does not work in the present dental services system.

1.4 The challenges to improving child oral health

Two key policy challenges confront those concerned about child oral health. First, extending and improving the effectiveness of efforts to prevent dental caries in children. Second, organising and delivering dental services in a way that captures and services children who have an unfavourable pattern of dental visiting, and ensuring that they are provided clinical preventive services.

There is a lack of specific evidence to inform policy at a national or state and territory level to help shape new directions for policy that will achieve improved child oral health. Now is an opportune time to respond to the problem of oral health in children. There is a simultaneous interest in the problem, policy and politics surrounding oral health in children.

Oral health in children is seen as an outcome influenced by children and their families, the community and the dental health system. Therefore, we conducted a study of child oral health to evaluate the oral health outcomes associated individual, family and community characteristics, including use of dental services within and across different state and territory service delivery system models to inform policy and assist in planning future programs for the Australian child population.

The study has adopted a specific approach to the virtuous cycle of new knowledge, its transfer and translation into action through a systematic approach to the documentation, analysis of the problem and the prescription of solutions needed.

Multiple factors at an individual, family and community level are now recognised as being associated with oral health and disease. Exposure to these factors is shaped by the social context into which people are born, and in which they grow, live and work across their lifetime (Marmot 2003; 2007; 2011). Broadening our view of what shapes oral health and disease in the population brings more points of intervention into view. This includes interventions to alter the distribution in the population of risk or protective factors for oral disease, or even interventions to alter the social circumstances that shape and maintain those factors, the so-called 'causes of the causes' (Sheiham et al. 2011).

There are distinct advantages in taking the broadest view of the possible points of intervention. As our view moves from the individual to the population, less individual effort is required in bringing about change and interventions can have increasing population impact (Frieden 2010). Small shifts in the risk and protective factor balance for the many rather than for the few, what Rose referred to as the 'Preventive paradox' (Rose 1992), can provide great reward.

Individual preventive and risk behaviours among children and the social characteristics of families and community factors like water fluoridation are more commonly investigated in Australian dental research. However, dental services are also a determinant of child oral health (Fisher-Owens et al. 2007). Rather less emphasis has been placed on the dental services influence on use of dental services, mix of services received and child oral health outcomes.

Our examination of dental services has been influenced by the National Health Performance Framework (NHPC 2001) and chronic care models (Bodenheimer et al. 2002). The study has the potential to shape future policy and programs for child oral health. This includes shaping an appropriate balance on child and family behavioural change, community or population interventions, and structure and organisation of dental service delivery to children.

1.5 The purpose and specific aims of the study

The purpose of the study was to inform policy makers and dental service providers at the national and state/territory level in developing policy that extends and improves the effectiveness of efforts to prevent dental caries and shapes effective dental service delivery so as to improve child oral health.

A nationwide study was conducted that combines an oral epidemiological examination and a social survey of risk and preventive behaviours, dental service use and other determinants of oral health in line with current international standards for large-scale oral epidemiological studies.

The underlying aims of the study were:

1. To identify individual, family, community, and dental system factors associated with oral health outcomes of Australian children. Oral health outcomes included caries experience, e.g. dmfs/DMFS, as well as consequences of the way disease is managed, e.g. untreated decay, missing or filled teeth and self-rated oral health.

2. To compare oral health status of children across different aspects of the dental services system.

3. To interpret and reflect on the research findings for policy makers and dental service providers at the national and state/territory level. The research findings provide scientific evidence to enable policy makers and service providers to reform the directions being pursued to improve child oral health.

Management of the study

This study became possible through the development of a partnership with all Australian states and territories. Researchers at The University of Adelaide led the study design and data collection including sample selection, development of the questionnaire and procedures for oral epidemiologic examinations, as well as preparation of unit record files for states/territories. The University researchers provided materials and resources for training of oral epidemiological examiners who were seconded or employed by the state/territory partners. Partner states and territories managed the scheduling of examinations at a local level. Researchers at The University of Adelaide have analysed the study data. All the partners have participated in discussion on the interpretation of the findings.

1.6 Purpose of this book

The purpose of this book is to provide a descriptive 'snapshot' of child oral health in Australia. This satisfies the core information requirement out of the study. It describes the caries preventive factors such as toothbrushing, the use of fluoridated toothpastes and the use of dental services, as well as caries risk factors such as dietary exposures to sugars. It presents the information on child oral health using frameworks that emphasise variation by socioeconomic characteristics of children's households and their reported pattern of dental service use. States and territories allow 'ecological' comparisons of areas and systems.

It is not the intention of this book to present a more analytic approach to variation in child oral health. Such research activities will be reported in accompanying scientific articles published in scientific journals. However, this report provides a rich array of information on child oral health and how it varies. This information can readily be used to formulate hypotheses for future research either to be conducted by ARCPOH research staff at The University of Adelaide or by other researchers under policy on access to data. Therefore, this report also serves to document a data set that hopefully will be used extensively to investigate ways to improve child oral health.

1.7 Organisation of this book

This introductory chapter briefly outlines the context in which the Study was conducted and explains the focus of this report. Chapters 2, 3 and 4 outline the methodology of the Study and the reliability of the oral epidemiological data collected, the data weighting process and measurement of the representativeness of the population sample, and possible bias in estimates of child oral health. Chapters 5, 6 and 7 present the descriptive findings on child oral health, use of dental services and oral health behaviours. Chapter 8 presents key general health behaviours that are highly relevant to child oral health. Chapter 9 presents an examination of the social inequality in child oral health. Chapter 10 presents a specific description of Indigenous child oral health. Chapter 11 presents comparisons of key findings against existing surveillance or survey data to establish trends in oral health, use of dental services and dental behaviours. Chapter 12 presents an interpretation of the findings together with conclusions and recommendations.

References

Armfield JM, Slade G & Spencer AJ 2010. Dental health of Australia's teenagers and pre-teen children: the Child Dental Health Survey, Australia 2003–04. Cat. no. DEN 199. Dental statistics and research series no. 52. Canberra: Australian Institute of Health and Welfare.

Armfield JM & Spencer AJ 2004. Consumption of non-public water: implications for children's caries experience. Community Dentistry and Oral Epidemiology 32(4):283–96.

Armfield JM & Spencer AJ 2012. Dental health behaviours among children 2002–2004: the use of fluoride toothpaste, fluoride tablets and drops, and fluoride mouth rinse. Dental statistics and research series no. 56. Cat. no. DEN 215. Canberra: Australian Institute of Health and Welfare.

Arnljot HA, Barmes DE, Cohen LK, Hunter PBV & Ship I (Editors) 1987. Oral health care systems. An international collaborative study. Geneva: World Health Organization.

Australian Bureau of Statistics 2016. Australian Health Survey: consumption of added sugars, 2011–12. Canberra: Australian Bureau of Statistics.

Australian Health Ministers' Advisory Council Oral Health, Community Care and Population Health Principal Committee, Oral Health Monitoring Group 2016. Healthy mouths, healthy lives: Australia's National Oral Health Plan 2015–2024. Canberra: COAG Health Council.

Australian Health Ministers' Advisory Council, Steering Committee for National Planning for Oral Health 2001. Oral health of Australians: national planning for oral health improvement: final report. Adelaide: SA Department of Human Services on behalf of Australian Health Ministers' Conference.

Australian Institute of Health and Welfare 2005. A picture of Australia's children. AIHW cat. no. PHE 58. Canberra: Australian Institute of Health and Welfare.

Australian Institute of Health and Welfare 2009. Health expenditure Australia 2007–08. Health and Welfare Expenditure Series no. 37. Cat. no. HWE 46. Canberra: Australian Institute of Health and Welfare.

Barnard PD 1956. Dental survey of state school children in New South Wales, January 1954 – June 1955. Canberra: Commonwealth Government Printer.

Bodenheimer T & Wagner EH, et al. 2002. Improving primary care for patients with chronic illness. JAMA 288:1775–9.

Casamassimo PS, Thikkurissy S, Edelstein BL & Maiorini E 2009. Beyond the dmft: the human and economic cost of early childhood caries. J Am Dent Assoc 140:650–7.

Chen M, Andersen RM, Barmes DE, Leclercq MH & Lyttle CS (Editors) 1997. Comparing oral health care systems: a second international collaborative study. Geneva: World Health Organization.

Do LG, Spencer AJ, Slade GD, Ha DH, Roberts-Thomson KF & Liu P 2010. Trend of income-related inequality of child oral health in Australia. Sep;89(9):959–64.

Ellershaw AC & Spencer AJ 2009. Trends in access to dental care among Australian children. Cat. no. DEN 198. Dental statistics and research series no. 51. Canberra: Australian Institute of Health and Welfare.

Ellershaw AC & Spencer AJ 2011. Dental attendance patterns and oral health status. Cat. no. DEN 208. Dental statistics and research series no. 57. Canberra: Australian Institute of Health and Welfare.

Fisher-Owens SA, Gansky SA, Platt LJ, Weintraub JA, Soobader MJ, Bramlett MD & Newacheck PW 2007. Influences on children's oral health: a conceptual model. Pediatrics 120:e510–20.

Fletcher RH, Fletcher SW, & Wagner EH 1988. Clinical epidemiology: the essentials. 2nd edition. Baltimore: Williams and Wilkins.

Frieden TR 2010. A framework for public health action: the Health Impact Pyramid. Am J Pub Health 100(4):590–5.

Gaughwin A, Spencer AJ, Brennan DS & Moss J 1999. Oral health of children in South Australia by socio-demographic characteristics and choice of provider. Community Dent Oral Epidemiol 27(2):93–102.

Horowitz AM & Kleinman DV 2008. Oral health literacy: the new imperative to better oral health. Dent Clin North Am 52:333–44.

Marmot MG 2003. Understanding social inequalities in health. Perspectives in Biol and Medicine 46:S9–S23.

Marmot M 2007. For the commission on social determinants of health. Achieving health equity: from root causes to fair outcomes. Lancet: 370:1153–63.

Marmot M &Bell R 2011. Social determinants and dental health. Adv Dent Res 23:201–6.

Mount GJ 2003. Minimal intervention dentistry: rationale of cavity design. Oper Dent 28:92–9.

Mount GJ 2007. New paradigm for operative dentistry. Aust Dent J 52:264–70.

Moynihan PJ & Kelly SAM 2014. Effect on caries of restricting sugars intake: systematic review to inform WHO guidelines. Journal of Dental Research 93(1):8–18.

National Advisory Committee on Oral Health, Australian Health Ministers' Advisory Council 2004. Healthy mouths healthy lives: Australia's National Oral Health Plan 2004–2013. Adelaide: Government of South Australia on behalf of AHMAC.

National Health and Medical Research Council 2007. Public statement; the efficacy and safety of fluoridation 2007. Canberra: NHMRC. Accessed 9 August 2016 at: https://www.nhmrc.gov.au/guidelines-publications/eh41.

National Health and Medical Research Council 2013. Australian Dietary Guidelines summary. Canberra: Commonwealth of Australia.

National Health Performance Committee (NHPC) 2001. National Health Performance Framework Report. Brisbane: Queensland Health.

Nyvad B, Machiulskiene V & Baelum V 1999. Reliability of a new caries diagnostic system differentiating between active and inactive caries lesions. Caries Res 33:252–60.

Pitts NB 2004. 'ICDAS' — an international system for caries detection and assessment being developed to facilitate caries epidemiology, research and appropriate clinical management. Community Dent Health 21(3):193–8.

Rockhill B, Kawachi I & Colditz GA 2000. Individual risk prediction and population-wide disease prevention. Epidemiology Reviews 22:176–80.

Rockhill B 2005. Theorizing about causes at the individual level while estimating effects at the population level: implications for prevention. Epidemiology and Soc 16:124–9.

Rockhill B, Newman B, Weinberg C 1998. Use and misuse of population attributable fractions. Am J Public Health. Jan;88(1):15–9. Erratum in: Am J Public Health 2008 Dec;98(12):2119.

Rose G 1992. The strategy of preventive medicine. Oxford: Oxford University Press.

Sheiham A, Alexander D, Cohen L, Marinho V, Moysés S, Petersen PE, Spencer J, Watt RG & Weyant R 2011. Global oral health inequalities: task group-implementation and delivery of oral health strategies. Adv Dent Res 23:259–67.

Sheiham A & James WPT 2014. 'A new understanding of the relationship between sugars, dental caries and fluoride use: implications for limits on sugars consumption.' Public Health Nutrition 17(10): 2176–218.

Slade G, Spencer AJ & Roberts-Thomson KF (Editors) 2007. Australia's dental generations: The National Survey of Adult Oral Health 2004–06. Canberra: Australian Institute of Health and Welfare.

Spencer AJ 1984. Time trends in exposure to optimally fluoridated water supplies among Australian adolescents. Community Dent Oral Epidemiol 12:1–4.

Spencer AJ &Brown DF 1986. Transition from school-based to community-based dental services. Community Health Stud 10:12–18.

Spencer AJ 1983. Financing dental care in the community. Community Dental Health Monograph Series, Number Two. Melbourne: University of Melbourne, Department of Conservative Dentistry.

Tugwell P, Bennett K, Sackett D & Haynes B 1984. Relative risk, benefits and costs of intervention. Pp. 1097–113. In: Warren KS & Mahmoud AAF (Editors). Tropical and geographical medicine. New York: McGraw-Hill.

UK Department of Health 1994. An oral health strategy for England. London: Department of Health.

Weinstein P, Harrison R & Benton T 2006. Motivating mothers to prevent caries: confirming the beneficial effect of counselling. J Am Dent Assoc 137:789–93.

World Health Organization 2016. Report of the commission on ending childhood obesity. Geneva: World Health Organization.

World Health Organization 2015. Guideline: Sugars intake for adults and children. Geneva: World Health Organization.

2 Measuring child oral health and its influences

S Chrisopoulos, A Ellershaw, L Luzzi, KF Roberts-Thomson and LG Do

2.1   Study population and sampling

The target population for the Survey was Australian children aged 5–14 years. To draw a representative sample of children from this target population a stratified two-stage sample design was implemented within each state/territory. In the first stage, schools were selected from a sampling frame of schools located within each jurisdiction. In the second stage, children were sampled from each selected school.

The sampling strategy was designed to derive accurate population estimates of the oral health of Australian children, and to make valid comparisons between the oral health of children across regions within each state. For New South Wales, Victoria and Queensland, the geographical regions were based on Area Health Services/Health Districts, while in the remaining jurisdictions they were based on Capital City/Rest of State. As a consequence, the sampling methodology differed slightly for each jurisdiction.

To sample children across the age range of 5–14 years both primary and secondary schools were in scope of the Survey. A sampling frame of schools was created from a list provided by each jurisdiction which included all public, catholic and independent primary and secondary schools. Information provided on the sampling frame for each school included school code, school name and address, school type, school enrolment and health district.

Schools were excluded from the sampling frame if they were:
- located in very remote locations that would be difficult to access by the mobile dental clinic van
- special schools
- small school enrolment (usually <50 students).

New South Wales

In New South Wales (NSW), there were 2,995 schools that were considered in scope with 2,087 primary only, 567 secondary only and 341 combined primary/secondary schools. Schools on the sampling frame were stratified into 15 regions based on NSW Local Health Districts (LHD). The number of primary and secondary schools selected from each LHD was determined by the region's percentage share of total school enrolment. For primary schools, enrolment was defined as children enrolled in year levels Kindergarten to Year 6. For secondary schools, enrolment was defined as children enrolled in year levels 7–9.

Combined primary/secondary schools were grouped with secondary only schools for selection purposes.

Table 2-1 summarises the selection of schools by region. The allocation of the number of schools to each region was based on the school enrolment numbers in each region. A larger number of schools were selected in smaller regions to ensure those regions were adequately represented. To ensure selected schools were adequately spread across all geographic regions, 156 schools were selected with the aim of examining eight children in each year level per school. The 156 selected schools consisted of 62 primary schools, 57 secondary schools and 37 combined primary/secondary schools.

To achieve a good representation of schools, the sampling frame was first split by region and then by primary versus secondary/combined school, and then sorted by the Index of Community Socio-Economic Index for Areas (ICSEA, developed by the Australian Curriculum, Assessment and Reporting Authority (ACARA)) for each school. Schools were then selected with probability proportional to size. This was done by calculating a skip interval based on the total number of school enrolments within the region and school type divided by the required number of schools to be selected. A start number ranging from one to the skip interval was randomly chosen and schools were sampled by applying the skip interval to the compiled list. Where a school declined to participate, the adjacent school on the list was provided as a replacement.

To ensure that children had a similar chance of selection in the Survey, an equal number of children was sampled from each selected school irrespective of school enrolment size. The number of children selected per school was based on an expected consent rate of 50%. For primary only schools, approximately 112 children were selected across year levels Kindergarten to Year 6. For secondary only schools, approximately 48 children were initially selected from Year levels 7–9. For combined primary/secondary schools approximately 160 children were selected. These numbers were expected to yield approximately eight examinations in each year level per school. Where the target number of children exceeded the number of enrolments, all children were selected.

The selection of children within schools was either undertaken by NSW Health or by school administrative staff depending on the school's preference. For primary schools, a list of children in all year levels was compiled which contained the child's birth date and age. Children who were aged less than five years were excluded from the list. A skip interval was calculated based on the number of children on the list divided by the required number of children to be selected. A random start number ranging from one to the skip interval was randomly chosen and children were sampled by applying the skip interval to the compiled list. For secondary schools, a list of children in year levels 7–9 was compiled with children aged over 14 years excluded from the list. Children were sampled using the same selection method as that implemented in primary schools. For combined primary/secondary schools a list of children in year levels K to 9 was compiled.

Oral health of Australian children

Table 2-1: Selection of schools by region, New South Wales

Local Health District	% of total enrolment	Primary schools selected	Secondary schools selected
Central Coast	4.4%	5	5
Far West	0.4%	6	5
Hunter New England	12.0%	12	8
Illawarra Shoalhaven	5.7%	5	5
Mid North Coast	3.2%	5	5
Murrumbidgee	4.2%	5	5
Nepean Blue Mountains	5.4%	6	6
Northern NSW	4.1%	5	5
Northern Sydney	11.9%	8	8
South Eastern Sydney	9.4%	8	8
South Western Sydney	14.2%	10	10
Southern NSW	2.0%	5	5
Sydney	5.9%	5	5
Western NSW	5.1%	5	5
Western Sydney	12.0%	9	9
Total	100.0%	99	94

Victoria

In Victoria (Vic), there were 2,113 schools that were considered in scope with 1,544 primary only, 338 secondary only and 231 combined primary/secondary schools. Schools on the sampling frame were stratified into eight regions based on Victorian Local Health Districts (LHD). The number of primary and secondary schools selected from each LHD was determined by the region's percentage share of total school enrolment. For primary schools, enrolment was defined as children enrolled in year levels Prep to Year 6. For secondary schools, enrolment was defined as children enrolled in year levels 7–9.

Combined primary/secondary schools were grouped with secondary only schools for selection purposes. Table 2-2 summarises the selection of schools by region. The allocation of the number of schools to each region was based on the school enrolment numbers in each region. To ensure selected schools were adequately spread across all geographic regions, 156 schools were selected with the aim of examining six children in each year level per school. The 156 selected schools consisted of 59 primary schools, 58 secondary schools and 39 combined primary/secondary schools.

To achieve a good representation of schools, the sampling frame was first split by region and then by primary versus secondary/combined school and then sorted by the Index of Community Socio-Economic Index for Areas (ICSEA) for each school. Schools were then selected with probability proportional to size. This was done by calculating a skip interval based on the total number of school enrolments within the region and school type divided by the required number of schools to be selected. A random start number ranging from one to the skip interval was randomly chosen and schools were sampled by applying the skip interval to the compiled list. Replacement schools were provided when schools declined to participate.

Table 2-2: Selection of schools by region, Victoria

Local Health District	% of total enrolment	Primary schools selected	Secondary schools selected
Barwon-South Western	4.4%	9	9
Eastern Metro	0.4%	15	15
Gippsland	12.0%	9	9
Grampians	5.7%	8	8
Hume	3.2%	8	8
Loddon Mallee	4.2%	9	9
North and West Metro	5.4%	21	21
Southern Metro	4.1%	19	18
Total	100.0%	98	97

To ensure that children had a similar chance of selection in the Survey, an equal number of children was sampled from each selected school irrespective of school enrolment size. The number of children selected per school was based on an expected consent rate of 30%. For primary only schools, approximately 140 children were selected across year levels Prep to Year 6. For secondary only schools, 60 children were initially selected from year levels 7–9. For combined primary/secondary schools 200 children were selected. These numbers were expected to yield approximately six examinations in each year level per school. Where the target number of children exceeded the number of enrolments, all children were selected.

The selection of children within schools was either undertaken by the Victorian Department of Human Services or by school administrative staff depending on the school's preference. For primary schools, a list of children in all year levels was compiled which contained the child's birth date and age. Children who were aged less than 5 years were excluded from the list. A skip interval was calculated based on the number of children on the list divided by the required number of children to be selected. A random start number ranging from one to the skip interval was randomly chosen and children were sampled by applying the skip interval to the compiled list. For secondary schools, a list of children in Year levels 7–9 was compiled with children aged over 14 years excluded from the list. Children were sampled using the same selection method as that implemented in primary schools. For combined primary/secondary schools, a list of children in year levels Prep to 9 was compiled.

Oral health of Australian children

Queensland

Queensland (Qld) was separated into two zones based on water fluoridation status. Zone 1 was defined as all regions in Queensland including metropolitan areas, rural cities and rural towns that did not have water fluoridation in 2008, but were scheduled to be fluoridated by 2011. Zone 2 was defined as the Townsville region, which had been fluoridated since 1964, and was the largest region in Queensland with water fluoridation.

The sampling strategy was designed to derive accurate population estimates of the oral health of Queensland children, and to make valid comparisons between the oral health of children in fluoridated and non-fluoridated regions. As Zone 1 was a much larger geographical region than Zone 2, there were significantly more schools listed on the Zone 1 sampling frame. As a consequence, a different sampling methodology was implemented in each zone.

Zone 1

To sample children across the age range of 5–14 years both primary and secondary schools were in scope of the Survey. A sampling frame of schools was created from a list provided by Queensland Health which included all public, catholic and independent primary and secondary schools.

Schools were excluded from the sampling frame if they were:
- located in very remote locations that would be difficult to access by the mobile dental clinic van
- special schools
- located in the few towns with fluoride already added to the water supply
- located in towns with enough natural fluoride in the local water
- located in towns with a small population size.

There were 1,310 schools on the sampling frame with 916 primary only, 218 secondary only and 176 combined primary/secondary schools. Schools on the sampling frame were stratified into three broad regions based on geographic information provided by Queensland Health — Northern, Central and Southern. The number of primary and secondary schools selected from each region was determined by the region's percentage share of total school enrolment. For primary schools, enrolment was defined as children enrolled in year levels Prep to Year 7. For secondary schools, enrolment was defined as children enrolled in year levels 8–10.

Combined primary/secondary schools were grouped with secondary only schools for selection purposes. To ensure selected schools were adequately spread across all geographic regions, 172 schools were sampled from Zone 1 with the aim of examining between five to seven children in each year level per school. Table 2-3 summarises the selection of schools by region. A larger number of schools was selected in the Northern region than that suggested by the allocation to ensure the region was adequately represented. The 172 selected schools consisted of 79 primary only, 66 secondary only and 27 combined primary/secondary.

Table 2-3: Selection of schools by region

Region	% of total enrolment	Primary schools selected	Secondary schools selected
Northern	11.0%	9	14
Central	41.4%	15	38
Southern	47.6%	8	41
Total	100.0%	96	93

To ensure that children from Zone 1 had a similar chance of selection in the Survey, an equal number of children was sampled from each selected school irrespective of school enrolment size. The number of children selected per school was based on an expected consent rate of 60%. For primary only schools, approximately 84 children were selected across year levels Prep to Year 7. For secondary only schools, approximately 24 children were initially selected from year levels 8–10, but this was subsequently increased to 42 due to lower than expected consent rates. For combined primary/secondary schools approximately 108 children were initially selected from year levels Prep to Year 10 but this was subsequently increased to 114 children. These numbers were expected to yield approximately five to seven examinations in each year level per school. The selection of children within schools was either undertaken by Queensland Health or by school administrative staff depending on the school's preference.

Zone 2

There were 46 schools on the sampling frame in-scope of fluoridated areas within the Townsville region. Of these 46 schools, 32 were primary only, 9 were secondary only and 5 were combined primary/secondary schools. Due to the small number of schools on the sampling frame every school was selected. To ensure children in Zone 2 had a similar chance of selection in the Survey, the number of children sampled in each school was proportional to the number of children aged 5–14 years enrolled in the school.

The selection of children was undertaken by either Queensland Health or by school administrative staff depending on the school's preference. A list of children in the school was compiled which contained the child's birthdate and age. Children who were aged less than 5 years or older than 14 years were excluded. To be able to examine approximately 4,000 children within the Townsville region every third child was selected from each schools list using a random start number ranging from 1 to 3.

Oral health of Australian children

Western Australia

In Western Australia (WA), there were 836 schools that were considered in scope with 595 primary only, 86 secondary only and 115 combined primary/secondary schools. Schools on the sampling frame were stratified into two regions based on ABS Statistical Division (SD), where SD 505 was assigned to Metropolitan and the remaining SDs were assigned Rest of State. The number of primary and secondary schools selected from each region was determined by the region's percentage share of total school enrolment. For primary schools, enrolment was defined as children enrolled in year levels Reception to Year 7. For secondary schools, enrolment was defined as children enrolled in year levels 8–9.

Combined primary/secondary schools were grouped with secondary schools for selection purposes. Table 2-4 summarises the selection of schools by region. The allocation of the number of schools to each region was based on the school enrolment numbers in each region. To ensure selected schools were adequately spread across all geographic regions, 103 schools were selected with the aim of examining six children in each year level per school. The 103 selected schools consisted of 40 primary schools, 30 secondary schools and 33 combined primary/secondary schools. Replacement schools were provided when schools declined to participate.

Table 2-4: Selection of schools by region, Western Australia

Region	% of total enrolment	Primary schools selected	Secondary schools selected
Metropolitan	78.2%	62	50
Rest of State	21.8%	11	13
Total	**100.0%**	**73**	**63**

To ensure that children had a similar chance of selection in the Survey, an equal number of children was sampled from each selected school irrespective of school enrolment size. The number of children selected per school was based on an expected consent rate of 50%. For primary only schools, approximately 96 children were selected across year levels Prep to Year 7. For secondary only schools, 24 children were initially selected from year levels 8–9. For combined primary/secondary schools, 120 children were selected. These numbers were expected to yield approximately six examinations in each year level per school. Where the target number of children exceeded the number of enrolments, all children were selected. The selection of children within schools was either undertaken by the WA Department of Human Services or by school administrative staff depending on the school's preference.

South Australia

In South Australia (SA), there were 669 schools that were considered in scope with 465 primary only, 88 secondary only and 116 combined primary/secondary schools. Schools on the sampling frame were stratified into two regions based on ABS Statistical Division (SD), where SD 405 was assigned to Metropolitan and the remaining SDs were assigned Rest of State. The number of primary and secondary schools selected from each region was determined by the region's percentage share of total school enrolment. For primary schools, enrolment was defined as children enrolled in year levels Reception to Year 7. For secondary schools, enrolment was defined as children enrolled in year levels 8–9.

Combined primary/secondary schools were grouped with secondary only schools for selection purposes. Table 2-5 summarises the selection of schools by region. The allocation of the number of schools to each region was based on the school enrolment numbers in each region. To ensure selected schools were adequately spread across all geographic regions, 108 schools were selected with the aim of examining six children in each year level per school. The 108 selected schools consisted of 40 primary schools, 33 secondary schools and 35 combined primary/secondary schools. Replacement schools were provided when schools declined to participate.

Table 2-5: Selection of schools by region, South Australia

Region	% of total enrolment	Secondary schools selected	Primary schools selected
Metropolitan	72.4%	52	47
Rest of State	27.6%	23	21
Total	100.0%	75	68

To ensure that children had a similar chance of selection in the Survey, an equal number of children was sampled from each selected school irrespective of school enrolment size. The number of children selected per school was based on an expected consent rate of 40%. For primary only schools, approximately 115 children were selected across year levels Reception to Year 7. For secondary only schools, 30 children were initially selected from year levels 8–9. For combined primary/secondary schools, 135 children were selected. These numbers were expected to yield approximately six examinations in each year level per school. Where the target number of children exceeded the number of enrolments, all children were selected. The selection of children within schools was either undertaken by the SA Health Department or by school administrative staff depending on the school's preference.

Oral health of Australian children

Tasmania

In Tasmania (Tas), there were 251 schools that were considered in scope with 163 primary only, 34 secondary only and 54 combined primary/secondary schools. Schools on the sampling frame were stratified into 2 regions based on ABS Statistical Division (SD), where SD 605 was assigned to Metropolitan and the remaining SDs were assigned Rest of State. The number of primary and secondary schools selected from each region was determined by the region's percentage share of total school enrolment. For primary schools, enrolment was defined as children enrolled in year levels Kindergarten to Year 6. For secondary schools, enrolment was defined as children enrolled in year levels 7–8.

Combined primary/secondary schools were grouped with secondary only schools for selection purposes. Table 2-6 summarises the selection of schools by region. The allocation of the number of schools to each region was based on the school enrolment numbers in each region. To ensure selected schools were adequately spread across all geographic regions, 57 schools were selected with the aim of examining 8 children in each year level per school. The 57 selected schools consisted of 22 primary schools, 20 secondary schools and 15 combined primary/secondary schools. Replacement schools were provided when schools declined to participate.

Table 2-6: Selection of schools by region, Tasmania

Region	% of total enrolment	Primary schools selected	Secondary schools selected
Metropolitan	44.2%	19	18
Rest of State	55.8%	18	17
Total	100.0%	37	35

To ensure that children had a similar chance of selection in the Survey, an equal number of children was sampled from each selected school irrespective of school enrolment size. The number of children selected per school was based on an expected consent rate of 50%. For primary only schools, approximately 128 children were selected across year levels Kindergarten to Year 6. For secondary only schools, 32 children were initially selected from year levels 7–8. For combined primary/secondary schools, 160 children were selected. These numbers were expected to yield approximately eight examinations in each year level per school. Where the target number of children exceeded the number of enrolments, all children were selected. The selection of children within schools was either undertaken by the Tasmanian Department of Human Services or by school administrative staff depending on the school's preference.

Australian Capital Territory

In the Australian Capital Territory (ACT), there were 110 schools that were considered in scope with 76 primary only, 16 secondary only and 16 combined primary/secondary schools. As all schools were considered Metropolitan, no stratification by region was performed. For primary schools, enrolment was defined as children enrolled in years Kindergarten to Year 6. For secondary schools, enrolment was defined as children enrolled in year levels 7–9.

Combined primary/secondary schools were grouped with secondary only schools for selection purposes. Table 2-7 summarises the selection of schools. The allocation of the number of schools to each region was based on the school enrolment numbers in each region. To ensure selected schools were adequately spread across the ACT, 76 schools were selected with the aim of examining ten children in each year level per school. The 33 selected schools consisted of 11 primary schools, 11 secondary schools and 11 combined primary/secondary schools. Replacement schools were provided when schools declined to participate.

Table 2-7: Selection of schools by region, Australian Capital Territory

Region	% of total enrolment	Primary schools selected	Secondary schools selected
Metropolitan	100.0%	22	22
Total	**100.0%**	**22**	**22**

To ensure that children had a similar chance of selection in the Survey, an equal number of children was sampled from each selected school irrespective of school enrolment size. The number of children selected per school was based on an expected consent rate of 50%. For primary only schools, approximately 140 children were selected across year levels Kindergarten to Year 6. For secondary only schools, 60 children were initially selected from year levels 7–9. For combined primary/secondary schools, 200 children were selected. These numbers were expected to yield approximately ten examinations in each year level per school. Where the target number of children exceeded the number of enrolments, all children were selected. The selection of children within schools was either undertaken by the ACT Department of Health or by school administrative staff depending on the school's preference.

Northern Territory

In the Northern Territory (NT), there were 82 schools that were considered in-scope with 51 primary only, 15 middle/secondary only and 16 combined primary/secondary schools. Schools on the sampling frame were stratified into two regions based on ABS Statistical Division (SD), where SD 705 was assigned to Metropolitan and the remaining SDs were assigned Rest of State. Regional NT was restricted to the Palmerston, Katherine, Alice Springs and Tennant Creek regions.

The allocation of the number of primary schools to each region was based on the school enrolment numbers in each region. Due to the small number of schools in the NT, all high schools and combined schools were selected. Further, due to smaller enrolment numbers in schools outside of the metropolitan area, an additional five primary schools were selected. Table 2-8 summarises the selection of schools by region. In total, 49 schools were selected with the aim of examining eight children in each year level per school. The 49 selected schools consisted of 25 primary schools, 14 secondary schools and ten combined primary/secondary schools. Replacement schools were provided when schools declined to participate.

Table 2-8: Selection of schools by region, Northern Territory

Region	% of total enrolment	Primary schools selected	Secondary schools selected
Darwin region	51.0%	16	11
Rest of State	49.0%	19	13
Total	100.0%	30	35

To ensure that children had a similar chance of selection in the Survey, an equal number of children was sampled from each selected school irrespective of school enrolment size. The number of children selected per school was based on an expected consent rate of 50%. For primary only schools, approximately 112 children were selected across year levels Kindergarten to Year 6. For secondary only schools, 36 children were initially selected from year levels 7–9. For combined primary/secondary schools 160 children were selected. These numbers were expected to yield approximately eight examinations in each year level per school. Where the target number of children exceeded the number of enrolments, all children were selected. The selection of children within schools was either undertaken by the NT Department of Health or by school administrative staff depending on the school's preference.

2.2 Sample size

Table 2-9: Proposed sample sizes by state/territory

State	NSW	Vic	Qld	WA	SA	Tas	ACT	NT	Total
Sample size	7,200	5,800	5,300	3,600	3,100	2,500	2,200	2,200	**31,800**

The minimum required sample size was calculated to address the specific aims of this study using standard methods (Cohen 1988; Roy et al. 2007). The existing data on child oral health status and distribution of children using different dental service models in states and territories were used for the estimates. Sample size was calculated to detect a difference of 0.2 between slopes — considered a small effect size (Cohen 1988) — of explanatory variables in multivariable regression models for age-adjusted caries experience with alpha level of 0.05 and statistical power of 80%, to achieve the Survey aims. The sample size varies between jurisdictions according to distribution of children using a service model (insured versus uninsured; publicly-subsidised private care versus privately funded care). The minimally required sample size is 2,200 children aged 5–14 years for the states with the most favourable distribution of the service use groups. The state/territory sample size was further upwardly adjusted to address jurisdiction objectives. The specific sample size of state/territories is displayed above (Table 2-9). It was also estimated that this sample size would be adequately powered to perform the planned multilevel analyses (Goldstein et al. 2002).

2.3 Parental self-complete questionnaires *(primary and secondary)*

Questions in the questionnaire were primarily based on those used in previous surveys conducted by ARCPOH, namely the Child Fluoride Study Mark I (1991–96) (Slade et al. 1995a; Slade et al. 1996a; Slade et al. 1996b), Child Fluoride Study Mark II (2002–05) and the National Dental Telephone Interview Surveys 1994, 1999, 2002 and 2010.

One section that was newly developed for this Survey was the evaluation of dental services. This section was based on the National Health Performance Committee's 2001 National Health Performance Framework Report (NHPC 2001). The Report asserted that health care services should be effective, appropriate, efficient, responsive, accessible, safe, continuous, capable and sustainable. To measure performance in the dental service setting, a set of indicators was developed representing each of these nine dimensions.

The main aim of the parent questionnaire was to identify contribution of decay-protective and decay-risk-factors to dental decay. These factors included sources of fluoride, dental care, dental visiting and dietary intake. The main sections of the questionnaire covered dental practices, dietary intake, the child's health, use of dental services, evaluation of the child's dental services, and use of orthodontic services, birthplace and residential movements, and characteristics of the household.

The main decay-protective-factor measured was exposure to fluoride. Lifetime exposure to fluoridated water was assessed through a number of questions on water sources at all stages of life, the use of filters that remove fluoride from drinking water and place of residence during the child's lifetime. The questionnaire also assessed additional fluoride exposure from other sources over the child's lifetime, such as toothpaste use, fluoride drops, fluoride mouth rinse, the application of fluoride at the dentist and home fluoride treatments prescribed by an oral health professional.

Use of dental services reflected the decay-protective and decay-risk-factor of dental care visiting habits. This section asked questions about the child's first dental visit, last dental visit and usual dental visits.

Current food and drink intake was included to reveal diet-related decay-risk-factors, such as consumption of sugar and soft drinks. Consumption of tap/public water and bottled water was also collected.

Additional information relevant to dental health outcomes and dental health perception was collected. This included perceived general and dental health, evaluation of dental services received at the child's last dental visit and use of orthodontic services. Household demographic information was collected, including parental socioeconomic information and household income.

2.4   Oral epidemiological examination

Information about clinical oral status was collected during standardised oral epidemiological (dental) examinations conducted by dental practitioners who undertook training in the Survey procedures. Only Survey participants who had a signed parental consent form for participation and a signed medical history form were examined. Schedules for examinations were organised by the dental examination teams and Survey co-ordinators. Examinations were conducted mostly onsite in participating schools in mobile dental clinics or fixed dental clinics if available. A small number of children were examined at a site not at their school. In such instances, children were brought to the examination by their parents/guardians according to arranged examination appointments.

Survey participants who attended the examination first confirmed their identity. The team then explained the procedures to the child. The examiners followed a standardised protocol to record oral mucosal lesions, levels of tooth loss, dental decay experience, dental fluorosis and other types of enamel opacity, enamel hypoplasia and dental trauma. During data collection, replicate examinations were conducted for approximately five study participants per examiner to evaluate the consistency of their findings when judged against the principal Survey examiners.

Selection and training of examiners and recorders

An examination team comprised of a dental examiner and a data recorder. The Survey co-ordinators in each state/territory worked with local health districts to initially select a group of dental examiners and data recorders/chairside assistants.

All selected teams undertook a special two-day training program conducted by oral epidemiologists from The University of Adelaide, namely Associate Professor Loc Do, Emeritus Professor John Spencer, Professor Kaye Roberts-Thomson, and Drs Diep Ha, Gloria Mejia and Peter Arrow. Training sessions were held in each state/territory locations convenient to a small group of examination teams.

Prior to the scheduled training session, examiners and recorders received the Examination Manual and the Data Recorder Manual and a specially prepared DVD detailing the Survey protocol, coding and procedures involved in the examination, and data recording and back-up processes. The manuals were written by the oral epidemiologists at ARCPOH, based on accepted protocols. The DVD, which had been filmed at the Australian Dental Association (NSW Branch) Centre for Professional Dental Development, illustrated the intra-oral procedures and demonstrated how criteria should be applied to make diagnoses and to code oral conditions.

For most of the first day of training, the teams underwent didactic learning and discussion with ARCPOH investigators. This included presentation of PowerPoint slides, viewing of the DVD and demonstration of the data entry screen. All aspects of the examination were verbally and visually presented and discussed in detail with the teams. Later on the first day and for the whole second day, time was spent on practising on volunteer children organised by local staff. The examiners practised all aspects of the examination on the volunteers under supervision of the trainers. The data recorders practised data entry. Each child volunteer was examined at least twice by different examiners. Areas of difference were discussed, and the rationale for decisions was explored by the trainers and examiners. Difficult decisions or interesting problems were shown to the whole group. This facilitated calibration between examiners, although inter-examiner reliability was not assessed during this training. At the conclusion of each day a tutorial was held to clarify any outstanding issues.

Scope of examination

Survey participants were examined in a supine position in standard dental chairs with illumination provided by the chair's overhead dental light. Examiners used an intra-oral mirror that additionally had its own battery-powered light source. A periodontal probe with 2mm markings was used to remove plaque and debris or to assess the contour and texture of a surface, for example when assessing non-cavitated lesions (described further below). However, sharp explorers were not used, and no radiographs were taken.

The following overview summarises criteria used to assess the main oral health variables reported in this report.

Tooth loss because of dental caries

For all children, examiners identified teeth absent in the dentition and distinguished between tooth loss because of dental caries and tooth loss for any other reasons (unerupted teeth, exfoliated teeth, teeth extracted for orthodontic reasons or lost because of trauma). Only teeth lost because of dental caries were counted in the decayed, missing or filled indices (dmf/DMF).

Dental caries experience of tooth surfaces

All teeth present were subdivided into five tooth surfaces: mesial, buccal, distal, lingual, and either occlusal (for premolars or molars) or incisal (for incisors and canines). Each coronal surface was assessed and categorised using visual criteria (no explorer was used) and one of the following codes was assigned:

- decay: cavitation of enamel, or dentinal involvement, or both are present

- recurrent caries: visible caries that is contiguous with a restoration

- filled unsatisfactorily: a filling placed for any reason in a surface that requires replacement but that has none of the above conditions

- filling to treat decay: a filling placed to treat decay in a surface that had none of the above conditions

- filling placed for reasons other than decay in a surface that has none of the above conditions (incisors and canines only)

- fissure sealant: fissure sealant visible on a surface where none of the above conditions were found

- sound: when none of the above conditions was found

Dental fluorosis experience

Dental fluorosis was assessed on the two permanent maxillary central incisors. Examiners first assessed exclusion criteria. If present, enamel opacities were differentiated between dental fluorosis and non-fluorotic opacities using the Russell Differential Diagnostic Criteria (Russell 1961). Diagnosed dental fluorotic opacities were assessed for severity using the Thylstrup and Fejectskov Index (TFI) (Fejerskov et al. 1988), which is a 'dry' index. Teeth were dried with compressed air prior to scoring. Scores ranged from 0 to 5. If a non-fluorotic opacity was diagnosed, a score of 9 was assigned and analysed separately.

Oral mucosal lesions

Examiners systematically assessed all sections of the mouth cavity to observe presence of oral mucosal lesions. If present, oral mucosal lesions were classified as 'Ulcerated', 'Odontogenic abscess' or 'Non-ulcerated' lesion. Location and further clinical diagnosis were not recorded.

Enamel hypoplasia

Examiners assessed all teeth for presence of enamel hypoplasia that was associated with loss of enamel structure. Enamel hypoplasia was recorded as present for the primary dentition only, permanent dentition only or both dentitions.

Trauma

Evidence and history of dental trauma was assessed visually on the six permanent maxillary anterior teeth. A history of trauma was confirmed by interview.

Occlusal traits

Ten occlusal traits were measured for children aged 12 years and over using the Dental Aesthetic Index (DAI) (Cons et al. 1986). DAI score was calculated for each individual examined and used to classify children into groups by severity level of malocclusion. The case definition used in this report is the prevalence of handicapping malocclusion (DAI of 36 or higher).

Data recording for examinations

Each code called by an examiner was recorded directly onto laptop computers using a Microsoft Access database specifically designed for the purpose. The database included logic checks and skip sequences to reduce the probability of recording errors. Recording was performed by data recorders, primarily dental assistants. Recorders were trained to use the database during the two-day training session for examination teams.

Procedures following the examination

At the end of the examination, study participants received a written report completed by the Survey examiner that described the main clinical findings. The report included general advice regarding dental treatment.

2.5 Data analysis

The aim of the data analysis was to generate summary statistics describing oral health, use of dental services and dental behaviours for the Australian child population. To achieve this, data files were constructed from the examination data entry database and the database of the questionnaire data. Data checking and cleaning were performed as necessary and the data files were merged. Summary measures of disease were computed and response categories were combined to create oral health outcome variables of interest. As described above, unit record weights were computed for each analytic data file.

Data files were managed and summary variables were computed using SAS software version 9.4. For the results presented in Chapters 5 to 10, percentages, means and their associated 95% CIs were generated using SAS callable procedures from SUDAAN software release 11.0.1. The SUDAAN procedures used sampling weights to generate population estimates and calculated 95% CIs that allowed for the complex sampling design used in this Survey. To do so, 'with replacement' sampling was specified with two levels of stratification: broader regions (Capital City/Rest of State) and schools of the study participants.

Cross-sectional findings

Tables in Chapters 5 to 8 present estimates of the frequency of oral health conditions, oral health and general health behaviours and dental service use. Dental caries and dental fluorosis status were presented separately for the primary and permanent dentitions. The experience of dental caries in the primary dentition was presented for three age groups: 5–6, 7–8 and 9–10 years, while the experience of dental caries in the permanent dentition was presented for the 6–8, 9–11 and 12–14-year age groups. Dental fluorosis was presented for the three age groups 6–8, 9–11 and 12–14 years. All other analyses were presented for five age groups: 5–6, 7–8, 9–10, 11–12, and 13–14 years.

Chapter 10 presents findings specific for Indigenous children. Because there were a low number of Indigenous children in the Survey, summary findings were estimated for all children or for two age groups: 5–8 years and 9–14 years.

If a cell in a table had low count (<5) value for that cell was omitted as 'statistically not reliable'. A dash (−) was used in the cell to mark it as empty.

The tables use two measures to express frequency of oral health conditions, use of dental services and dental behaviours:

- Prevalence was expressed as the percentage of children with a characteristic of interest. This included percentages for some characteristics that were dichotomous (for example, presence versus absence of natural teeth) and for other characteristics that were counts or multiple categories collapsed to create a single category of interest (for example, presence of one or more decayed tooth surfaces.

- Disease severity was expressed as the mean number, per person, of anatomical sites that had a condition of interest. Sites were teeth or tooth surfaces. To compute severity, the number of affected sites was first counted for each examined person. The mean number of counted sites per person was then computed, together with its 95% CI.

Seven grouping variables were used to classify children into different sub-groups. These characteristics are described below.

Sex

Sex was classified as 'Male' or 'Female'.

Indigenous identity

Indigenous identity was based on responses to the question 'Are you of Aboriginal or Torres Strait Islander origin?' People who responded 'Yes, Aboriginal', 'Yes, Torres Strait Islander' or 'Yes, Torres Strait Islander & Aboriginal' were classified as Indigenous. People who responded 'no' were classified as non-Indigenous. Some 449 children did not have a definitive answer to this question and were excluded from this analysis.

Parent country of birth

Parents/guardians were asked to indicate their country of birth. Responses were collated to 'Australian born' and 'overseas born' for each parent. Then it was collated between the two parents/guardians, if applicable. If either of the parents were born overseas, then the combined response would be 'overseas born'. Otherwise, the child was classified as having parental country of birth as 'Australian born'. Some 276 children did not have a definitive answer to this question and were excluded from this analysis.

Parental education

Parents/guardians were asked to indicate their highest level of educational attainment. Six response options were collapsed to form three categories:

'School only': if parental responses were either 'incomplete' or 'complete school';

'Vocational training': if parental responses were either 'partial' or 'complete' vocational training;

'Tertiary education': if parental responses were either 'partial' or 'complete' tertiary education.

The highest reported level of education attainment of the parents/guardians was chosen for this variable. Some 1319 respondents did not provide a valid response on this item and were not included in this analysis.

Household income

Parents/guardians were asked to choose a most appropriate category for their total household income before tax. This income included all types of incomes of all people in the household. The ten available categories were collapsed to form three groups: 'Low' (<$60,000/year), 'Medium' ($60,000 to $120,000/year), or 'High' (more than $120,000/year). Some 1491 respondents did not provide a valid response on this item and were not included in this analysis.

Residential location

Residential location was classified as 'Major city', 'Inner regional', 'Outer regional' or 'Remote/Very remote', based on the residential postcode of children reported in the parental questionnaire. This classification was based on the Remoteness Area Structure of the Australian Statistical Geography Standard (ASGS) developed by the Australian Bureau of Statistics (Australian Bureau of Statistics 2013).

Reason for the last dental visit

Parents/guardians were asked to provide the reason for the last dental visit of the child. The valid responses were collapsed into two categories: 'check-up' and 'dental problem'.

Analysis of trends between surveys

Chapter 11 presents an analysis of trends between this current Survey and several existing surveys of child oral health in Australia. The available surveys are the National Oral Health Survey of Australia (NOHSA) 1987–88, a series of Child Dental Health Surveys (CDHS) across time and a series of National Dental Telephone Interview Surveys (NDTIS) conducted periodically at ARCPOH. The CDHS collected data from children attending the school dental service in a number of states/territories in Australia. Two specific studies, the Child Fluoride Study (CFS) Mark 1 (1991–92) and Mark 2 (2003–04) collected social survey and oral health status data among children attending school dental services. The CFS Mark I was conducted in SA and Qld while the CFS Mark II was conducted in SA, Qld, Vic and Tas. Therefore, those surveys covered just more than half of the child population in the participating states. Those details should be taken into account in interpreting results of this Survey.

The CDHS data have been presented for the 5–6-year age group and the 12-years-age group. The NDTIS data were used to report patterns of dental service use among Australian children aged 5–14 years. The CFS Mark 1 and Mark 2 data were used to report patterns of dental behaviours among children in Qld.

Age group analysis aims to describe the amount of change in population health for selected age groups. Direction and magnitude of changes in oral health status, use of dental services or dental behaviours are described by comparing estimates between the surveys. Trend of the changes are discussed.

Data of the previous surveys are housed at ARCPOH. Comparable data items were extracted and managed and summary variables were computed using SAS 9.3 in a similar manner as described for National Child Oral Health Study (NCOHS) data. Percentages, means and their associated 95% CIs were generated using SAS-callable procedures for complex sampling from SUDAAN software release 11.1.

References

Australian Bureau of Statistics 2013. Australian Statistical Geography Standard (ASGS): Volume 5 — Remoteness Structure, Australia, July 2011. ABS Cat. No. 1270.0.55.005. Canberra: Australia.

Cohen J 1988. Statistical power analysis for the behavioral sciences. New Jersey: Lawrence Erlbaum Associates.

Cons NC, Jenny J & Kohout F 1986. DAI: the Dental Aesthetic Index. Iowa City: College of Dentistry University of Iowa.

Fejerskov O, Manji F & Baelum V 1988. Dental fluorosis: a handbook for health workers. Copenhagen: Munksgaard.

Goldstein H, Browne W & Rasbash J 2002. Multilevel modelling of medical data. Stat Med 21(21):3291-315.

NHPC 2001. National Health Performance Framework report: Aug; 2001 Canberra: Australian Institute of Health and Welfare.

Roy A, Bhaumik DK, Aryal S & Gibbons RD 2007. Sample size determination for hierarchical longitudinal designs with differential attrition rates. Biometrics 63(3):699–707.

Russell AL 1961. The differential diagnosis of fluoride and nonfluoride enamel opacities. J Public Health Dent 21:143–6.

Slade GD, Davies MJ, Spencer AJ & Stewart JF 1995. Associations between exposure to fluoridated drinking water and dental caries experience among children in two Australian states. J Public Health Dent 55(4):218–28.

Slade GD, Spencer AJ, Davies MJ & Burrow D 1996a. Intra-oral distribution and impact of caries experience among South Australian school children. Aust Dent J 41(5):343–50.

Slade GD, Spencer AJ, Davies MJ & Stewart JF 1996b. Caries experience among children in fluoridated Townsville and unfluoridated Brisbane. Aust N Z J Public Health 20(6):623–9.

3 Data weighting, consideration and estimation procedures

A Ellershaw, C Koster and LG Do

Sample surveys are conducted to make informed inferences about a target population. In order to produce reliable estimates of population parameters a sample should reflect the characteristics of the target population from which it is drawn. This rarely happens in practice as sample designs commonly select participants with unequal probabilities of selection leading to certain groups within the target population being over- or under-represented in the sample. Similarly, survey response rates often vary significantly by sociodemographic status leading to samples that are unrepresentative of the target population and therefore biased population estimates. These concerns can be addressed by the application of survey weights that adjust the sociodemographic composition of the sample to reflect the target population. Consequently, population estimates derived from the weighted sample more closely reflect the true population parameters.

The National Child Oral Health Study (NCOHS) sampled 24,664 children from primary and secondary schools across Australia to estimate the oral health status of children aged 5–14 years. To produce reliable state and territory survey estimates, children from less populated jurisdictions were oversampled and therefore had a higher chance of selection in the Survey. Similarly, children from fluoridated areas of Queensland were oversampled to ensure a sufficient sample size to produce reliable survey estimates by fluoride exposure in that state. As the oral health status of Australian children varies significantly by geographic region (Centre for Oral Health Strategy 2009; Centre for Oral Health Strategy 2013; Do & Spencer 2014; Mejia et al. 2012), it was paramount that the weighting strategy accounted for these differential probabilities of selection.

Furthermore, analysis of the NCOHS sample highlighted differences in response rates by type of school attended and across a range of child, parent and household sociodemographic characteristics. Children from parents with a high level of education were over-represented in the sample. Conversely, Indigenous children and children from single parent families were under-represented. Response rates also varied by geographic region with participation lower in capital cities than other regions. As the association between sociodemographic status and children's oral health is well established (Centre for Oral Health Strategy 2009; Centre for Oral Health Strategy 2013; Do & Spencer 2014; Mejia et al. 2012; Armfield et al. 2006), the weighting strategy was designed to correct for the differential response rates inherent in the Survey.

Child examination and questionnaire data was weighted separately for each state and territory by deriving survey weights that adjusted the sociodemographic composition of the sample in each jurisdiction to reflect the state and territory population distributions. This ensured the weighting strategy was consistent across all jurisdictions and therefore the state and territory datasets could be combined to form a national weighted dataset. Details of the processes used to derive the final survey weights are described in the following sections.

3.1 Weighting adjustment by type of school attended

The aim of the first weighting process was to ensure that the percentage of children attending public, catholic and independent schools in the sample reflected the population percentage distribution derived from school enrolment data.

Population distributions were derived separately by region (Capital City/Rest of State) and grade (primary/secondary) and compared with the corresponding sample distributions. The initial weight assigned to each child was dependent on the type of school they attended and was derived as the school type population percentage divided by the corresponding sample percentage. This ensured that the weighted sample distribution for type of school attended reflected the corresponding population distribution.

To illustrate the weighting process, the following example refers to children attending primary schools located within a Capital City region. The percentage of children in the sample attending a public primary school (50%) was compared with the population percentage (70%) derived from school enrolment numbers. As children from public primary schools were under-represented in the sample, an initial weight of 1.4 (70% divided by 50%) was assigned to these children to increase the sample representation of public school children. Conversely, children attending Independent and catholic primary schools were over-represented in the sample and therefore the initial weight assigned to these children was less than one to ensure the sample representation of private school children was proportionate to their population distribution.

3.2 Weighting adjustment by sociodemographic characteristics

The aim of the next weighting process was to ensure that the sociodemographic characteristics of the sample reflected those of the population of Australian children aged 5–14 years. Population distributions for a range of child, parental and household sociodemographic characteristics were derived from Australian Bureau of Statistics (ABS) Census data and compared with the corresponding weighted sample distributions. Comparisons were undertaken for the following sociodemographic characteristics, which were all treated as categorical variables:

Child characteristics

- child's age
- child's sex
- child's Indigenous status
- child's remoteness area
- child's regional location

Oral health of Australian children

- parents'/guardians' country of birth
- parents'/guardians' education level
- parents'/guardians' employment status

Household characteristics

- household income
- family composition

Due to large differences in the sociodemographic composition of Capital City and Rest of State/Territory regions, separate population totals were derived for these geographic regions based on the ABS classification Greater Capital City Statistical Areas (GCCSA). Details of the data sources used to derive the population and sample distributions for each sociodemographic characteristic are described below.

Derivation of population percentage distributions

a) Child characteristics

The population percentage distributions for child's age and sex were derived from 2011 Estimated Residential Population (ERP) counts provided in ABS catalogue number 3235.0, Population by Age and Sex, Regions of Australia. Population counts for children aged 5–14 years were aggregated across Statistical Area Level 2 (SA2) regions to derive ABS GCCSA level population totals by single year age and sex respectively for each state and territory.

Population counts in some remote parts of the Northern Territory were excluded as children were not examined in these regions. To derive the population distribution for the rest of Northern Territory GCCSA region, postcode level population counts were obtained from the ABS 2011 Census TableBuilder product, table reference: Postal area (POA) by Sex (SEXP) and Age (AGEP), Counting: Persons, Place of Usual Residence. Population counts of children aged 5–14 years who resided in the remote or very remote postcodes 840, 846, 854, 862, 872, 885 and 886 were excluded from population totals (approximately 4,000 children).

The population percentage distribution for child's Indigenous status was sourced from the ABS 2011 Census TableBuilder product, table reference: GCCSA by Indigenous status (INGP) and AGEP, Counting: Persons, Place of Usual Residence. For GCCSA region rest of Northern Territory, postcode level population counts were obtained from table reference: POA by INGP and AGEP, Counting: Persons, Place of Usual Residence. Population counts of children aged 5–14 years who resided in postcodes 840, 846, 854, 862, 872, 885 and 886 were excluded from population totals.

The population percentage distribution for remoteness area was sourced from the ABS 2011 Census TableBuilder product, table reference: Remoteness area (RA) by AGEP, Counting: Persons, Place of Usual Residence. For GCCSA region rest of Northern Territory, postcode level population counts were obtained from table reference: POA by RA and AGEP, Counting: Persons, Place of Usual Residence. Population counts of children aged 5–14 years who resided in postcodes 840, 846, 854, 862, 872, 885 and 886 were excluded from population totals.

The geographic areas used to derive the regional population percentage distributions varied by state and territory. For New South Wales, the regional geographic areas were defined as the 16 Local Health Districts (LHD) and for Victoria the nine Dental Health Service (DHS) regions. Regional population counts of children aged 5–14 years were supplied by the New South Wales and Victorian Dental Health Services (DHS) by single year age. To maintain consistency with the 2011 ABS ERP counts, a factor was applied to the DHS population counts to ensure they summed to the total New South Wales ERP and total Victorian ERP for children aged 5–14 years respectively.

For the remaining states and territories, the regional geographic areas were defined as the ABS statistical area level 4 (SA4) regions. ERP counts were obtained from ABS catalogue number 3235.0, Population by Age and Sex, Regions of Australia, which provided single year age population counts. SA2 level population counts of children aged 5–14 years were aggregated to derive SA4 level population totals. For the Australian Capital Territory and Northern Territory, the SA4 regions were equivalent to the GCCSA regions.

b) **Parental characteristics**

Population percentage distributions for the sociodemographic characteristics of parents (or guardians) of examined children were derived from 2011 Census data supplied by the ABS consultancy service. Population counts of children aged 5–14 years who were living in families were provided by parents' country of birth (BPLP), level of education (QALLP) and employment status (LFSP). Postcode level population counts were aggregated to GCCSA regions to derive the GCCSA level population totals for each sociodemographic characteristic. For GCCSA region rest of Northern Territory, children aged 5–14 years who resided in postcodes 840, 846, 854, 862, 872, 885 and 886 were excluded from population totals.

For parents' country of birth, the population distribution was derived for the classification categories 'neither parent born overseas' and 'either parent born overseas'. For parents' level of education, the population distribution was derived for the classification categories 'neither parent has completed a Bachelor degree or higher' or 'either parent has completed a Bachelor degree or higher'. For parents' employment status population distributions were derived for the classification categories 'neither parent employed' or 'either parent employed'.

c) **Household characteristics**

Population percentage distributions for family composition and family income were sourced from 2011 Census data supplied by the ABS consultancy service. Population counts of children aged 5–14 years who were living in families were provided by family composition (FMCF) and weekly family income (FINF). Postcode level population counts were aggregated to GCCSA regions to derive the GCCSA level population totals for each sociodemographic characteristic. For GCCSA region rest of Northern Territory, children aged 5–14 years who resided in postcodes 840, 846, 854, 862, 872, 885 and 886 were excluded from population totals.

For family composition, the population distribution was derived for the classification categories 'couple family' and 'single parent family'. For family income, the weekly income categories provided by the ABS were converted to equivalent annual income categories. The annual income categories '<$60,000', '$60,000–$120,000' and '>$120,000' were referred to as low, medium and high income categories respectively.

The Census population counts provided by the ABS for several of these sociodemographic characteristics included a 'not stated' category. Population counts in this category were small for all characteristics (0.5%–1.5%) except family income (11%). All population percentage distributions were derived excluding the 'not stated' category.

Derivation of weighted sample percentage distributions

To derive the corresponding weighted sample percentage distributions, children were assigned to the appropriate classification category for each sociodemographic characteristic based on information provided in the survey questionnaire. Children who could not be assigned to a category due to incomplete questionnaire information were treated as missing data.

Allocation of children to ABS remoteness area and to regional geographic areas was based on the child's postcode of usual residence. Children were assigned to a remoteness category using the ABS correspondence file '1270055006C190 Postcode 2012 to Remoteness Area 2011' available on the ABS website (Australian Statistical Geography Standard Correspondences). For postcodes that did not map to a single remoteness area, children were assigned to the most populated area if more than 90% of the postcodes population resided within that remoteness area. For the remaining postcodes, the child's residential suburb/locality was used to allocate the correct remoteness category. The ABS correspondence file, 'Locality 2011 to Remoteness Areas 2011' (Australian Statistical Geography Standard Correspondences) was used to map suburb/locality to a remoteness area.

For regional geographic areas, children from New South Wales and Victoria were allocated to LHD and DHS regions respectively using correspondence files provided by the Dental Health Services. For the remaining states and territories, children were allocated to SA4 regions using the ABS correspondence file 'Postcode to SA4' (Australian Statistical Geography Standard Correspondences). For postcodes that did not map to a single SA4 region, children were assigned to the most populated region if more than 90% of the postcodes population resided within that SA4 region. For the remaining postcodes, the child's residential suburb/locality was used to allocate the correct SA4 region. The ABS correspondence file 'Locality to SA2' (Australian Statistical Geography Standard Correspondences) was used to map suburb/locality to a SA2 region and consequently a SA4 region.

The weighted sample percentage distributions for each sociodemographic characteristic were then derived using the child's initial weight. Missing data was excluded from the derivation of these distributions.

Comparison of population and weighted sample distributions

Comparison of the population and corresponding weighted sample distributions identified significant differences for a number of key sociodemographic characteristics. Distributional variations were evident for all states and territories and GCCSA regions within each state and territory.

Table 3-1 presents a comparison of the percentage distributions at the state/territory level. Comparisons are not presented if differences between the distributions are small.

Children from more educated families where at least one parent had completed a Bachelor degree or higher were significantly over-represented in the sample. This finding was consistent across all states and territories with differences ranging from 13–26 percentage points. Children from families with at least one parent employed were also over-represented in most states and territories although differences were smaller ranging from 5–12 percentage points.

Conversely, children from one-parent families were under-represented in several states and territories with differences ranging from 5–9 percentage points, and Indigenous children were under-represented in the Northern Territory and Western Australia.

Comparisons by remoteness area identified that children living in Major city areas of New South Wales, Queensland, South Australia and Victoria were under-represented in the sample with differences ranging from 13–23 percentage points. There were also significant differences by regional location although these differences are not presented in the Table.

A common weighting strategy to improve the representativeness of a sample is to benchmark the sample to known population totals; for example, survey data is commonly weighted to geographic region by age and by sex population totals. However, when a sample requires weighting to a large number of sociodemographic variables, the population totals for the cross-classification of these variables are generally not available due to confidentiality reasons. Furthermore, the large number of cross-classification weighting cells can lead to the sample being spread too thinly.

To overcome these weighting issues an iterative weighting procedure known as raking ratio estimation was used to weight the NCOHS sample data (Deming 1943). The advantage of this procedure is that population totals are only required for single categorical variables rather than the cross-classification of a range of categorical variables. A description of the raking ratio estimation procedure is provided below.

Table 3-1: Comparison of population and weighted sample distributions

State/Territory	Weighted sample %	Population %
Parent completed a Bachelor degree[1]		
ACT	65.0	51.6
NSW	50.1	33.1
NT	44.5	22.2
Qld	40.1	27.8
SA	49.0	28.0
Tas	49.5	23.2
Vic	50.7	35.0
WA	52.2	30.7
Parent employed[2]		
NSW	89.2	84.2
NT	91.9	80.2
Qld	90.6	84.6
SA	92.3	84.1
Tas	87.8	81.5
Vic	91.0	86.4
WA	92.2	85.9
Parent born overseas[3]		
NSW	31.5	39.0
NT	32.7	26.0
Qld	40.6	32.8
One parent families		
NT	18.8	24.2
Qld	17.8	22.3
SA	14.0	22.7
Tas	18.8	24.9
Child Indigenous		
NT	20.2	38.2
WA	3.4	6.0
Major cities remoteness area		
NSW	54.1	72.0
Qld	42.2	59.3
SA	57.1	70.2
Vic	51.3	73.8

1 Children were classified to the parent completed a Bachelor degree category if they had at least one parent who had completed a Bachelor degree or higher.
2 Children were classified to the parent employed category if they had at least one parent who was employed.
3 Children were classified to the parent born overseas category if they had at least one parent who was born overseas.

Raking ratio estimation

In contrast to standard weighting procedures, raking ratio estimation usually progresses one variable at a time. The process commences with the first variable by summing the initial weights for all children belonging to the first classification category of the variable. The weighted sample total is then compared with the corresponding population total and an adjustment, defined as the ratio of the population total to the weighted sample total, is applied to the child's initial weight.

The process is then repeated for the remaining classification categories of the first variable to derive weight adjustments for children in each classification category. Once completed, the weighted sample totals derived from the adjusted weights correspond to the population totals, or equivalently, the weighted sample and population distributions are equivalent.

The raking procedure then moves to the next variable applying the same process to derive weight adjustments for each classification category of this variable. The first iteration of the procedure is completed when weight adjustments have been applied for all variables included in the raking process.

As the raking procedure is performed for one variable at a time, the process of adjusting the weights for the next variable may mean the weighted sample distributions for previously adjusted variables no longer correspond with the population distributions. Despite this, as the process continues over numerous iterations alternating between the different variables the weight adjustments become progressively smaller. Convergence of the process occurs when the weighted sample totals correspond to the population totals for all variables specified in the raking process.

While this weighting technique ensures equivalence between the weighted sample totals and corresponding population totals for individual variables used in the raking process, the same equivalence is not required for the cross-classification of all variables. Due to the rapid decline in response rates over the last decade this weighting procedure has become popular among research organisations worldwide (Hidiroglou & Patak 2006; DeBell & Krosnick 2009; British Social Attitudes Survey 2012; Pennay 2010).

To illustrate the raking ratio estimation procedure, a simplified example using two sociodemographic variables, parent education status and child Indigenous status, is presented in Table 3-2. The weighted sample total in this Table refers to the sum of weights for all children assigned to a particular cross-classification cell.

Table 3-2: Example of the raking ratio estimation procedure with two variables

	Non-Indigenous	Indigenous	Population total
Neither parent has completed a Bachelor degree	weighted sample total=W_{11}	weighted sample total=W_{12}	N_{1+}
Either parent has completed a Bachelor degree	weighted sample total =W_{21}	weighted sample total=W_{22}	N_{2+}
Population total	N_{+1}	N_{+2}	N_{++}

The raking process starts with the first variable, parent education status. The weighted sample total for the classification category 'neither parent has completed a Bachelor degree' ($W_{11}+W_{12}$) is compared with the corresponding population total (N_{1+}). The ratio $N_{1+} / (W_{11}+W_{12})$ is applied to the child's initial weight to derive an adjusted weight for children in this category.

Similarly, the weighted sample total for the category 'either parent has completed a Bachelor degree' ($W_{21}+W_{22}$) is compared with the corresponding population total (N_{2+}). The weight adjustment $N_{2+} / (W_{21}+W_{22})$ is applied to derive a new weight for children in this second category. Once this process is completed the weighted sample totals for parental education correspond to the population totals.

The procedure moves to the second variable, child Indigenous status, and the ratios $N_{+1} /(W_{11}+ W_{21})$ and $N_{+2} / (W_{12}+ W_{22})$ are applied to the child's current weight for children in the 'non-Indigenous' and 'Indigenous' categories respectively. The weighted sample totals for child Indigenous status are now equivalent to the corresponding population totals but equivalence may no longer apply for the parental education variable. Consequently, the procedure is repeated over several iterations alternating between each variable until agreement is reached between the weighted sample totals and corresponding population totals for both variables.

A more comprehensive explanation of the raking ratio estimation procedure is provided in the paper 'A SAS macro for balancing a weighted sample' (Izrael et al. 2000). To perform this procedure, sample data was submitted to the SAS® macro 'Rake_and_Trimm' developed by Izrael et al. (2009). One of the constraints of this macro was that each child must be assigned to a valid classification category for each sociodemographic variable used in the raking process. The percentage of children in the NCOHS sample who were missing a classification category due to incomplete questionnaire data is presented in Table 3-3.

Table 3-3: Percentage of children missing a classification category

Sociodemographic characteristic	% missing
Child's age	0.0
Child's sex	0.0
Child's Indigenous status	1.8
Child's remoteness area	0.0
Child's regional location	0.0
Parents'/guardians' country of birth	1.1
Parents'/guardians' education level	5.3
Parents'/guardians' employment status	3.2
Household income	6.0
Family composition	1.5

Missing data was imputed using the SAS procedure MI with singular imputation and age by sex stratification specified. As the sociodemographic variables were categorical, missing data was imputed using a discriminant function (Yim 2015). Imputation was undertaken for one variable at a time and children within an age by sex stratum were assigned to a classification category in order to maintain similar pre-and-post imputation distributions. After completion of the weighting process imputed values were reset to missing on the weighted dataset.

A second constraint of the macro was that population totals for each raking variable must sum to the same overall population total. Consequently, the population percentage distributions derived from ABS Census data were applied to the ABS estimated residential population totals for each state and territory.

The 'Rake_and_Trimm' macro also required a tolerance level be specified which enabled the raking process to converge if the combined difference between the weighted sample totals and corresponding population totals did not exceed the specified level. If a tolerance level of one unit was specified, the macro did not converge until all corresponding totals were equivalent. To ensure convergence in the raking process a tolerance level of ten units was specified for all states and territories except Queensland, where the level was set to 50 units.

The variables included in the raking procedure were consistent across all states and territories and are provided in the Appendix. Details of the classification categories specified for each variable and the corresponding population totals input to the raking procedure are also provided. There were minor variations in the classification categories used for certain jurisdictions. Due to the large Indigenous population in the Northern Territory, the variables Indigenous status and age were combined to create more detailed raking categories defined by GCCSA region, by Indigenous status and by two-year age group. There was also some variation in the remoteness area categories due to the small sample size in the Inner regional area of the Australian Capital Territory and the Remote/Very remote areas of Tasmania. These variations are explained in the Appendix.

A final requirement of the macro was that an initial weight be specified for the first iteration of the raking procedure. The initial weight input to the macro was the weight derived in the first weighting process, which corrected sample representation by type of school attended. Output from the macro included each child's raked weight, the minimum and maximum raked weight, the coefficient of variation and a comparison of the weighted sample totals and corresponding population totals for each sociodemographic variable.

3.3 Benchmarking to geographic region by age population counts

The final weighting process applied an adjustment to the weights derived from the raking process to ensure they summed to the regional by age population totals for each state and territory. The regional areas were identical to those used in the raking process and age was defined as the two-year age groups 5-6 years, 7-8 years, 9-10 years, 11-12 years and 13-14 years.

The regional by age population totals for NSW and Vic were provided by the respective Dental Health Services. For the remaining jurisdictions, the population totals were obtained from ABS catalogue number 3235.0, Population by Age and Sex, Regions of Australia.

Children were assigned to a regional by age group weighting cell and weighted sample totals were derived for each weighting cell by summing the raked weights for children belonging to the same cell. The weighted sample totals were then compared to the corresponding population totals to derive a separate adjustment for each weighting cell. The adjustment, defined as the ratio of the population total to the weighted sample total, was then applied to the child's raked weight. The weighting formula to derive the final weight is provided below.

$$w_i = \frac{N_{s,r,a}}{\sum\limits_{i \in s,r,a} r_i} * r_i \qquad \text{Where:} \qquad \begin{array}{l} i = \text{child} \\ s = \text{state or territory} \\ r = \text{region} \\ a = \text{age group} \\ r_i = \text{raked weight for child } i \\ N_{s,r,a} = \text{ERP for state/territory } s, \text{ region } r, \\ \qquad \text{age group } a \end{array}$$

Where the sample size was insufficient in a weighting cell similar regions were combined. In Queensland, the SA4 regions Brisbane-West and Brisbane Inner City were combined for children aged 13-14 years. Similarly, the Toowoomba and Ipswich SA4 regions were combined for children in this age group. For children aged 11-12 years, the Queensland-Outback and Cairns SA4 regions were combined. In

Western Australia, the SA4 regions Western Australia–Wheat Belt and Western Australia–Outback were combined for children aged 13–14 years.

If the largest weights in a particular state or territory were significantly larger than other high weights, they were designated as outliers and individually reduced. The process of benchmarking to regional by age population totals was then repeated to derive new weights. Although the outlier weights were reduced to limit their impact on survey estimates they still remained among the largest weights. A maximum of ten weights were adjusted in each jurisdiction although it was usually less than five.

The weighted state and territory samples were then combined to form the national dataset used to derive population estimates published in this report. The overall weighting strategy ensured that the joint regional by age group distributions, derived from the final weights, reflected the corresponding population distributions in each jurisdiction and therefore Australia. The weighting strategy also ensured that the marginal weighted sample distributions for the other sociodemographic characteristics were very similar to the corresponding population distributions at both the jurisdictional and national level. Comparisons of these distributions are provided in Chapter 4.

Summary

The NCOHS weighting strategy was developed to account for the differential probabilities of selection inherent in the sample design and to address significant variation in response rates by sociodemographic status.

Sample weights were derived to adjust the sociodemographic composition of the sample to reflect the state/territory population distributions for the following characteristics:

- type of school attended
- child's age, sex, Indigenous status and regional location
- parent's (guardian's) education level, employment status and country of birth
- family income and composition

This ensured that the sociodemographic composition of the weighted national dataset was representative of the target child population at both the jurisdictional and national level. Consequently, the application of these sample weights significantly improves the reliability of national and jurisdictional population estimates derived from the Survey, and enables valid comparisons between state and territory estimates despite variations in sample design, operational procedures and response rates.

Oral health of Australian children

References

Armfield JM, Slade GD & Spencer AJ 2006. Socioeconomic differences in children's dental health: The Child Dental Health Survey, Australia 2001. Dental Statistics and Research Series No. 33. AIHW cat. no. DEN 152. Canberra: Australian Institute of Health and Welfare.

Australian Statistical Geography Standard Correspondences, 2011. Accessed June 2016: http://www.abs.gov.au/websitedbs/d3310114.nsf/home/correspondences.

Centre for Oral Health Strategy NSW 2009. The New South Wales Child Dental Health Survey 2007. Available at: www.health.nsw.gov.au/cohs.

Centre for Oral Health Strategy NSW, NSW Ministry of Health 2013. The New South Wales Teen Dental Survey 2010. Sydney: NSW Ministry of Health.

DeBell M & Krosnick JA 2009. Computing weights for American National Election Study Survey Data. ANES Technical Report series, no. nes012427. Ann Arbor, MI, & Palo Alto, CA: American National Election Studies. Available at: http://www.electionstudies.org/resources/papers/nes012427.pdf.

Deming WE 1943. Statistical Adjustment of Data. New York: Wiley.

Do LG & Spencer AJ (Editors) 2014. The beginning of change: Queensland Child Oral Health Survey 2010–2012. Adelaide: Australian Research Centre for Population Oral Health.

Hidiroglou MA & Patak Z 2006. Raking Ratio Estimation: An application to the Canadian Retail Trade Survey. Journal of Official Statistics 22(1):71–80.

Izrael D, Hoaglin DC & Battaglia MP 2000. A SAS macro for balancing a weighted sample. Paper 258-25. Proceedings of the Twenty-Fifth Annual SAS Users Group International Conference, SAS Institute Inc., Cary, NC.

Izrael D, Battaglia MP & Frankel MR 2009. Extreme Survey Weight Adjustment as a Component of Sample Balancing (a.k.a. Raking). Paper 247-2009. SAS Global Forum: Washington, D.C.

Mejia GC, Amarasena N, Ha DH, Roberts-Thomson KF & Ellershaw AC 2012. Child Dental Health Survey Australia 2007: 30-year trends in child oral health. Dental statistics and research series no. 60. Cat. no. DEN 217. Canberra: Australian Institute of Health and Welfare.

Park A, Clery E, Curtice J, Phillips M & Utting D (Editors) 2012. British social attitudes: the 29th Report, London: NatCen Social Research. Available at: www.bsa-29.natcen.ac.uk.

Pennay DW 2010. Profiling the 'mobile phone only' population. Results from a dual-frame telephone survey presented at the ACSPRI Social Science Methodology Conference December 2010.

Yim C 2015. Paper 3295-2015 Imputing missing data using SAS®. San Luis Obispo: California Polytechnic State University.

4 Measuring representativeness of the study participants

L Luzzi, DH Ha, A Ellershaw, C Koster, DS Brennan and S Chrisopoulos

This Survey gathered information from a representative sample of the Australian child population aged 5–14 years to describe the oral health status of the population and factors related to use of dental services and dental behaviours, as well as associated individual, family, and community factors such as the sociodemographic characteristics of the child's household.

Surveys provide a means of measuring a population's characteristics, self-reported and observed behaviour, and needs. Unlike a census, where all members of a population are studied, sample surveys gather information from only a portion of a population of interest. In a statistically valid survey, the sample is objectively chosen so that each member of the population will have a known non-zero chance of selection. Only then can the results be reliably projected from the sample to the population.

Surveys, however, are not exempt of errors (or bias), which can occur when some segments of the population do not participate in the survey. As not all Australian children were included in this Survey, there is potential that the sample does not accurately represent the population of interest.

Errors due to sampling depend on the sample selection strategy and can be measured statistically. Variability inherent to the sampling process is expressed using the 95% confidence interval. On the other hand, non-sampling error or bias is more problematic because it is more difficult to measure and control. Bias due to non-participation occurs when the participants differ from the non-participants or the targeted population in one or more characteristics. The potential for bias due to non-participation or non-response can be explored by examining key sociodemographic characteristics of the Survey sample, and comparing them with known characteristics of the target population.

As outlined in Chapter 3, this Survey employed rigorous sampling procedures to achieve a representative sample of the Australian child population aged 5–14 years. The procedures used to derive survey weights for this Survey reflect the standards of best practice for weighting complex survey data, and are procedures used by leading statistical agencies. Procedures used to derive survey weights ensure valid estimates and inferences of the target child population can be made. The methodologies employed in the Survey will minimise any potential bias, which will be assessed in this chapter. Minimising potential bias is critical as this will determine whether results of this study can be generalised to the larger population.

This chapter presents sociodemographic characteristics of the population, both at a state/territory level and national level. Firstly, to examine the potential for bias, school and child participation rates by school characteristics will be examined. Secondly, response rates and non-participation bias will be examined by area-level socioeconomic indicators, and key characteristics of the sample (such as child's sex, child's Indigenous identity, child's residential location, parents' country of birth, parents' Indigenous identity, parents' employment status, household composition, household income) will be compared to Census population benchmarks. Lastly, a comparison of observed and adjusted estimates of oral health indicators will be discussed.

4.1 Sociodemographic characteristics

This section describes the characteristics of the study population, which includes child's sex, child's Indigenous identity, child's residential location, child's reason for their last dental visit, parents' country of birth, parental education and household income. These characteristics are used in the following chapters to describe variation in oral health outcomes of the population.

For parents' country of birth, if a child had at least one parent who was born overseas, the child was assigned to the parents' born overseas category otherwise they were assigned to the Australian born category. For parental education, the child was assigned to the category that reflected the parents' highest education level. For example, if a child had at least one parent with some tertiary education, the child was assigned to the tertiary education category. For the characteristic of household income, children were assigned to an income category based on the total income of the household in which they resided. Children were excluded from the analysis when the characteristic of interest was unknown.

Characteristics of children in Australia

Table 4-1 presents the estimated percentage distribution of Australian children aged 5–14 years derived from weighted Survey data by sociodemographic characteristics.

There were minor variations in the distribution of Australian children by sex. The largest difference was observed amongst children aged 7–8 years in which there was a higher proportion (5.0 percentage points) of males than females.

Indigenous children represented 5.5% of the total child population with a slightly higher proportion of Indigenous children in the 7–8 years (6.0%) and 11–12 years (6.0%) age groups.

The percentage of children with at least one parent born overseas comprised 36.4% of the sample and did not vary markedly between age groups.

Almost half of children (48.1%) had a parent with some tertiary education and a further 22.3% of children had a parent with some level of vocational training. Differences by parental education across age groups were generally small and not statistically significant.

Children were more likely to live in medium level income households (38.4%) than in low (32.5%) or high (29.1%) income level households. The slight variations in the percentage of children in each income category across age groups were not statistically significant.

Some 68.0% of all Australian children lived in a Major city area, while a further 19.7% lived in an Inner regional area, 9.8% lived in an Outer regional area, and 2.5% lived in a Remote/Very remote region. Variations in the distribution of residential location across age groups were not statistically significant.

Although the majority of children made their last dental visit for the purpose of a check-up (79.9%), one-fifth of children (20.1%) last visited for a dental problem. Prevalence of problem visiting was highest among children aged 7–8 years (24.0%) and lowest amongst children aged 13–14 years (15.0%).

Comparisons at the national level indicated that the study population had a similar proportion of females and males and the majority of children were non-Indigenous. Just over 36% of children had a parent who was born overseas, almost 50% of children (48.1%) had a parent with some tertiary education and almost 40% of children lived in medium level income households. Although there was some variation in the distribution of characteristics across age groups, in almost all instances these differences were not statistically significant.

Oral health of Australian children

Table 4-1: Percentage of children by selected characteristics — Australia

	Population: children aged 5–14 years					
	All ages	5–6	7–8	9–10	11–12	13–14
Sex						
Male	51.2	51.4	52.5	50.4	51.7	50.2
	49.8–52.6	49.3–53.4	50.5–54.5	48.1–52.7	49.4–54.0	46.6–53.7
Female	48.8	48.7	47.5	49.6	48.3	49.8
	47.4–50.2	46.6–50.7	45.5–49.5	47.3–51.9	46.0–50.6	46.3–53.4
Indigenous identity						
Non-Indigenous	94.6	94.2	94.0	94.6	94.0	95.9
	93.6–95.3	92.6–95.4	92.6–95.2	93.4–95.6	92.6–95.2	94.8–96.8
Indigenous	5.5	5.9	6.0	5.4	6.0	4.1
	4.7–6.4	4.6–7.4	4.8–7.4	4.4–6.6	4.8–7.4	3.2–5.2
Parents' country of birth						
Australian born	63.6	64.1	63.5	63.4	63.1	63.9
	61.7–65.4	61.1–66.9	60.5–66.3	60.7–66.0	60.6–65.4	60.4–67.3
Overseas born	36.4	36.0	36.5	36.6	36.9	36.1
	34.6–38.3	33.1–38.9	33.7–39.5	34.0–39.3	34.6–39.4	32.7–39.6
Parental education						
School	29.6	29.5	28.2	28.3	31.9	30.0
	28.0–31.3	26.7–32.5	25.6–31.0	26.0–30.8	29.6–34.3	27.2–32.9
Vocational training	22.3	21.2	21.2	23.0	21.7	24.3
	21.2–23.4	19.4–23.2	19.3–23.2	21.0–25.1	19.9–23.5	22.0–26.6
Tertiary education	48.1	49.2	50.6	48.7	46.4	45.8
	46.1–50.1	45.9–52.6	47.5–53.7	45.7–51.7	43.9–48.9	42.5–49.1
Household income						
Low	32.5	32.4	30.8	32.1	34.0	33.1
	30.6–34.5	29.5–35.5	28.0–33.8	29.3–35.0	31.5–36.5	30.1–36.3
Medium	38.4	37.4	38.2	39.7	37.8	38.8
	37.0–39.8	35.0–39.9	35.9–40.6	37.3–42.2	35.7–39.9	36.5–41.3
High	29.1	30.2	31.0	28.2	28.2	28.0
	27.2–31.1	27.0–33.5	28.1–34.1	25.6–30.9	25.9–30.7	25.1–31.1
Residential location						
Major city	68.0	69.4	68.4	67.6	67.3	67.1
	65.1–70.7	65.3–73.3	64.3–72.2	63.6–71.4	64.0–70.5	62.5–71.3
Inner regional	19.7	19.2	19.2	20.0	20.4	19.9
	17.4–22.3	16.0–22.9	16.0–22.7	16.9–23.5	17.7–23.4	16.4–23.9
Outer regional	9.8	8.9	9.7	9.7	9.8	10.7
	8.2–11.6	6.9–11.3	7.7–12.2	7.7–12.0	8.1–11.9	8.6–13.3
Remote/Very remote	2.5	2.5	2.7	2.7	2.4	2.3
	1.6–3.9	1.3–4.6	1.6–4.7	1.5–4.8	1.5–4.0	1.4–3.7
Reason for last dental visit						
Check-up	79.9	80.7	76.0	77.8	79.5	85.0
	78.8–81.0	78.2–83.1	73.7–78.1	75.9–79.6	77.7–81.3	83.2–86.6
Dental problem	20.1	19.3	24.0	22.2	20.5	15.0
	19.0–21.2	16.9–21.8	21.9–26.3	20.4–24.1	18.7–22.3	13.4–16.8

Row 1: Proportions were computed using weighted data.
Row 2: 95% CI: Confidence intervals for estimates were computed using weighted data.
Columns are arranged by age at time of Survey.

Table 4-2 presents the estimated percentage distribution of children aged 5–14 years derived from weighted Survey data by sociodemographic characteristics and by state/territory. Similar patterns were observed for comparisons at the jurisdictional level although differences varied across jurisdictions.

The distribution of children by sex across different jurisdictions was very similar to the national distribution.

As expected, for Northern Territory there was a high proportion of Indigenous children (38.7%) sampled. Queensland had a higher proportion of Indigenous children (9.4%) compared to the national proportion of Indigenous children in the Survey (5.5%), while Victoria and Australian Capital Territory had a lower proportion of Indigenous children (1.3% and 2.8%, respectively).

South Australia, Northern Territory and Tasmania had a lower proportion of children with an overseas born parent compared to the national proportion of children with a parent who was born overseas (36.4%), while this proportion was higher in Western Australia (45.5%).

In the Australian Capital Territory, just over two-thirds of children (67.4%) had a parent with some tertiary education, which was significantly higher than the national proportion of 48.1%.

Just over half of children in the Australian Capital Territory (52.7%) and over one-third of children in Western Australia (36.8%) lived in high level income households. These proportions were significantly higher than the national estimate of 29.1%. In contrast, a significantly lower proportion of children from Tasmania and South Australia lived in high level income households (16.9% and 22.1%, respectively).

For most jurisdictions, the distribution of children by residential location was very similar to the national distribution. However, variations existed for Northern Territory and Western Australia. Children in the Northern Territory lived in either Remote/Very remote (44.0%) or Outer regional areas (56.0%). In Western Australia, there was a higher proportion of children living in Remote/Very remote areas when compared to the national estimate of 2.5%.

A significantly higher proportion of children in South Australia and Western Australia made their last dental visit for the purpose of a check-up (85%). This is compared to the national estimate of 79.9%.

Oral health of Australian children

Table 4-2: Percentage of children by selected characteristics, states and territories, Australia

	Population: children aged 5–14 years								
	Australia	ACT	NSW	NT	Qld	SA	Tas	Vic	WA
Sex									
Male	51.2	51.2	51.2	51.2	51.1	51.5	51.7	51.2	51.4
	49.8–52.6	45.9–56.5	48.1–54.3	46.6–55.8	48.9–53.3	48.0–54.9	47.2–56.2	47.9–54.4	48.7–54.2
Female	48.8	48.8	48.8	48.8	48.9	48.5	48.3	48.8	48.6
	47.4–50.2	43.5–54.1	45.7–51.9	44.2–53.4	46.7–51.1	45.1–52.0	43.8–52.8	45.6–52.1	45.8–51.3
Indigenous identity									
Non-Indigenous	94.6	97.3	95.1	61.3	90.6	96.5	92.4	98.7	93.7
	93.6–95.3	95.9–98.2	93.7–96.2	47.3–73.7	87.5–93.0	94.8–97.7	89.4–94.6	97.9–99.1	89.9–96.1
Indigenous	5.5	2.8	4.9	38.7	9.4	3.5	7.6	1.3	6.3
	4.7–6.4	1.8–4.1	3.8–6.3	26.3–52.7	7.0–12.5	2.3–5.2	5.4–10.6	0.9–2.1	3.9–10.1
Parents' country of birth									
Australian born	63.6	64.0	61.3	73.5	67.9	71.0	84.2	62.2	54.6
	61.7–65.4	58.3–69.4	57.1–65.4	65.8–80.0	65.4–70.3	67.7–74.0	80.6–87.1	57.7–66.4	51.0–58.1
Overseas born	36.4	36.0	38.7	26.5	32.1	29.0	15.8	37.8	45.5
	34.6–38.3	30.6–41.7	34.6–42.9	20.0–34.2	29.7–34.6	26.0–32.3	12.9–19.4	33.6–42.3	41.9–49.0
Parental education									
School	29.6	15.3	28.9	34.6	33.9	31.2	26.4	29.0	25.7
	28.0–31.3	11.9–19.4	25.5–32.6	25.4–45.1	30.9–37.1	26.6–36.2	22.3–30.9	25.6–32.6	22.2–29.5
Vocational training	22.3	17.3	21.1	23.4	23.7	24.9	29.9	20.1	25.7
	21.2–23.4	14.5–20.5	18.9–23.5	18.1–29.7	21.7–25.7	21.3–28.8	26.2–34.0	18.0–22.4	22.8–28.7
Tertiary education	48.1	67.4	50.0	42.0	42.4	43.9	43.7	51.0	48.6
	46.1–50.1	61.4–72.9	45.6–54.4	34.3–50.0	39.2–45.7	38.9–49.1	39.0–48.5	46.8–55.1	44.2–53.1

Continued ...

The National Child Oral Health Study 2012–14

Table 4-2: (continued) Percentage of children by selected characteristics, states and territories, Australia

	Population: children aged 5–14 years								
	Australia	ACT	NSW	NT	Qld	SA	Tas	Vic	WA
Household income									
Low	32.5	17.7	32.6	33.4	33.3	35.6	40.0	32.9	27.5
	30.6–34.5	*13.0–23.7*	*28.5–36.9*	*21.1–48.6*	*29.7–37.0*	*30.9–40.6*	*33.8–46.5*	*28.7–37.5*	*23.6–31.7*
Medium	38.4	29.7	36.3	34.7	40.3	42.3	43.1	39.6	35.7
	37.0–39.8	*25.5–34.2*	*33.4–39.3*	*26.2–44.3*	*37.9–42.7*	*38.8–45.8*	*38.3–48.0*	*36.5–42.9*	*33.0–38.5*
High	29.1	52.7	31.1	31.9	26.5	22.1	16.9	27.5	36.8
	27.2–31.1	*44.6–60.5*	*26.9–35.6*	*23.9–41.0*	*23.5–29.7*	*18.5–26.2*	*13.7–20.8*	*23.6–31.7*	*32.2–41.7*
Residential location									
Major city	68.0	100	72.2	—	59.9	70.2	—	73.8	73.8
	65.1–70.7	—	*66.2–77.5*	—	*54.1–65.4*	*63.1–76.4*	—	*68.5–78.5*	*64.7–81.3*
Inner regional	19.7	—	20.4	—	22.2	11.7	64.6	21.2	10.0
	17.4–22.3	—	*15.7–26.1*	—	*17.3–28.0*	*6.9–19.1*	*52.0–75.4*	*16.6–26.6*	*6.3–15.4*
Outer regional	9.8	—	6.8	56.0	15.3	13.7	35.4	4.9	7.2
	8.2–11.6	—	*4.1–11.2*	*46.4–65.2*	*11.8–19.5*	*9.4–19.5*	*24.6–48.0*	*2.9–8.2*	*3.5–14.2*
Remote/Very remote	2.5	—	0.6	44.0	2.7	4.5	—	0.1	9.1
	1.6–3.9	—	*0.2–1.6*	*34.8–53.6*	*0.8–8.4*	*1.9–10.0*	—	*0.0–0.6*	*4.2–18.5*
Reason for last dental visit									
Check-up	79.9	81.0	78.1	73.8	77.7	85.1	81.6	81.0	84.8
	78.8–81.0	*78.0–83.6*	*75.4–80.5*	*66.5–80.1*	*75.5–79.6*	*83.2–86.8*	*78.8–84.1*	*78.9–83.0*	*82.6–86.7*
Dental problem	20.1	19.0	21.9	26.2	22.4	14.9	18.4	19.0	15.2
	19.0–21.2	*16.4–22.0*	*19.5–24.6*	*19.9–33.5*	*20.4–24.5*	*13.2–16.8*	*15.9–21.2*	*17.0–21.1*	*13.3–17.4*

Row 1: Proportions were computed using weighted data.
Row 2: 95% CI: Confidence intervals for estimates were computed using weighted data.
Columns are arranged by age at time of Survey.

Oral health of Australian children

4.2 Participation in the Survey

Response rates are analysed at two levels, firstly by analysing the participation of schools selected in the Survey, and secondly by analysing the participation of children sampled through the selected schools.

School Participation

Across Australia, a total of 876 schools were selected from the sampling frame of 10,450 schools in scope for the Survey. In-scope schools consisted of 5,929 primary only schools, 1,371 secondary only schools and 3,150 combined primary/secondary schools.

The number of schools that consented to participate in the Survey was 841. Of the original schools selected, 432 consented to participate in the Survey and 409 schools were replaced. Replacement schools were provided on a case-by-case basis to ensure that they were from the same region and same school socioeconomic characteristics as the original school selected. This strategy was possible for the majority of schools that were replaced.

Analysis of the schools selected and the schools which participated in the Survey is provided by region of the school and school type (Table 4-3).

Table 4-3: School participation by region of school and school type, states and territories, Australia

	AUS	ACT	NSW	NT	Qld	SA	Tas	Vic	WA
	Number of schools selected								
Region of school									
Capital city	492	33	83	25	76	76	27	89	83
Rest of State	384	—	73	24	138	32	30	67	20
School type									
Catholic	172	6	30	6	44	27	12	33	14
Independent	134	8	28	10	25	13	6	24	20
Public	570	19	98	33	145	68	39	99	69
Total	**876**	**33**	**156**	**49**	**214**	**108**	**57**	**156**	**103**
	Number of schools participated								
Region of school									
Capital city	459	33	70	22	83	62	28	83	78
Rest of State	382	—	90	17	121	35	27	71	21
School type									
Catholic	142	5	20	5	42	20	12	25	13
Independent	110	3	21	6	19	13	6	27	15
Public	589	25	119	28	143	64	37	102	71
Total	**841**	**33**	**160**	**39**	**204**	**97**	**55**	**154**	**99**

Child Participation

There were 24,664 children examined across Australia. The number of children selected in each school was over-sampled to account for an estimated percentage of parents who would not consent to their child being examined.

The child participation rate, calculated as a percentage, is provided by region of school and school type. It is calculated as the number of children examined divided by the number of children selected for each region and school type. To derive child participation rates by region, children were assigned to a region based on the location of the school they attended.

The overall participation rate for children selected across Australia was 31.0%. Participation ranged from 20.6% in the Northern Territory to 49.4% in the Australian Capital Territory. Participation rates varied across region with participation rates higher in Capital cities compared to Rest of State (32.6% compared with 29.4%). Participation rates also varied by school type with participation highest for children selected from catholic schools (34.5%) and lowest for children selected from public schools (31.3%).

Table 4-4: Child participation by region of school and school type, states and territories, Australia

	AUS	ACT	NSW	NT	Qld	SA	Tas	Vic	WA
				Number of children examined					
Region of school									
Capital city	13,701	2,213	2,231	421	1,732	1,937	869	2,287	2,011
Rest of State	10,963		2,503	444	3,675	1,059	680	2,066	536
School type									
Catholic	4,587	287	663	132	1,124	742	396	716	527
Independent	4,086	298	801	201	659	566	214	828	519
Public	15,991	1,628	3,270	532	3,624	1,688	939	2,809	1,501
Total	**24,664**	**2,213**	**4,734**	**865**	**5,407**	**2,996**	**1,549**	**4,353**	**2,547**
				Child participation rate (%)					
Region of school									
Capital city	32.6	51.7	30.8	19.9	30.8	32.7	34.5	25.3	37.7
Rest of State	29.4	—	25.5	21.2	33.4	28.2	32.7	28.3	43.6
School type									
Catholic	34.5	53.1	33.1	22.3	33.9	32.5	32.8	31.8	47.7
Independent	27.0	49.7	22.2	23.7	34.9	31.7	30.5	19.8	34.6
Public	31.3	48.7	28.5	19.2	31.7	30.1	34.9	28.4	37.9
Total	**31.0**	**49.4**	**27.7**	**20.6**	**32.5**	**31.0**	**33.7**	**26.6**	**38.8**

Oral health of Australian children

4.3 Assessment of non-participation bias

Despite the many advantages of studies based on a sample of individuals, surveys are not exempt of errors. Errors occur when the results obtained from the survey data which uses a sample of the population are different from the results that would have been obtained if data were gathered from the total population (i.e. a census). These errors (or bias) may result when some segments of the population do not participate in a survey. Bias due to non-participation occurs when the participants differ from the non-participants or the target population in one or more characteristics. Nonetheless, low participation rates are not necessarily indicative of biased estimates, for example, when participation is not systematically limited to a segment of the population in such instances, despite low participation the sample continues to appropriately represent the target population.

Several approaches can be taken to determine the potential for and extent of bias. For this Survey, two approaches were adopted. The first approach was to examine participation rates at the small area level to determine whether participation in the Survey was correlated to an area's socioeconomic characteristics. The second approach was to compare the population estimates derived from the sample with the known sociodemographic characteristics.

Relationship between small area socioeconomic indicators and participation rates

To examine variation in participation rates at the small area level, children were assigned to a postcode based on the location of the school they were selected from. Participation at postcode level was defined as the number of children examined in a postcode divided by the number of children selected in the postcode.

This variability in participation rates provided the opportunity to examine if characteristics of small geographic areas were associated with participation in the Survey. The Australian Bureau of Statistics (ABS) Socio-economic Indexes for Areas (SEIFA), defined at the postcode level, was used to examine if Survey participation rates differed systematically between advantaged and disadvantaged postcodes.

This analysis focused on the Index of Relative Socio-economic Advantage and Disadvantage (IRSAD) (Australian Bureau of Statistics 2013). The IRSAD is a continuum in which lower values indicate more disadvantaged areas (areas with a relatively higher proportion of people with low income and more people with unskilled occupations) and higher values indicate more advantaged areas (areas with a relatively high proportion of people with high income and skilled occupations). For this analysis, the IRSAD were assigned to the postcode of each school's location.

Figure 4–1 presents the correlation between participation rates at the postcode level and the corresponding IRSAD score.

The ABS 2011 SEIFA IRSAD values for Australian postcodes ranged between 588 and 1,191 with only 38 of 2,418 postcodes having a score below 800 (1.5%). The IRSAD values for postcodes where children were selected from ranged between 689 and 1,151 with 5 of 556 postcodes (0.9%) having an IRSAD score below 800.

Participation rates were not similarly distributed across the range of IRSAD scores. As can be seen from Figure 4-1, data points were not randomly dispersed. This Figure shows a significant relationship between IRSAD score and postcode participation rate, with participation rate lower among lower IRSAD scores. A correlation coefficient of 0.23 and its associated p-value of <0.0001 further indicates a small, yet significant, correlation between participation in the Survey and level of socioeconomic advantage/disadvantage of areas.

The potential impact of the bias found in participation rates by area level socioeconomic factors on estimates relating to the oral health of children will be examined in the section 'Direct standardisation using population benchmarks' within this chapter.

Oral health of Australian children

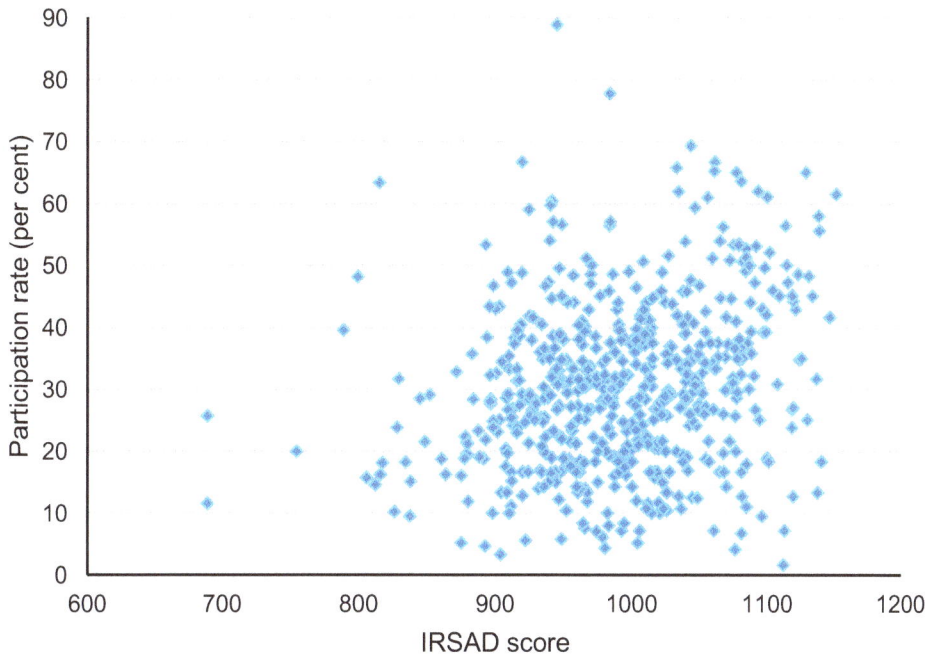

Figure 4-1: Participation in the examination among postcodes classified by the Index of Socio-economic Advantage and Disadvantage (IRSAD)

Comparison with population benchmarks

Although the weighting strategy was designed to ensure the sociodemographic composition of the sample closely reflected that of the population of Australian children aged 5–14 years, it is important to present comparisons at both the national and jurisdictional levels to investigate any potential for bias. The following tables compare the estimated population distributions derived from the weighted national dataset with the known population distributions for a range of sociodemographic characteristics relating to the child, the child's parents (or guardians) and the child's household.

The known population distributions for child's age and sex were derived from the ABS 2011 estimated residential population counts provided in catalogue number 3235.0, Population by Age and Sex, Regions of Australia. For child's Indigenous identity and remoteness area the population distributions were derived from the ABS 2011 Census TableBuilder product. The population distributions for regional location in NSW and Victoria were supplied by the respective Dental Health Services. For the remaining States and Territories the regional population distributions were derived from the ABS 2011 estimated residential population counts provided in catalogue number 3235.0. The known population distributions for parental and household characteristics were sourced from the 2011 Census via an ABS consultancy service. More details of the data sources used to derive these distributions are provided in Chapter 3

For each sociodemographic characteristic, the estimated percentage derived from the survey is compared with the actual population percentage. If the 95% confidence interval for the survey estimate does not contain the actual population percentage this indicates the sample is unrepresentative of the child population for that sociodemographic characteristic.

Comparisons at the national level indicated the estimated and actual population distributions were almost identical for all sociodemographic characteristics (Table 4-5). Differences were largest for parent education status, where the estimated percentage of children with at least one parent with a Bachelor degree or higher was 0.8 percentage points higher than the actual population percentage.

A similar pattern was observed for comparisons at the jurisdictional level although differences were slightly larger in some jurisdictions. With the exception of remoteness area for Tasmania and the Australian Capital Territory, all 95% confidence intervals for survey estimates derived from the national dataset contained the known population percentage. In Tasmania, 1.8% of the child population lived in Remote/Very remote areas but the survey estimated 0% as examinations were not conducted in these areas (Table 4-11). Similarly, children were not examined in the Inner regional areas of the Australian Capital Territory but 0.2% of the child population lived in these areas (Table 4-6).

The jurisdiction with the largest differences between the estimated and actual population distributions was the Northern Territory (Table 4-8). The survey underestimated the percentage of children with at least one Indigenous parent by 3.0 percentage points. Differences were also observed for the sociodemographic characteristics parent education status and parent labour force status. The percentage of children with a parent who had completed a Bachelor degree or higher was overestimated by 1.9 percentage points and the percentage of children with an employed parent (either full-time or part-time) was overestimated by 1.3 percentage points.

In New South Wales, differences between the estimated and actual population distributions were largest for the sociodemographic characteristics parent education status and household income (Table 4-7). The percentage of children with a highly educated parent was overestimated by 1.1 percentage points and the percentage of children living in high income households was overestimated by 1.0 percentage point. The opposite result was observed in Queensland, where the percentage of children living in high income households was underestimated by 0.8 percentage points (Table 4-9).

Differences between the estimated and actual population distributions in South Australia were largest for parent education status, with the Survey overestimating the percentage of children with a parent who had completed a Bachelor degree or higher by 0.9 percentage points (Table 4-10). In Tasmania, variations by remoteness area have been described previously. For all other sociodemographic characteristics, differences between the estimated and actual population distributions were less than 0.8 percentage points. Similar results were observed in Victoria, where the maximum difference between distributions was less than 0.5 percentage points (Table 4-12).

For Western Australia, the survey overestimated the percentage of children living in Remote/Very remote areas by 1.8 percentage points and underestimated the percentage living in Outer regional areas by 1.6 percentage points (Table 4-13). Other differences between the estimated and actual population distributions were observed for parent education status (1.1 percentage points).

The above comparisons indicate that differences between the estimated and actual population distributions were minor at both jurisdictional and national level and therefore we can conclude that the sociodemographic composition of the weighted national dataset closely reflected that of the target child population.

Table 4-5: Population benchmark comparison — Australia

	Survey estimate		Population benchmark
	% of children	(95% CI)	% of children
Child characteristics			
Child age			
5–6 years	20.5	(19.4–21.6)	20.4
7–8 years	19.7	(18.7–20.7)	19.6
9–10 years	19.7	(18.7–20.6)	19.7
11–12 years	20.0	(19.2–20.8)	20.0
13–14 years	20.1	(17.9–22.6)	20.3
Child sex			
Male	51.2	(49.8–52.6)	51.3
Female	48.8	(47.4–50.2)	48.7
Child Indigenous identity			
Non-Indigenous	95.1	(94.3–95.8)	95.1
Indigenous	4.9	(4.2–5.7)	4.9
Parent/guardian characteristics			
Parents' country of birth			
Australian born	63.6	(61.7–65.4)	63.5
Overseas born[1]	36.4	(34.6–38.3)	36.5
Parent Indigenous identity			
Non-Indigenous	95.9	(95.1–96.6)	95.9
Indigenous[2]	4.1	(3.4–4.9)	4.1
Parent labour force status			
Employed	85.2	(83.7–86.6)	85.0
Not employed[3]	14.8	(13.4–16.3)	15.0
Parent education status			
Completed Bachelor degree	32.6	(30.7–34.5)	31.8
No Bachelor degree[4]	67.4	(65.5–69.3)	68.2
Household characteristics			
Type of household			
One parent household	20.9	(19.8–22.2)	21.0
Two parent household	79.1	(77.8–80.2)	79.0
Household income			
Low	32.5	(30.6–34.5)	32.6
Medium	38.4	(37.0–39.8)	38.4
High	29.1	(27.2–31.1)	29.0

Oral health of Australian children

Table 4-5: Population benchmark comparison — Australia (continued)

	Survey estimate		Population benchmark
	% of children	(95% CI)	% of children
		Geographic characteristics	
Child remoteness area			
Major cities	68.0	(65.1–70.7)	67.8
Inner regional	19.7	(17.4–22.3)	19.8
Outer regional	9.8	(8.2–11.6)	9.9
Remote/Very remote	2.5	(1.6–3.9)	2.5

1 Children were classified to the overseas born category if they had at least one parent who was born overseas.
2 Children were classified to the Indigenous category if they had at least one parent who was Indigenous.
3 Children were classified to the employed category if they had at least one parent who was employed.
4 Children were classified to the completed Bachelor degree category if they had at least one parent who had completed a Bachelor degree or higher.

Table 4-6: Population benchmark comparison — Australian Capital Territory

	Survey estimate		Population benchmark
	% of children	(95% CI)	% of children
Child characteristics			
Child age			
5–6 years	21.3	(17.2–26.1)	21.3
7–8 years	19.8	(15.9–24.4)	19.8
9–10 years	19.2	(15.9–22.9)	19.2
11–12 years	19.9	(17.1–23.1)	19.9
13–14 years	19.8	(11.9–31.1)	19.8
Child sex			
Male	51.2	(45.9–56.5)	51.2
Female	48.8	(43.5–54.1)	48.8
Child Indigenous identity			
Non-Indigenous	97.3	(95.9–98.2)	97.3
Indigenous	2.7	(1.8–4.1)	2.7
Parent/guardian characteristics			
Parents' country of birth			
Australian born	64.0	(58.3–69.4)	63.9
Overseas born[1]	36.0	(30.6–41.7)	36.1
Parent Indigenous identity			
Non-Indigenous	97.5	(96.1–98.3)	97.7
Indigenous[2]	2.5	(1.7–3.9)	2.3
Parent labour force status			
Employed	91.9	(88.7–94.3)	92.0
Not employed[3]	8.1	(5.7–11.3)	8.0
Parent education status			
Completed Bachelor degree	51.7	(44.8–58.6)	51.6
No Bachelor degree[4]	48.3	(41.4–55.2)	48.4
Household characteristics			
Type of household			
One parent household	18.4	(14.6–22.8)	18.3
Two parent household	81.6	(77.2–85.4)	81.7
Household income			
Low	17.7	(13.0–23.7)	17.7
Medium	29.6	(25.5–34.2)	29.5
High	52.7	(44.6–60.5)	52.8

Oral health of Australian children

Table 4-6: Population benchmark comparison — Australian Capital Territory (continued)

	Survey estimate		Population benchmark
	% of children	(95% CI)	% of children
		Geographic characteristics	
Child remoteness area			
Major cities	100.0	(–)	99.8
Inner regional	–	(–)	0.2
Outer regional	–	(–)	–
Remote/Very remote	–	(–)	–
Child SA4 region			
Australian Capital Territory	100.0	(–)	100.0

1 Children were classified to the overseas born category if they had at least one parent who was born overseas.
2 Children were classified to the Indigenous category if they had at least one parent who was Indigenous.
3 Children were classified to the employed category if they had at least one parent who was employed.
4 Children were classified to the completed Bachelor degree category if they had at least one parent who had completed a Bachelor degree or higher.

Table 4-7: Population benchmark comparison — New South Wales

	Survey estimate		Population benchmark
	% of children	(95% CI)	% of children
Child characteristics			
Child age			
5–6 years	20.8	(18.4–23.4)	20.5
7–8 years	20.0	(17.9–22.2)	19.7
9–10 years	19.6	(17.6–21.7)	19.7
11–12 years	19.8	(18.3–21.5)	20.0
13–14 years	19.8	(15.1–25.5)	20.1
Child sex			
Male	51.2	(48.1–54.3)	51.5
Female	48.8	(45.7–51.9)	48.5
Child Indigenous identity			
Non-Indigenous	95.1	(93.7–96.2)	95.1
Indigenous	4.9	(3.8–6.3)	4.9
Parent/guardian characteristics			
Parents' country of birth			
Australian born	61.3	(57.1–65.4)	61.0
Overseas born[1]	38.7	(34.6–42.9)	39.0
Parent Indigenous identity			
Non-Indigenous	95.8	(94.6–96.8)	95.9
Indigenous[2]	4.2	(3.2–5.4)	4.1
Parent labour force status			
Employed	84.5	(81.0–87.4)	84.2
Not employed[3]	15.5	(12.6–19.0)	15.8
Parent education status			
Completed Bachelor degree	34.2	(29.9–38.7)	33.1
No Bachelor degree[4]	65.8	(61.3–70.1)	66.9
Household characteristics			
Type of household			
One parent household	20.8	(18.7–23.2)	21.1
Two parent household	79.2	(76.8–81.3)	78.9
Household income			
Low	32.6	(28.5–36.9)	33.5
Medium	36.3	(33.4–39.3)	36.4
High	31.1	(26.9–35.6)	30.1

Oral health of Australian children

Table 4-7: Population benchmark comparison – New South Wales (continued)

	Survey estimate		Population benchmark
	% of children	(95% CI)	% of children
		Geographic characteristics	
Child remoteness area			
Major cities	72.2	(66.2–77.5)	72.0
Inner regional	20.4	(15.7–26.1)	20.7
Outer regional	6.8	(4.1,11.2)	6.7
Remote/Very remote	0.6	(0.2,1.6)	0.6
Child local health district			
Sydney	5.8	(2.8–11.8)	5.8
South Western Sydney	14.0	(9.9–19.4)	14.0
South Eastern Sydney	9.4	(5.7–14.9)	9.4
Illawarra Shoalhaven	5.3	(2.9–9.5)	5.3
Western Sydney	12.8	(8.7–18.4)	12.8
Nepean Blue Mountains	5.3	(3.4–8.1)	5.3
Northern Sydney	11.5	(7.1–17.9)	11.5
Central Coast	4.6	(3.2–6.7)	4.6
Hunter New England	12.5	(9.5–16.2)	12.5
Northern NSW	4.0	(2.7–6.0)	4.0
Mid North Coast	2.9	(1.8–4.8)	2.9
Southern NSW	2.8	(2.0–3.8)	2.8
Murrumbidgee	3.6	(2.1–6.2)	3.6
Western NSW	4.3	(2.4–7.4)	4.3
Far West	0.4	(0.2–1.0)	0.4
Network with Vic	0.7	(0.3–1.5)	0.7

1 Children were classified to the overseas born category if they had at least one parent who was born overseas.
2 Children were classified to the Indigenous category if they had at least one parent who was Indigenous.
3 Children were classified to the employed category if they had at least one parent who was employed.
4 Children were classified to the completed Bachelor degree category if they had at least one parent who had completed a Bachelor degree or higher.

Table 4-8: Population benchmark comparison — Northern Territory

	Survey estimate		Population benchmark
	% of children	(95% CI)	% of children
Child characteristics			
Child age			
5–6 years	20.8	(16.5–25.7)	20.8
7–8 years	20.3	(16.3–24.9)	20.2
9–10 years	20.2	(16.1–25.2)	20.3
11–12 years	19.3	(14.6–25.0)	19.3
13–14 years	19.4	(11.9–30.0)	19.4
Child sex			
Male	51.2	(46.6–55.8)	50.9
Female	48.8	(44.2–53.4)	49.1
Child Indigenous identity			
Non-Indigenous	61.3	(47.3–73.7)	61.8
Indigenous	38.7	(26.3–52.7)	38.2
Parent/guardian characteristics			
Parents' country of birth			
Australian born	73.5	(65.8–80.0)	74.0
Overseas born[1]	26.5	(20.0–34.2)	26.0
Parent Indigenous identity			
Non-Indigenous	61.9	(47.9–74.2)	64.9
Indigenous[2]	38.1	(25.8–52.1)	35.1
Parent labour force status			
Employed	81.5	(69.7–89.4)	80.2
Not employed[3]	18.5	(10.6–30.3)	19.8
Parent education status			
Completed Bachelor degree	24.1	(17.8–31.7)	22.2
No Bachelor degree[4]	75.9	(68.3–82.2)	77.8
Household characteristics			
Type of household			
One parent household	24.2	(17.5–32.4)	24.2
Two parent household	75.8	(67.6–82.5)	75.8
Household income			
Low	33.4	(21.1–48.6)	34.4
Medium	34.7	(26.2–44.3)	34.4
High	31.9	(23.9–41.0)	31.2

Oral health of Australian children

Table 4.8: Population benchmark comparison — Northern Territory (continued)

	Survey estimate		Population benchmark
	% of children	(95% CI)	% of children
		Geographic characteristics	
Child remoteness area			
Major cities	–	(–)	–
Inner regional	–	(–)	–
Outer regional	56.0	(46.4–65.2)	57.1
Remote/Very remote	44.0	(34.8–53.6)	42.9
Child SA4 region			
Darwin	56.0	(46.4–65.2)	56.0
NT Outback	44.0	(34.8–53.6)	44.0

1 Children were classified to the overseas born category if they had at least one parent who was born overseas.
2 Children were classified to the Indigenous category if they had at least one parent who was Indigenous.
3 Children were classified to the employed category if they had at least one parent who was employed.
4 Children were classified to the completed Bachelor degree category if they had at least one parent who had completed a Bachelor degree or higher.

Table 4-9: Population benchmark comparison — Queensland

	Survey estimate		Population benchmark
	% of children	(95% CI)	% of children
Child characteristics			
Child age			
5–6 years	20.5	(18.7–22.3)	20.5
7–8 years	19.5	(17.7–21.4)	19.5
9–10 years	19.9	(18.4–21.5)	19.9
11–12 years	19.9	(18.5–21.4)	19.9
13–14 years	20.2	(16.3–24.8)	20.2
Child sex			
Male	51.1	(48.9–53.3)	51.3
Female	48.9	(46.7–51.1)	48.7
Child Indigenous identity			
Non-Indigenous	93.1	(90.4–95.1)	93.1
Indigenous	6.9	(4.9–9.6)	6.9
Parent/guardian characteristics			
Parents' country of birth			
Australian born	67.9	(65.4–70.3)	67.2
Overseas born[1]	32.1	(29.7–34.6)	32.8
Parent Indigenous identity			
Non-Indigenous	94.2	(91.3–96.1)	94.2
Indigenous[2]	5.8	(3.9–8.7)	5.8
Parent labour force status			
Employed	84.7	(81.3–87.5)	84.6
Not employed[3]	15.3	(12.5–18.7)	15.4
Parent education status			
Completed Bachelor degree	28.3	(25.3–31.5)	27.8
No Bachelor degree[4]	71.7	(68.5–74.7)	72.2
Household characteristics			
Type of household			
One parent household	22.6	(20.0–25.5)	22.3
Two parent household	77.4	(74.5–80.0)	77.7
Household income			
Low	33.3	(29.7–37.0)	32.5
Medium	40.3	(37.9–42.7)	40.3
High	26.5	(23.5–29.7)	27.3

Oral health of Australian children

Table 4.9: Population benchmark comparison — Queensland (continued)

	Survey estimate		Population benchmark
	% of children	(95% CI)	% of children
		Geographic characteristics	
Child remoteness area			
Major cities	59.9	(54.1–65.4)	59.5
Inner regional	22.2	(17.3–28.0)	21.6
Outer regional	15.2	(11.8–19.5)	15.7
Remote/Very remote	2.7	(0.8–8.4)	3.4
Child SA4 region			
Brisbane East	5.1	(3.1–8.1)	5.1
Brisbane North	3.8	(2.3–6.3)	3.8
Brisbane South	6.3	(4.1–9.7)	6.3
Brisbane West	3.5	(2.1–5.7)	3.8
Brisbane Inner City	3.7	(1.9–7.1)	3.4
Cairns	5.9	(3.8–9.1)	5.6
Darling Downs–Maranoa	3.1	(1.1–8.3)	3.1
Fitzroy	5.3	(4.1–6.8)	5.3
Gold Coast	10.8	(7.9–14.6)	10.8
Ipswich	7.8	(5.4–11.0)	7.3
Logan–Beaudesert	7.6	(5.1–11.1)	7.6
Mackay	4.0	(2.0–7.7)	4.0
Moreton Bay North	5.2	(3.1–8.5)	5.2
Moreton Bay South	4.4	(2.3–8.2)	4.4
Queensland Outback	2.0	(0.4–9.0)	2.3
Sunshine Coast	6.9	(4.8–10.0)	6.9
Toowoomba	3.0	(1.0–8.8)	3.4
Townsville	5.3	(4.7–5.9)	5.3
Wide Bay	6.4	(3.6–11.2)	6.4

1 Children were classified to the overseas born category if they had at least one parent who was born overseas.
2 Children were classified to the Indigenous category if they had at least one parent who was Indigenous.
3 Children were classified to the employed category if they had at least one parent who was employed.
4 Children were classified to the completed Bachelor degree category if they had at least one parent who had completed a Bachelor degree or higher.

Table 4-10: Population benchmark comparison — South Australia

	Survey estimate		Population benchmark
	% of children	(95% CI)	% of children
Child characteristics			
Child age			
5–6 years	19.8	(17.5–22.4)	19.8
7–8 years	19.4	(17.2–21.8)	19.4
9–10 years	19.6	(17.6–21.8)	19.6
11–12 years	20.4	(18.0–23.1)	20.4
13–14 years	20.7	(15.7–26.8)	20.7
Child sex			
Male	51.5	(48.0–54.9)	51.1
Female	48.5	(45.1–52.0)	48.9
Child Indigenous identity			
Non-Indigenous	96.5	(94.8–97.7)	96.2
Indigenous	3.5	(2.3–5.2)	3.8
Parent/guardian characteristics			
Parent country of birth			
Australian born	71.0	(67.7–74.0)	70.3
Overseas born[1]	29.0	(26.0–32.3)	29.7
Parents' Indigenous identity			
Non-Indigenous	97.4	(95.5–98.5)	97.1
Indigenous[2]	2.6	(1.5–4.5)	2.9
Parent labour force status			
Employed	84.7	(80.6–88.1)	84.1
Not employed[3]	15.3	(11.9–19.4)	15.9
Parent education status			
Completed Bachelor degree	28.9	(24.8–33.3)	28.0
No Bachelor degree[4]	71.1	(66.7–75.2)	72.0
Household characteristics			
Type of household			
One parent household	22.6	(19.3–26.4)	22.7
Two parent household	77.4	(73.6–80.7)	77.3
Household income			
Low	35.6	(30.9–40.6)	35.8
Medium	42.3	(38.8–45.8)	41.8
High	22.1	(18.5–26.2)	22.3

Oral health of Australian children

Table 4.10: Population benchmark comparison — South Australia (continued)

	Survey estimate		Population benchmark
	% of children	(95% CI)	% of children
		Geographic characteristics	
Child remoteness area			
Major cities	70.2	(63.1–76.4)	70.2
Inner regional	11.7	(6.9–19.1)	11.9
Outer regional	13.7	(9.4–19.5)	13.7
Remote/Very remote	4.4	(1.9–10.0)	4.1
Child SA4 region			
Adelaide Central and Hills	16.2	(11.2–22.8)	16.2
Adelaide North	26.3	(19.3–34.6)	26.3
Adelaide South	20.8	(14.0–29.9)	20.8
Adelaide West	11.8	(7.6–18.0)	11.8
Barossa–Yorke–Mid North	7.1	(4.4–11.4)	7.1
South Australia Outback	6.1	(4.3–8.6)	6.1
South Australia South East	11.7	(8.4–15.9)	11.7

1 Children were classified to the overseas born category if they had at least one parent who was born overseas.
2 Children were classified to the Indigenous category if they had at least one parent who was Indigenous.
3 Children were classified to the employed category if they had at least one parent who was employed.
4 Children were classified to the completed Bachelor degree category if they had at least one parent who had completed a Bachelor degree or higher.

Table 4-11: Population benchmark comparison — Tasmania

	Survey estimate		Population benchmark
	% of children	(95% CI)	% of children
Child characteristics			
Child age			
5–6 years	19.7	(15.8–24.4)	19.7
7–8 years	18.8	(16.0–22.1)	18.8
9–10 years	19.8	(16.5–23.5)	19.8
11–12 years	20.7	(17.9–23.9)	20.7
13–14 years	20.9	(13.8–30.4)	20.9
Child sex			
Male	51.7	(47.2–56.2)	51.7
Female	48.3	(43.8–52.8)	48.3
Child Indigenous identity			
Non-Indigenous	92.4	(89.4–94.6)	92.5
Indigenous	7.6	(5.4–10.6)	7.5
Parent/guardian characteristics			
Parents' country of birth			
Australian born	84.2	(80.6–87.1)	84.2
Overseas born[1]	15.8	(12.9–19.4)	15.8
Parent Indigenous identity			
Non-Indigenous	92.7	(89.9–94.9)	93.4
Indigenous[2]	7.3	(5.1–10.1)	6.6
Parent labour force status			
Employed	81.2	(75.0–86.1)	81.5
Not employed[3]	18.8	(13.9–25.0)	18.5
Parent education status			
Completed Bachelor degree	23.1	(19.1–27.6)	23.2
No Bachelor degree[4]	76.9	(72.4–80.9)	76.8
Household characteristics			
Type of household			
One parent household	25.0	(21.0–29.4)	24.9
Two parent household	75.0	(70.6–79.0)	75.1
Household income			
Low	40.0	(33.8–46.5)	40.4
Medium	43.1	(38.3–48.0)	42.4
High	16.9	(13.7–20.8)	17.2

Oral health of Australian children

Table 4.11: Population benchmark comparison — Tasmania (continued)

	Survey estimate		Population benchmark
	% of children	(95% CI)	% of children
		Geographic characteristics	
Child remoteness area			
Major cities	–	(–)	–
Inner regional	64.6	(52.0–75.4)	64.8
Outer regional	35.4	(24.6–48.0)	33.4
Remote/Very remote	–	(–)	1.8
Child SA4 region			
Hobart	41.3	(32.5–50.6)	41.3
Launceston and North East	28.0	(19.6–38.2)	28.0
South East	7.6	(4.0–14.0)	7.6
West and North West	23.2	(16.8–31.1)	23.2

1 Children were classified to the overseas born category if they had at least one parent who was born overseas.
2 Children were classified to the Indigenous category if they had at least one parent who was Indigenous.
3 Children were classified to the employed category if they had at least one parent who was employed.
4 Children were classified to the completed Bachelor degree category if they had at least one parent who had completed a Bachelor degree or higher.

Table 4-12: Population benchmark comparison — Victoria

	Survey estimate		Population benchmark
	% of children	(95% CI)	% of children
Child characteristics			
Child age			
5–6 years	20.4	(18.3–22.7)	20.5
7–8 years	19.7	(17.7–21.8)	19.8
9–10 years	19.6	(17.6–21.8)	19.6
11–12 years	20.0	(18.5–21.6)	19.9
13–14 years	20.3	(15.8–25.6)	20.2
Child sex			
Male	51.2	(47.9–54.4)	51.3
Female	48.8	(45.6–52.1)	48.7
Child Indigenous identity			
Non-Indigenous	98.7	(97.9–99.1)	98.6
Indigenous	1.3	(0.9–2.1)	1.4
Parent/guardian characteristics			
Parents' country of birth			
Australian born	62.2	(57.7–66.4)	62.5
Overseas born[1]	37.8	(33.6–42.3)	37.5
Parent Indigenous identity			
Non-Indigenous	99.1	(98.6–99.5)	98.9
Indigenous[2]	0.9	(0.5–1.4)	1.1
Parent labour force status			
Employed	86.5	(83.5–88.9)	86.4
Not employed[3]	13.5	(11.1–16.5)	13.6
Parent education status			
Completed Bachelor degree	35.4	(31.8–39.3)	35.0
No Bachelor degree[4]	64.6	(60.7–68.2)	65.0
Household characteristics			
Type of household			
One parent household	19.3	(16.9–22.0)	19.4
Two parent household	80.7	(78.0–83.1)	80.6
Household income			
Low	32.9	(28.7–37.5)	32.8
Medium	39.6	(36.5–42.9)	39.9
High	27.5	(23.6–31.7)	27.3

Oral health of Australian children

Table 4.12: Population benchmark comparison — Victoria (continued)

	Survey estimate		Population benchmark
	% of children	(95% CI)	% of children
		Geographic characteristics	
Child remoteness area			
Major cities	73.8	(68.5–78.5)	73.8
Inner regional	21.2	(16.6–26.6)	21.3
Outer regional	4.9	(2.9–8.2)	4.8
Remote/Very remote	0.1	(0.0–0.6)	0.1
Child dental health service			
Barwon South West	7.1	(5.1–9.6)	7.1
Grampians	4.4	(2.8–6.8)	4.4
Loddon Mallee	6.2	(4.6–8.4)	6.2
Hume	5.4	(3.4–8.6)	5.4
Gippsland	4.9	(3.4–7.1)	4.9
Western Metro	14.5	(10.7–19.2)	14.5
Northern Metro	15.5	(10.4–22.4)	15.5
Eastern Metro	18.1	(13.3–24.1)	18.1
Southern Metro	24.0	(18.2–30.9)	24.0

1 Children were classified to the overseas born category if they had at least one parent who was born overseas.
2 Children were classified to the Indigenous category if they had at least one parent who was Indigenous.
3 Children were classified to the employed category if they had at least one parent who was employed.
4 Children were classified to the completed Bachelor degree category if they had at least one parent who had completed a Bachelor degree or higher.

Table 4-13: Population benchmark comparison — Western Australia

	Survey estimate		Population benchmark
	% of children	(95% CI)	% of children
Child characteristics			
Child age			
5–6 years	20.4	(18.1–22.8)	20.4
7–8 years	19.6	(17.6–21.7)	19.6
9–10 years	19.6	(17.5–21.8)	19.6
11–12 years	20.2	(17.8–22.9)	20.2
13–14 years	20.3	(15.6–25.8)	20.3
Child sex			
Male	51.4	(48.7–54.2)	51.0
Female	48.6	(45.8–51.3)	49.0
Child Indigenous identity			
Non-Indigenous	93.7	(89.9–96.1)	94.0
Indigenous	6.3	(3.9–10.1)	6.0
Parent/guardian characteristics			
Parents' country of birth			
Australian born	54.5	(51.0–58.1)	54.3
Overseas born[1]	45.5	(41.9–49.0)	45.7
Parent Indigenous identity			
Non-Indigenous	95.2	(92.2–97.1)	94.9
Indigenous[2]	4.8	(2.9–7.8)	5.1
Parent labour force status			
Employed	86.0	(83.0–88.6)	85.9
Not employed[3]	14.0	(11.4–17.0)	14.1
Parent education status			
Completed Bachelor degree	31.8	(27.5–36.5)	30.7
No Bachelor degree[4]	68.2	(63.5–72.5)	69.3
Household characteristics			
Type of household			
One parent household	19.6	(17.0–22.4)	19.6
Two parent household	80.4	(77.6–83.0)	80.4
Household income			
Low	27.5	(23.6–31.7)	27.6
Medium	35.7	(33.0–38.5)	36.3
High	36.8	(32.2–41.7)	36.1

Oral health of Australian children

Table 4.13: Population benchmark comparison — Western Australia (continued)

	Survey estimate		Population benchmark
	% of children	(95% CI)	% of children
		Geographic characteristics	
Child remoteness area			
	73.8	(64.7–81.3)	73.8
	10.0	(6.3–15.4)	10.1
	7.2	(3.5–14.2)	8.8
	9.0	(4.2–18.5)	7.2
Child SA4 region			
Bunbury	7.7	(4.7–12.4)	7.7
Mandurah	3.7	(1.8–7.2)	3.7
Perth Inner	5.6	(3.2–9.4)	5.6
Perth North East	10.0	(5.8–16.9)	10.0
Perth North West	22.0	(16.4–28.9)	22.0
Perth South East	18.3	(13.0–25.1)	18.3
Perth South West	16.0	(11.1–22.6)	16.0
Western Aust.Outback	9.0	(4.1–18.5)	10.5
Western Aust.Wheat Belt	7.7	(3.9–14.5)	6.2

1 Children were classified to the overseas born category if they had at least one parent who was born overseas.
2 Children were classified to the Indigenous category if they had at least one parent who was Indigenous.
3 Children were classified to the employed category if they had at least one parent who was employed.
4 Children were classified to the completed Bachelor degree category if they had at least one parent who had completed a Bachelor degree or higher.

Assessment of inter-examiner reliability

In this Survey, examiners were dental professionals who were employees in the state/territory dental service. A total of 62 dental examiners were involved. Whenever there are multiple examiners, there is potential for variation between examiners in their diagnostic criteria and recording of oral health indices. In order to minimise this variation three approaches were adopted. First, each examiner was given a clinical manual describing the examination protocol and a DVD that demonstrated intra-oral procedures. Each contained simple and clear codes for each component of the examination. Second, a two-day calibration training program was undertaken by all examiners. Third, within a few weeks of beginning Survey examinations, each examiner was tested against the 'gold standard examiners' to measure the degree of inter-examiner reliability. The first two approaches are described above. The remainder of this section presents the results of inter-examiner reliability.

Gold standard examiners conducted the repeated examinations. Arrangement was made with the state/territory Survey co-ordinator and examination teams to organise field visits by one of the gold standard examiners. The repeated examinations were conducted on a day when the examiner was conducting real examinations at a location. The gold standard examiner conducted a masked examination after the field examiner had completed examining a child. The repeated examinations were conducted in the same way as described above except that plaque and gingival indices were not re-scored because plaque and gingival changes after an examination were expected. Repeated examinations were also recorded on to the data entry screen and extracted for analysis. Data of the gold standard examiners were pooled together.

Reliability of each examiner relative to a gold standard examiner was measured by calculating the intra-class correlation coefficient (ICC). The ICC can range from negative values to a maximum of 1.0, with higher values demonstrating greater agreement. Guidelines for interpreting the related kappa statistic propose that values of 0.2 or less represent 'poor or slight' agreement, values from >0.2–0.4 represent 'fair' agreement, values from >0.4–0.6 represent 'moderate' agreement, values from >0.6–0.8 represent 'substantial' agreement, and values greater than 0.8 represent 'almost perfect' agreement (Landis & Koch 1977).

Oral health of Australian children

Table 4-14: Summary of findings from assessment of inter-examiner reliability

Index	No. of examiners evaluated	No. of replicate pairs evaluated	Median reliability[a]
Number of primary teeth present per person	62	984	0.997
Number of permanent teeth present per person	62	984	0.995
Number of decayed primary tooth surfaces per person	62	984	0.941
Number of filled primary tooth surfaces per person	62	984	0.931
Number of missing primary tooth surfaces per person	62	984	0.905
Number of decayed, missing and filled primary tooth surfaces per person	62	984	0.954
Number of decayed permanent tooth surfaces per person	62	984	0.674
Number of filled permanent tooth surfaces per person	62	984	0.680
Number of missing permanent tooth surfaces per person	62	984	0.844
Number of decayed, missing and filled permanent tooth surfaces per person	62	984	0.689
Dental fluorosis of maxillary permanent incisors status of individual teeth	62	733	0.810

(a)   Numbers are intra-class correlation coefficients, except for dental fluorosis, where the kappa statistic is presented.

Direct standardisation using population benchmarks

The previous analysis on the distribution of key sociodemographic characteristics of the Australian sample indicated that the study sample closely reflected the Census distributions, and therefore no bias was present.

However, Figure 4-1 showed a significant relationship between IRSAD score and postcode participation rate, with participation rate lower among lower IRSAD scores. Participation rates were not similarly distributed across the range of IRSAD scores, which indicated a significant correlation between participation in the Survey and level of socioeconomic advantage/disadvantage of areas. Consequently, there was a need to investigate the potential impact of this bias on the main outcome variables relating to children's oral health. This potential bias was assessed using a statistical method called direct standardisation. This method involves the calculation of oral health estimates by adjusting the Survey distribution of the characteristic in question to be the same as the corresponding Census distribution. For this analysis, SUDAAN statistical software was used to perform direct standardisation by specifying the Census distribution for the SEIFA IRSAD variable in the standard weight (stdwgt) statement.

The difference between the adjusted oral health estimate and the observed Survey estimate provides a measure of the degree of bias due to variations in participation.

Table 4-15 compares the observed estimates derived from the Survey with the adjusted estimates for seven important oral health indicators by area level characteristics.

The observed estimate and adjusted estimates for the last four oral health indicators (i.e., average number of dmft, average number of dmfs, average number of DMFT and, average number of DMFS) were identical. For the first three oral health indicators (% children with dmft>0, and % children with DMFT>0, % children with good or excellent oral health), the difference between the observed and adjusted Survey estimates was small.

For standardisation by SEIFA IRSAD, there was a slight increase in the percentage of children with dmft>0 increasing from 41.5% to 42.0% (i.e., the adjusted Survey estimate was 0.5 percentage points higher than the observed estimate) and the percentage of children with DMFT>0 increasing from 23.3% to 23.6% (i.e., the adjusted Survey estimate was 0.3 percentage points higher than the observed estimate). Standardisation also yielded a slight decrease in children with good or excellent oral health, with the percentage of children decreasing from 87.9% to 87.3%, 0.6 percentage points lower. However, all variations between the observed estimate and corresponding standardised estimate were not statistically significant.

Oral health of Australian children

Table 4-15: Observed and adjusted estimates of oral health indicators standardised to 2011 Census benchmarks for SEIFA IRSAD — Australia

Oral health indicator	Observed estimate	Estimate and 95%CI adjusted for: SEIFA IRSAD
% children with dmft>0	41.5 (39.9-43.1)	42.0 (40.6-43.3)
% children with DMFT>0	23.3 (22.2-24.5)	23.6 (22.5-24.7)
% children with good or excellent oral health	87.9 (87.1-88.7)	87.3 (86.6-88.1)
Average number of dmft	1.5 (1.4-1.6)	1.5 (1.4-1.6)
Average number of dmfs	3.1 (2.9-3.3)	3.1 (3.0-3.3)
Average number of DMFT	0.5 (0.5-0.5)	0.5 (0.5-0.5)
Average number of DMFS	0.7 (0.6-0.7)	0.7 (0.7-0.8)

Summary

Chapter 4 presents sociodemographic and state/territory characteristics of the sample and then uses several approaches to evaluate the potential for bias including area-level socioeconomic factors in relation to participation rates and comparison of the sample estimates to the child population as characterised by the 2011 Census, as well as methods of direct standardisation of Survey estimates to Census data.

The sociodemographic characteristics of the study population were described for Australia overall and by states and territories.

The data for the study population (Australian children aged 5–14 years) indicated a similar proportion of females and males and the majority of children were non-Indigenous. Just over 36% of children had a parent who was born overseas, and almost 50% of children (48.1%) had a parent with some tertiary education. Children were more likely to live in medium level income households (38.4%) than in low (32.5%) or high (29.1%) income level households. Although there was some variation in the distribution of characteristics across age groups, in almost all instances these differences were not statistically significant.

As in all studies that are limited to a sample of the population (as opposed to a population census), there exists the possibility of bias in the Survey estimates. We employed various methods to investigate the potential that bias might be present.

Firstly, response rates were examined by area-level socioeconomic indicators. The correlation between participation rates at the level of school postcodes and SEIFA IRSAD scores (Australian Bureau of Statistics 2011) for the corresponding geographic areas indicated that response rates were not similarly distributed across the range of IRSAD scores and the data points on the graph were not randomly dispersed indicating a significant relationship between IRSAD and postcode response rates. Hence, potential bias was found in participation rates by area level socioeconomic factors. Consequently, NCOHS estimates were standardised to reflect the Census distributions of this particular factor. Differences between observed estimates and adjusted estimates were small (and not statistically significant) after standardisation of SEIFA IRSAD to its Census distribution. Hence, standardising by SEIFA IRSAD had little impact on the measures of children's oral health indicating that the bias due to differential response rates across sociodemographic groups was negligible. Small changes in the standardised estimates indicates that the weighting strategy which adjusted for differential response rates across a range of sociodemographic factors has largely accounted for the fluctuations in response rates across postcodes.

Secondly, key characteristics of the sample were compared to Census population benchmarks. NCOHS survey estimates were comparable to the total Australian child population regarding key sociodemographic characteristics with no statistically significant differences found for the sociodemographic characteristics examined (evidenced by the Census estimate laying within the 95% confidence interval of the survey estimate). Survey estimates were also comparable at state and territory level.

The use of rigorous sampling and weighting procedures has ensured that bias within the survey was negligible. Therefore, estimates derived from NCOHS data are accurate estimates of the true population parameters.

Oral health of Australian children

References

Australian Bureau of Statistics 2013. Census of Population and Housing: Socio-Economic Indexes for Areas (SEIFA), Australia, 2011. Catalogue number 2033.0.55.001.

Landis JR & Koch GG 1977. The measurement of observer agreement for categorical data. Biometrics 33(1):159–74.

5 Children's oral health status in Australia, 2012–14

DH Ha, KF Roberts-Thomson, P Arrow, KG Peres and LG Do

5.1 Introduction

Dental caries is the most common chronic infectious disease in childhood, caused by a complex interaction over time between acid-producing bacteria and fermentable carbohydrates (sugars and other carbohydrates from food and drink that can be fermented by bacteria), as well as many host factors including teeth condition and saliva (Fejerskov 2004; Fisher-Owens et al. 2007). Dental caries is characterised by the loss of mineral ions from the tooth (demineralisation), stimulated largely by the presence of bacteria and their by-products. Remineralisation occurs when partly dissolved crystals are induced to grow by the redepositing of minerals via saliva. The demineralisation of the tooth surface can be limited by the use of fluorides. Normally, a balance occurs between the demineralisation and remineralisation of the tooth surface (enamel). However, this balance is disturbed under some conditions, and the subsequent chronic demineralisation leads to the formation of holes or cavities in the tooth surface. In its early stages the damage can be reversed with the use of fluoride. Cavitation (a hole in the tooth) beyond the outer enamel covering of the tooth into the tissues can lead to a bacterial infection, which may cause considerable pain and require surgery or the removal of the tooth. Once the cavity has formed a filling is needed to restore the form and function of the tooth. Childhood caries is a serious public health problem in both developing and industrialised countries (Casamassimo et al. 2009).

At about the age of 5 or 6 years, children start losing their primary (deciduous/baby) teeth, which are replaced by their permanent teeth. Most children have lost all their primary teeth and have gained their permanent teeth (with the exception of wisdom teeth, which may erupt several years, or even decades, later) by the age of 12 years. Therefore, analyses of dental caries in adolescents only report the level of disease in permanent teeth. Younger children generally have a mixture of primary and permanent teeth, from ages 5 to 12 years. The convention is to report on these two sets of teeth separately.

5.2 Methods

Dental caries experience and other oral conditions were collected through oral epidemiological examinations. Didactic and clinical training for the examination teams was conducted. Frequent refresher sessions were also provided. Examinations were held in fixed or mobile dental clinics under standardised conditions.

Key findings in this chapter are presented as two measurements.

- Prevalence was expressed as the percentage of children with a defined outcome, within a defined population.
- Disease severity was expressed as the mean number, per child, of anatomical sites that had condition of interest. Sites were teeth or tooth surfaces.

These unadjusted means and prevalence give an indication of the burden of oral health outcomes in the whole population and population subgroups.

5.3 Experience of dental caries

Caries experience is typically assessed in surveys by the dmft (in primary teeth) and DMFT (in permanent teeth) index, which has been in use for decades. The dmft/DMFT index requires that the condition of each tooth is classified based on experience of decay. The index contains three components related to whether teeth, or tooth surfaces, have untreated caries, have already had fillings for caries, or have been removed because of caries. The components are:

- Untreated caries, which at the tooth level is referred to as dt/DT (this includes teeth that were filled in the past but which needed further treatment)
- Filled teeth, referred to as (ft/FT), with no recurrent decay present
- Teeth missing (extracted) due to decay referred to as (mt/MT).

Primary dentition

Primary teeth (also known as baby teeth, milk teeth or deciduous teeth), are the first set of teeth that each person has. Children have a maximum of 20 primary teeth, and these are gradually replaced by the permanent teeth usually at about age 6. This section reports on caries experience in the primary dentition among children aged 5 to 10 years at the time of the Survey. For children aged 11 years or older, caries experience in the primary dentition is not reported. Natural exfoliation of primary teeth means that dmf scores can be less sensitive after the age of 10 years.

Untreated dental caries

The prevalence of untreated dental caries in the primary dentition is reported in Table 5-1 among children aged 5–10 years. Untreated dental caries reflects both the prevalence of dental caries in the population and access to dental care for treatment.

The percentage of all children aged 5–10 years who had at least one tooth with untreated caries in the primary dentition was 27.1%; that is, more than one in every four children in this age group had untreated caries. The prevalence among the specific two-year age groups varied little from that figure.

Among all children in the 5–10-year age group the lowest proportion with untreated caries in the primary dentition was 18.3% in children from households with the highest income, and the highest (44.0%) was among Indigenous children.

More Indigenous children (44.0%) had untreated caries compared with non-Indigenous children (25.9%), Differences were seen in each age group.

A greater proportion of children with an overseas born parent (29.8%) had untreated caries in their primary dentition compared to children of Australian born parent (25.6%). This pattern was also seen in children aged 5–6 years where those of overseas born parents had 1.4 times the prevalence of untreated caries in the primary dentition relative to children of Australian born parents (31.8% versus 22.9%).

More children whose parents had school-level education had untreated caries in the primary dentition (35.6%) compared with children of parents with vocational (25.1%) and tertiary level (22.3%) education. Differences between children from households where parents had school-level education and households with tertiary-educated parents were apparent in the 5–6-years and 7–8-year age groups and between those with school educated parents and vocationally educated parents in the 5–6-year and 7–8-year age groups.

Children in households with a low income had almost twice the prevalence of untreated caries in the primary dentition (35.9%) compared with children in households with the highest incomes (18.3%) and 1.5 times that of children in medium income households (24.6%). A difference between children from low income households and high income households was apparent in each two-year age group and between those from low income households and medium income households in the 5–6-year and 7–8-year age groups.

A higher proportion of children living in remote or very remote locations had untreated caries in the primary dentition (37.8%) compared with children in all other locations. Among children aged 5–6 years there was a higher proportion of children with untreated decay in remote areas compared with those in Major cities.

Children whose reason for last dental visit was a dental problem had almost twice the prevalence of untreated caries in the primary dentition (42.2%) compared to children who visited for a check-up (21.5%). This pattern was seen across all age groups.

In summary, prevalence of untreated caries in the primary dentition was related to Indigenous identity, country of birth, parental education, household income, residential location and reason for last dental visit.

Oral health of Australian children

Table 5-1: Percentage of children with untreated decayed teeth in the primary dentition in the Australian child population

	Population: children aged 5–10 years			
	All ages	5–6	7–8	9–10
All	27.1	26.1	28.4	27.0
	25.6–28.6	*23.9–28.3*	*26.0–30.8*	*24.9–29.1*
Sex				
Male	28.1	26.8	29.6	28.0
	26.2–30.0	*23.9–29.8*	*26.7–32.5*	*25.1–31.0*
Female	26.1	25.3	27.1	25.9
	24.3–27.9	*22.6–28.2*	*24.2–30.0*	*23.3–28.7*
Indigenous identity				
Non-Indigenous	25.9	24.9	26.6	26.4
	24.5–27.4	*22.6–27.2*	*24.3–28.9*	*24.3–28.6*
Indigenous	44.0	44.1	50.2	37.2
	37.6–50.7	*34.8–53.7*	*40.5–59.9*	*29.3–45.6*
Parents' country of birth				
Australian born	25.5	22.9	27.3	26.4
	23.9–27.1	*20.7–25.2*	*24.7–30.0*	*23.9–29.0*
Overseas born	29.8	31.8	29.6	28.0
	27.4–32.3	*28.0–35.8*	*26.0–33.4*	*24.9–31.1*
Parental education				
School	35.6	37.6	38.0	30.9
	32.7–38.5	*33.2–42.2*	*33.8–42.4*	*26.7–35.4*
Vocational training	25.1	23.9	28.3	23.3
	22.8–27.5	*20.4–27.7*	*24.1–32.8*	*20.1–26.8*
Tertiary education	22.3	19.8	21.2	25.9
	20.7–23.8	*17.3–22.5*	*18.6–24.1*	*23.2–28.8*
Household income				
Low	35.9	39.0	37.8	30.8
	33.4–38.5	*35.1–43.0*	*33.9–41.9*	*27.4–34.4*
Medium	24.6	21.5	24.8	27.6
	22.9–26.5	*18.9–24.4*	*21.9–27.8*	*24.6–30.8*
High	18.3	15.3	18.4	21.5
	16.5–20.2	*12.4–18.8*	*14.9–22.5*	*18.0–25.3*
Residential location				
Major city	25.7	25.1	26.6	25.5
	23.7–27.7	*22.3–28.1*	*23.7–29.7*	*22.7–28.3*
Inner regional	29.2	25.3	31.3	31.2
	26.6–32.0	*21.7–29.2*	*26.7–36.2*	*27.6–35.0*
Outer regional	29.9	30.6	31.9	27.4
	25.9–34.3	*25.0–36.7*	*26.4–37.8*	*23.6–31.4*
Remote/Very remote	37.8	42.3	39.7	31.7
	32.4–43.5	*31.6–53.7*	*29.1–51.4*	*23.1–41.7*
Reason for last dental visit				
Check-up	21.5	19.8	21.6	22.7
	20.0–23.0	*17.4–22.5*	*19.3–24.2*	*20.4–25.1*
Dental problem	42.2	47.3	43.4	37.4
	39.2–45.1	*41.2–53.4*	*39.0–47.9*	*33.2–41.8*

Row 1: Proportions were computed using weighted data.
Row 2: 95% CI: Confidence intervals for estimates were computed using weighted data.
Columns are arranged by age at time of Survey.

Table 5-2 shows the average number of tooth surfaces with untreated decay by sociodemographic factors. The average number of tooth surfaces with untreated decay gives an indication of the severity of the disease and the burden it has on the child. Each tooth was divided into five surfaces. Each surface was assessed for the presence of untreated decay, which was defined as a cavity in the surface enamel caused by the caries process. Higher numbers of surfaces with untreated decay reflect both new disease and access to dental treatment services.

Among all children the average number of untreated decayed surfaces was 1.3. The number was highest among children in the youngest age group and lowest in the oldest age group. The average number of untreated surfaces varied by sociodemographic factors with the highest number seen in children whose reason for their last dental visit was a dental problem (2.5 surfaces) and the lowest in children from households with a high income (0.6 surfaces).

Indigenous children had higher numbers of untreated decayed surfaces than non-Indigenous children, in all children (3.4 versus 1.2 surfaces) and in all age groups. Children aged 5–6 years with an overseas-born parent, had a higher average number of untreated decayed surfaces (2.0 surfaces) compared to children with Australian-born parents (1.3 surfaces).

Children whose parents had a school-only education only had more untreated decayed tooth surfaces (2.2 surfaces) compared to children with vocationally educated parents (1.0 surface) and tertiary-educated parents (0.9 surfaces). This pattern was seen among children in the 5–6-years and 7–8-years age groups.

Differences in average numbers of untreated decayed surfaces were also seen by household income. Among all children there was a gradient in the average number of surfaces by household income with children from low income households having a higher average number (2.0 surfaces) than those from medium income households (1.0 surface) who, in turn, had more than children from high income households (0.6 surfaces). In the specific two-year age groups children from low income households consistently had higher average numbers of untreated decayed surfaces than those from medium and high income households.

Children who last made a dental visit because of a problem had over 3 times the average number of untreated decayed tooth surfaces than those who last visited for a check-up (2.5 versus 0.8 surfaces). Among children aged 5–6 years, the difference between those who visited for a problem and those who visited for a check-up was 3.5-fold (3.5 versus 0.9 surfaces), in children aged 7–8 years it was 3.4-fold (2.7 versus 0.8 surfaces) and in those aged 9–10 years a 2.1-fold difference (1.5 versus 0.7 surfaces).

In summary, the average number of untreated decayed tooth surfaces varied by age group, Indigenous identity, country of birth, parental education, household income and reason for last dental visit.

Table 5-2: Average number of untreated decayed tooth surfaces per child in the primary dentition in the Australian child population

| | Population: children aged 5–10 years | | | |
	All ages	5—6	7—8	9—10
All	1.3	1.5	1.4	1.0
	1.2–1.4	*1.3–1.7*	*1.2–1.6*	*0.9–1.1*
Sex				
Male	1.4	1.5	1.5	1.1
	1.2–1.6	*1.2–1.8*	*1.3–1.7*	*0.9–1.3*
Female	1.2	1.5	1.3	0.8
	1.0–1.4	*1.2–1.8*	*1.0–1.5*	*0.7–1.0*
Indigenous identity				
Non-Indigenous	1.2	1.4	1.2	0.9
	1.0–1.3	*1.1–1.6*	*1.0–1.4*	*0.8–1.0*
Indigenous	3.4	4.0	3.6	2.6
	2.4–4.4	*2.1–5.8*	*2.6–4.6*	*1.5–3.7*
Parents' country of birth				
Australian born	1.2	1.3	1.3	1.0
	1.0–1.3	*1.0–1.5*	*1.0–1.5*	*0.8–1.2*
Overseas born	1.5	2.0	1.6	1.0
	1.3–1.7	*1.6–2.3*	*1.3–1.8*	*0.9–1.2*
Parental education				
School	2.2	2.7	2.4	1.3
	1.8–2.5	*2.2–3.3*	*2.0–2.9*	*1.0–1.6*
Vocational training	1.0	1.2	1.0	0.8
	0.8–1.2	*0.8–1.6*	*0.8–1.2*	*0.5–1.0*
Tertiary education	0.9	0.8	0.9	0.9
	0.8–1.0	*0.7–1.0*	*0.7–1.1*	*0.7–1.0*
Household income				
Low	2.0	2.6	2.1	1.4
	1.8–2.3	*2.1–3.1*	*1.7–2.6*	*1.1–1.7*
Medium	1.0	1.1	1.0	0.9
	0.9–1.2	*0.8–1.4*	*0.8–1.2*	*0.7–1.1*
High	0.6	0.6	0.7	0.6
	0.5–0.7	*0.4–0.8*	*0.5–0.9*	*0.5–0.7*
Residential location				
Major city	1.2	1.4	1.3	0.9
	1.0–1.4	*1.2–1.7*	*1.1–1.5*	*0.7–1.0*
Inner regional	1.4	1.4	1.5	1.4
	1.1–1.7	*0.9–1.8*	*1.1–2.0*	*1.0–1.7*
Outer regional	1.5	2.0	1.5	1.0
	0.9–2.1	*1.1–3.0*	*1.0–2.0*	*0.6–1.5*
Remote/Very remote	2.1	2.9	1.8	1.5
	1.2–3.0	*1.6–4.3*	*1.0–2.7*	*0.2–2.9*
Reason for last dental visit				
Check-up	0.8	0.9	0.8	0.7
	0.7–0.9	*0.7–1.1*	*0.7–1.0*	*0.6–0.8*
Dental problem	2.5	3.5	2.7	1.5
	2.1–2.8	*2.6–4.3*	*2.2–3.2*	*1.2–1.8*

Row 1: Means were computed using weighted data.
Row 2: 95% CI: Confidence intervals for estimates were computed using weighted data.
Columns are arranged by age at time of Survey.

Tooth loss due to dental caries

Tooth loss in the primary dentition only includes teeth lost due to dental caries and does not include tooth loss due to exfoliation.

Table 5-3 shows the percentage of children who have lost at least one primary tooth due to dental caries. The lowest percentage was among children from high income households (2.9%) and the highest percentage was among children whose last dental visit was for a problem (16.6%).

Overall, 5.6% of children had lost at least one tooth, but this varied across age groups with the highest percentage of children in the 7–8-year age group (7.5%), which was higher than the younger age group (3.8%) and the older age group (5.5%).

More Indigenous children had a missing tooth due to caries than non-Indigenous children among all children (9.7% versus 5.3%). This was also seen among children aged 7–8 years (13.6% versus 6.9%).

A higher proportion of children whose parents had school-only education had missing teeth compared to children of parents who had vocational level education (8.8% versus 4.9%). There was a 2.4-fold relative difference in the percentage of children with missing teeth between children whose parents' highest education was school-level and children of tertiary-educated parents (8.8% versus 3.7%). This pattern was seen across all age groups.

There was a gradient in the percentage of children with missing teeth due to dental caries across household income groups with 9.3% of children from low income households having missing teeth compared to children from medium income households (4.3%) — a 2.2-fold relative difference. The relative difference between children from low and high income households was 3.2 times (9.3% versus 2.9%) and 1.6 times between children from medium and high income households (4.3% versus 2.9%). In each specific two-year age group, there were more children with missing teeth in low income households relative to the medium and high income households.

The highest percentage of children with missing teeth was in those who had last made a dental visit for a problem. Among all children who last visited for a problem, there were 4.7 times more children with missing teeth compared to children who last visited for a check-up. This difference was 7.2-fold in the 5–6-year age group, 4.5-fold in the 7–8-year age group and 3.8 times in the 9–10-year age group.

In summary, the prevalence of tooth loss among children in the primary dentition was related to age group, Indigenous identity, parental education, household income and reason for last dental visit.

Table 5-3: Percentage of children with missing teeth due to dental caries in the primary dentition in the Australian child population

	Population: children aged 5–10 years			
	All ages	5—6	7—8	9—10
All	5.6	3.8	7.5	5.5
	4.9–6.2	*3.0–4.7*	*6.3–8.8*	*4.6–6.5*
Sex				
Male	5.7	3.5	8.0	5.7
	5.0–6.5	*2.6–4.6*	*6.7–9.6*	*4.6–7.1*
Female	5.4	4.1	6.9	5.3
	4.5–6.3	*3.1–5.3*	*5.4–8.7*	*4.1–6.8*
Indigenous identity				
Non-Indigenous	5.3	3.5	6.9	5.4
	4.6–5.9	*2.7–4.4*	*5.8–8.2*	*4.4–6.4*
Indigenous	9.7	7.2	13.6	8.2
	7.1–13.0	*3.8–13.1*	*9.2–19.6*	*4.7–13.8*
Parents' country of birth				
Australian born	5.3	3.4	7.3	5.4
	4.6–6.1	*2.6–4.4*	*6.0–8.7*	*4.3–6.8*
Overseas born	5.9	4.3	7.7	5.7
	4.8–7.1	*3.0–6.1*	*5.9–9.9*	*4.2–7.5*
Parental education				
School	8.8	6.3	12.6	7.9
	7.5–10.4	*4.7–8.4*	*10.0–15.8*	*6.0–10.2*
Vocational training	4.9	2.6	6.8	5.4
	3.9–6.1	*1.5–4.3*	*4.9–9.4*	*3.7–7.8*
Tertiary education	3.7	2.3	4.5	4.4
	3.1–4.5	*1.6–3.3*	*3.7–5.6*	*3.3–6.0*
Household income				
Low	9.3	7.1	12.5	8.6
	8.0–10.8	*5.3–9.4*	*10.2–15.3*	*6.7–11.0*
Medium	4.3	2.8	5.6	4.4
	3.6–5.0	*1.9–4.0*	*4.4–7.0*	*3.2–6.0*
High	2.9	1.2	3.8	3.8
	2.2–3.7	*0.6–2.5*	*2.7–5.1*	*2.6–5.5*
Residential location				
Major city	4.9	3.8	6.3	4.6
	4.1–5.7	*2.8–5.0*	*5.0–8.0*	*3.6–5.8*
Inner regional	7.3	3.3	10.6	8.2
	6.0–8.8	*2.2–4.9*	*8.0–14.0*	*5.9–11.1*
Outer regional	5.7	3.6	8.2	5.3
	4.5–7.2	*2.3–5.4*	*6.0–11.1*	*3.7–7.6*
Remote/Very remote	9.6	8.0	11.8	9.0
	6.3–14.3	*3.2–18.3*	*7.9–17.3*	*4.3–18.0*
Reason for last dental visit				
Check-up	3.5	2.2	4.5	3.6
	2.9–4.1	*1.6–3.1*	*3.6–5.6*	*2.8–4.5*
Dental problem	16.6	16.0	20.1	13.5
	14.4–19.0	*12.4–20.4*	*16.2–24.5*	*10.7–16.9*

Row 1: Proportions were computed using weighted data.
Row 2: 95% CI: Confidence intervals for estimates were computed using weighted data.
Columns are arranged by age at time of Survey.

In a population with somewhat lower levels of tooth loss due to dental decay it is more informative and sensitive to measure average numbers of missing tooth surfaces per child than missing teeth. Each missing tooth was considered to have three surfaces affected by decay, as counting five surfaces per tooth as missing would overestimate the average number of tooth surfaces affected by decay. Table 5-4 shows the average number of missing tooth surfaces per child in the primary dentition.

The average number of missing surfaces due to dental caries was 0.3 surfaces. This number was highest (1.0 surface) in children who last made a dental visit due to a problem and was lowest (0.1 surfaces) among children from high income households.

There were no differences by age group or sex, nor by country of birth. Among all ages, Indigenous children had 2.3 times the average number of missing tooth surfaces compared with non-Indigenous children (0.7 versus 0.3 surfaces).

All children of parents whose highest level of education was school level had 3 times the average number of missing surfaces compared to children from tertiary-educated parents and twice that of vocationally educated parents (0.6 versus 0.2 surfaces, and 0.6 versus 0.3 surfaces, respectively). This relative difference between children of school educated parents and both vocationally and tertiary-educated parents was five-fold among children aged 5–6 years (0.5 versus 0.1 surfaces). There was a relative difference of 2.7-fold between children of school educated parents and tertiary-educated parents among ages 7–8 years (0.8 versus 0.3 surfaces).

Children from low income households had a six-fold relative higher average number of missing tooth surfaces than children from high income households and twice the average number of children from medium income households (0.6 versus 0.1, and 0.6 versus 0.3 surfaces, respectively). Among children aged 5–6 years the relative difference was five-fold between those from low income households compared with high income households and 2.5-fold difference between children from medium income households and high income households (0.5 versus 0.1, and 0.5 versus 0.2 surfaces, respectively).

All children who last made a dental visit because of a problem had 5 times the average number of missing tooth surfaces compared to children who last visited for a check-up (1.0 versus 0.2 surfaces). This pattern was seen in the two-year age group. There was a 5.5-fold difference in children aged 5–6 years, a 3.7-fold among those aged 7–8 years and a 4.5-fold relative difference among those aged 9–10 years who made their last dental visit for a problem rather than a check-up.

In summary, Indigenous children, children of parents with school-only education, children from low income households and children whose last dental visit was for a problem had relatively more missing tooth surfaces than their counterparts.

Table 5-4: Average number of missing tooth surfaces due to dental caries per child in the primary dentition in the Australian child population

| | Population: children aged 5–10 years | | | |
	All ages	5—6	7—8	9—10
All	0.3	0.3	0.4	0.3
	0.3–0.4	*0.2–0.3*	*0.3–0.5*	*0.3–0.4*
Sex				
Male	0.4	0.3	0.5	0.4
	0.3–0.4	*0.2–0.3*	*0.3–0.6*	*0.2–0.5*
Female	0.3	0.3	0.4	0.3
	0.3–0.4	*0.2–0.3*	*0.3–0.5*	*0.2–0.4*
Indigenous identity				
Non-Indigenous	0.3	0.2	0.4	0.3
	0.3–0.4	*0.2–0.3*	*0.3–0.5*	*0.2–0.4*
Indigenous	0.7	0.8	0.8	0.6
	0.5–1.0	*0.3–1.3*	*0.4–1.3*	*0.3–1.0*
Parents' country of birth				
Australian born	0.3	0.2	0.4	0.4
	0.3–0.4	*0.2–0.3*	*0.3–0.5*	*0.2–0.5*
Overseas born	0.4	0.3	0.5	0.3
	0.3–0.4	*0.2–0.4*	*0.3–0.6*	*0.2–0.4*
Parental education				
School	0.6	0.5	0.8	0.6
	0.5–0.7	*0.3–0.7*	*0.5–1.0*	*0.3–0.8*
Vocational training	0.3	0.1	0.4	0.3
	0.2–0.4	*0.1–0.2*	*0.2–0.5*	*0.2–0.5*
Tertiary education	0.2	0.1	0.3	0.2
	0.2–0.3	*0.1–0.2*	*0.2–0.3*	*0.1–0.3*
Household income				
Low	0.6	0.5	0.8	0.6
	0.5–0.7	*0.3–0.7*	*0.6–1.0*	*0.4–0.8*
Medium	0.3	0.2	0.3	0.3
	0.2–0.3	*0.1–0.3*	*0.2–0.4*	*0.1–0.4*
High	0.1	0.1	0.2	0.2
	0.1–0.2	*0.0–0.1*	*0.1–0.2*	*0.1–0.4*
Residential location				
Major city	0.3	0.2	0.4	0.3
	0.2–0.4	*0.1–0.3*	*0.3–0.5*	*0.2–0.4*
Inner regional	0.5	0.3	0.6	0.5
	0.3–0.6	*0.2–0.5*	*0.4–0.8*	*0.3–0.6*
Outer regional	0.4	0.3	0.5	0.3
	0.3–0.5	*0.1–0.6*	*0.3–0.7*	*0.2–0.4*
Remote/Very remote	0.7	0.5	0.6	0.9
	0.3–1.1	*0.2–0.9*	*0.3–1.0*	*0.1–1.9*
Reason for last dental visit				
Check-up	0.2	0.2	0.3	0.2
	0.2–0.3	*0.1–0.2*	*0.2–0.3*	*0.2–0.3*
Dental problem	1.0	1.1	1.1	0.9
	0.8–1.2	*0.8–1.4*	*0.8–1.4*	*0.5–1.2*

Row 1: Means were computed using weighted data.
Row 2: 95% CI: Confidence intervals for estimates were computed using weighted data.
Columns are arranged by age at time of Survey.

Filled teeth due to dental caries

Fillings for the treatment of tooth decay leave a permanent mark on a tooth and are one measure of a person's experience of dental decay (Table 5-5). The presence of fillings gives an indication of access to and patters of dental treatment. Just over one-quarter of all children aged 5–10 years had at least one filling in their primary dentition. This percentage increased from 15.4% among children aged 5–6 years, to 30.1% among those aged 7–8 years and 33.7% among those aged 9–10 years. The prevalence among all children was highest amongst children who last made a dental visit for a problem (52.2%) and lowest in children from high income households (22.3%).

More Indigenous children had received a filling (36.1%) compared to non-Indigenous children (25.7%). This was seen in the 7–8 years (40.9% versus 29.4%) and 9–10 years (45.9% versus 33.1%) age groups.

Among all children and in all age groups a greater proportion of children whose parents only had school-level education had experienced a filling compared to children of tertiary-educated parents. In all children, the relative difference was 1.4-fold (31.7% versus 22.8%), in the 5–6-year age group 1.7-fold (20.4% versus 12.2%), in the 7–8-year age group 1.3-fold (36.3% versus 27.3%), and in the 9–10-year age group a 1.3-fold relative difference (39.5% versus 29.3%).

Children from low income households had a higher prevalence of fillings (29.6%) compared with children from high income households (22.3%). This difference was also seen in the 5–6-year age group (19.5% versus 11.3%) and the 9–10-year age group (36.8%versus 28.2%).

Among all children, those from locations outside Major cities had higher prevalence of fillings than children in Major cities. This prevalence was 35.1% for remote children, 31.9% for Outer regional children and 30.4% for Inner regional children compared with 23.9% for children in Major city locations. In the 5–6-year age group more Outer regional children had fillings (20.8%) compared to those from Major cities (13.8%). In the 9–10-year age group more remote children (48.6%) had fillings than children from Major cities (31.0%).

Among all children and in all age groups a greater proportion of children who last made a dental visit for a problem had experienced a filling compared to children who visited for a check-up. In all children, the relative difference was 2.1-fold (52.2% versus 24.5%), in the 5–6-year age group 3.4-fold (46.7% versus 13.9%), in the 7–8-year age group 2.1-fold (56.0% versus 27.0%) and in the 9–10-year age group a 1.7-fold relative difference (52.2% versus 31.0%).

In summary, prevalence of filled teeth was related to age group, Indigenous identity, parental education, household income, residential location and reason for last dental visit.

Oral health of Australian children

Table 5-5: Percentage of children with filled teeth due to dental caries in the primary dentition in the Australian child population

| | Population: children aged 5–10 years | | | |
	All ages	5—6	7—8	9—10
All	**26.2**	**15.4**	**30.1**	**33.7**
	24.9–27.6	*13.8–17.0*	*28.1–32.0*	*31.5–35.9*
Sex				
Male	26.3	15.5	30.8	33.2
	24.6–28.1	*13.5–17.7*	*28.2–33.6*	*30.6–35.8*
Female	26.1	15.2	29.2	34.3
	24.3–27.9	*13.2–17.4*	*26.6–32.0*	*31.1–37.5*
Indigenous identity				
Non-Indigenous	25.7	14.9	29.4	33.1
	24.3–27.0	*13.4–16.6*	*27.5–31.3*	*30.9–35.4*
Indigenous	36.1	22.6	40.9	45.9
	31.4–41.0	*16.1–30.7*	*33.1–49.2*	*37.3–54.7*
Parents' country of birth				
Australian born	26.1	14.8	29.2	35.0
	24.5–27.7	*13.1–16.7*	*26.8–31.7*	*32.1–37.9*
Overseas born	26.8	16.7	31.7	32.1
	24.8–28.8	*14.0–19.7*	*28.9–34.7*	*28.9–35.4*
Parental education				
School	31.7	20.4	36.3	39.5
	29.2–34.2	*17.3–23.7*	*32.4–40.3*	*35.3–43.7*
Vocational training	26.7	15.7	27.5	36.7
	24.2–29.3	*12.6–19.2*	*23.5–31.9*	*32.2–41.3*
Tertiary education	22.8	12.2	27.3	29.3
	21.2–24.3	*10.4–14.1*	*24.8–29.8*	*26.8–31.9*
Household income				
Low	29.6	19.5	33.2	36.8
	27.4–31.8	*16.5–22.8*	*29.8–36.7*	*33.1–40.7*
Medium	25.9	15.1	28.0	34.6
	24.2–27.7	*13.0–17.3*	*25.3–30.8*	*31.5–37.9*
High	22.3	11.3	28.2	28.2
	20.1–24.7	*9.0–14.2*	*24.6–32.0*	*24.0–32.6*
Residential location				
Major city	23.9	13.8	27.6	31.0
	22.3–25.6	*11.9–15.9*	*25.3–30.0*	*28.3–33.8*
Inner regional	30.4	17.3	35.1	39.0
	27.7–33.1	*14.4–20.5*	*30.7–39.7*	*34.6–43.6*
Outer regional	31.9	20.8	37.0	37.3
	29.1–34.7	*17.1–25.0*	*32.7–41.6*	*32.3–42.5*
Remote/Very remote	35.1	24.2	32.1	48.6
	28.6–42.2	*14.5–37.3*	*25.2–39.9*	*34.2–63.1*
Reason for last dental visit				
Check-up	24.5	13.9	27.0	31.0
	22.9–26.1	*12.0–16.0*	*24.8–29.3*	*28.4–33.6*
Dental problem	52.2	46.7	56.0	52.2
	49.1–55.2	*41.2–52.2*	*51.2–60.6*	*47.6–56.6*

Row 1: Proportions were computed using weighted data.
Row 2: 95% CI: Confidence intervals for estimates were computed using weighted data.
Columns are arranged by age at time of Survey.

Five tooth surfaces on each tooth was assessed for the presence of a filling in this Survey. The average number of filled tooth surfaces reflects both the history of tooth decay and adequacy of dental treatment. Fillings leave a permanent record of the experience of tooth decay on a tooth surface.

The average number of filled tooth surfaces per child among all children was 1.5 (Table 5-6). The highest average number was seen in children who last made a dental visit because of a problem (3.2 surfaces) and the lowest average number was found in children whose parent had a tertiary education and children from high income households (1.3 surfaces).

The average number of filled surfaces varied by age group. Children in the 5–6-year age group had, on average, fewer filled surfaces (0.9 surfaces) than children in the 7–8-year and 9–10-year age groups (1.8 surfaces).

Children whose parents only had school-level education had, on average, more filled tooth surfaces (1.8 surfaces) compared to children with a tertiary-educated parent (1.3 surfaces).

Children of all ages from low income households had, on average, more filled surfaces (1.8 surfaces) than children from high income households (1.3 surfaces).

Children who last visited for a dental problem had 2.3 times more filled surfaces than children who made a dental visit for a check-up (3.2 versus 1.4 surfaces). This pattern was seen across all age groups. The relative difference was 3.8-fold in the 5–6-year age group (3.0 surfaces versus 0.8 surfaces), 2.3-fold in the 7–8-year age group (3.5 versus 1.5 surfaces) and 1.8-fold in the 9–10-year age group (3.0 versus 1.7 surfaces).

In summary, the average number of filled tooth surfaces was related to age group, parental education, household income and reason for last dental visit.

Table 5-6: Average number of filled tooth surfaces due to caries in the primary dentition in the Australian child population

	Population: children aged 6–14 years			
	All ages	5—6	7—8	9—10
All	**1.5**	**0.9**	**1.8**	**1.8**
	1.4–1.6	*0.8–1.1*	*1.6–1.9*	*1.6–2.0*
Sex				
Male	1.5	0.9	1.8	1.8
	1.4–1.6	*0.7–1.0*	*1.6–2.0*	*1.6–2.1*
Female	1.5	1.0	1.7	1.8
	1.4–1.7	*0.8–1.2*	*1.5–2.0*	*1.6–2.1*
Indigenous identity				
Non-Indigenous	1.5	0.9	1.7	1.8
	1.4–1.6	*0.8–1.1*	*1.5–1.9*	*1.6–2.0*
Indigenous	2.1	1.1	2.7	2.6
	1.6–2.7	*0.6–1.7*	*1.7–3.7*	*1.5–3.7*
Parents' country of birth				
Australian born	1.5	0.9	1.7	1.9
	1.3–1.6	*0.7–1.0*	*1.4–1.9*	*1.6–2.1*
Overseas born	1.6	1.1	2.0	1.8
	1.4–1.8	*0.7–1.4*	*1.7–2.3*	*1.5–2.0*
Parental education				
School	1.8	1.2	2.0	2.2
	1.6–2.0	*0.9–1.5*	*1.7–2.2*	*1.8–2.6*
Vocational training	1.6	0.9	1.9	1.9
	1.3–1.8	*0.6–1.1*	*1.4–2.5*	*1.5–2.3*
Tertiary education	1.3	0.7	1.6	1.6
	1.2–1.4	*0.6–0.9*	*1.4–1.8*	*1.4–1.8*
Household income				
Low	1.8	1.2	2.1	2.1
	1.6–2.0	*0.9–1.5*	*1.7–2.4*	*1.7–2.4*
Medium	1.4	0.9	1.6	1.8
	1.3–1.6	*0.7–1.1*	*1.4–1.8*	*1.6–2.0*
High	1.3	0.7	1.6	1.6
	1.1–1.5	*0.4–1.0*	*1.3–2.0*	*1.3–1.9*
Residential location				
Major city	1.4	0.9	1.6	1.7
	1.3–1.5	*0.7–1.1*	*1.4–1.8*	*1.5–1.9*
Inner regional	1.7	1.0	2.1	2.1
	1.5–2.0	*0.7–1.3*	*1.7–2.6*	*1.7–2.6*
Outer regional	1.9	1.2	2.1	2.3
	1.5–2.2	*0.9–1.5*	*1.8–2.5*	*1.7–3.0*
Remote/Very remote	1.6	1.0	1.7	2.1
	1.1–2.1	*0.3–1.8*	*1.3–2.2*	*1.2–3.1*
Reason for last dental visit				
Check-up	1.4	0.8	1.5	1.7
	1.2–1.5	*0.7–1.0*	*1.3–1.8*	*1.4–1.9*
Dental problem	3.2	3.0	3.5	3.0
	2.9–3.5	*2.3–3.7*	*3.1–4.0*	*2.6–3.5*

Row 1: Means were computed using weighted data.
Row 2: 95% CI: Confidence intervals for estimates were computed using weighted data.
Columns are arranged by age at time of Survey.

Total caries experience in the primary dentition

The prevalence of caries experience in the primary dentition reflects a child's lifetime experience of decay in their primary dentition. This is because decay leaves a permanent mark on the tooth surface, either a cavity in the enamel or a filling or a missing surface due to extraction due to caries.

Among all children aged 5–10 years, 41.7% had experienced dental caries (Table 5-7). The highest proportion of children with decay experience was found in children who last made a dental visit because of a problem (68.3%) and the lowest proportion was found in children from households with high incomes (33.0%). More children in the 7–8-year and 9–10-year age groups had caries experience than those aged 5–6 years. Among all children, there were differences by Indigenous identity, parental education, household income, residential location and reason for last dental visit.

The proportion of Indigenous children who had experienced caries was 1.5 times the proportion of non-Indigenous children. A similar pattern was seen in each age group with a 1.6-fold relative difference among children aged 5–6 years, a 1.5-fold difference in those aged 7–8 years and a 1.4-fold difference in those aged 9–10 years.

More children of parents with school-level education had caries experience compared to children of vocationally and tertiary-educated parents among all children (50.7%versus 40.8% and 36.2%) and in the 5–6-year and 7–8-year age groups. In the 9-10-year age group there was only a difference between children of school-only educated parents compared with children of tertiary-educated parents.

The prevalence of dental caries was higher among children from low income households (50.4%) than children from medium income households (39.6%), which in turn was higher than for children in high income households (33.0%). This pattern was seen in the 5–6-year age group with a 2.1-fold relative difference between low and high income households and a 1.5-fold difference between the proportion of children from low and medium income households. In the 7–8-year and 9–10-year age group, there was a difference in the prevalence of caries between low and high income households.

Differences in the prevalence of caries experience were also seen related to residential location. In all children and in all age groups, children in Major cities had the lowest prevalence. Those in remote areas had 1.4 times the prevalence of caries than children in Major cities. In the 5–6-year age group the difference was 1.6-fold.

The largest relative differences between population groups were seen between children who last made a dental visit for a problem, where 1.9 times more children had experienced caries, compared with children who had visited for a check-up. More children who visited for a problem had experienced caries in each age group, with a 2.4-fold relative difference in the 5–6-year age group, a 1.9-fold relative difference in the 7–8-year age group and a 1.6-fold relative difference in the 9–10-year age group.

In summary, differences in prevalence of caries experience related to age group, Indigenous identity, parental education, household income residential location and reason for last dental visit. The greatest relative differences were seen consistently in all population groups (except age group) in the 5–6-year age group.

Oral health of Australian children

Table 5-7: Percentage of children with caries experience in the primary dentition in the Australian child population

	Population: children aged 5–10 years			
	All ages	5—6	7—8	9—10
All	41.7	34.3	45.1	46.2
	40.1–43.3	*31.9–36.6*	*42.6–47.4*	*43.7–48.6*
Sex				
Male	42.5	34.8	46.0	47.0
	40.4–44.6	*31.7–38.0*	*42.9–49.1*	*43.9–50.1*
Female	40.9	33.7	44.0	45.3
	38.9–42.9	*30.8–36.7*	*40.9–47.2*	*42.1–48.5*
Indigenous identity				
Non-Indigenous	40.5	33.1	43.3	45.3
	38.9–42.1	*30.7–35.5*	*41.0–45.7*	*42.9–47.7*
Indigenous	60.6	51.9	67.0	63.3
	54.5–66.3	*41.9–61.7*	*58.0–74.8*	*55.0–70.9*
Parents' country of birth				
Australian born	40.6	31.7	43.6	47.0
	38.8–42.4	*29.3–34.2*	*40.6–46.5*	*43.9–50.1*
Overseas born	43.7	39.0	47.2	45.2
	41.2–46.2	*34.9–43.1*	*43.7–50.5*	*41.9–48.5*
Parental education				
School	50.7	46.2	54.9	51.4
	47.8–53.5	*41.6–50.8*	*50.6–59.0*	*46.8–55.9*
Vocational training	40.8	32.6	42.5	47.2
	38.0–43.6	*28.7–36.8*	*37.8–47.4*	*42.7–51.7*
Tertiary education	36.2	27.5	39.1	42.5
	34.3–38.1	*24.7–30.4*	*36.1–42.1*	*39.5–45.5*
Household income				
Low	50.4	47.4	53.4	50.9
	47.9–52.9	*43.3–51.4*	*49.4–57.2*	*46.9–54.7*
Medium	39.6	30.7	41.0	46.9
	37.4–41.7	*27.9–33.7*	*37.8–44.2*	*43.3–50.6*
High	33.0	22.8	38.0	38.8
	30.7–35.3	*19.6–26.4*	*33.9–42.3*	*34.4–43.4*
Residential location				
Major city	39.1	32.4	42.2	43.3
	37.0–41.3	*29.4–35.4*	*39.2–45.2*	*40.1–46.4*
Inner regional	46.1	34.9	51.1	52.4
	43.3–48.8	*31.1–38.9*	*46.1–56.0*	*48.4–56.4*
Outer regional	48.3	43.1	52.0	49.5
	44.3–52.2	*37.2–49.1*	*46.8–57.0*	*44.2–54.8*
Remote/Very remote	53.3	50.5	49.4	60.0
	48.3–58.3	*39.8–61.0*	*36.2–62.6*	*48.2–70.8*
Reason for last dental visit				
Check-up	36.1	28.2	37.8	41.0
	34.2–37.9	*25.4–31.1*	*35.1–40.6*	*38.2–43.8*
Dental problem	68.3	68.1	71.4	65.5
	65.6–70.9	*62.4–73.2*	*66.9–75.5*	*61.3–69.5*

Row 1: Proportions were computed using weighted data.
Row 2: 95% CI: Confidence intervals for estimates were computed using weighted data.
Columns are arranged by age at time of Survey.

The number of decayed, missing and filled tooth surfaces reflects the child's lifetime experience of dental decay in the primary dentition. This is because decay leaves a permanent mark on the tooth surface, either a cavity in the enamel or a filling, or a missing surface due to extraction due to caries. In this Survey, each tooth was regarded as having five surfaces, however if a tooth was missing because of decay only three surfaces were counted as this more accurately reflects the average disease experience in a tooth extracted due to decay.

The average number of decayed, missing and filled tooth surfaces per child in the primary dentition of Australian children aged 5–10 years was 3.1 (Table 5-8). The highest number was 6.7 in children who last made a dental visit because of a problem. The lowest number was 2.1 in children from high income households.

The largest relative difference between population groups was between children who last made a dental visit for a problem who had 2.8 times the number of surfaces with decay experience than children who last visited for a check-up (6.7 versus 2.4 surfaces). Among all children, Indigenous children had 2.2 times the tooth surfaces with caries experience than non-Indigenous children (6.3 versus 2.9 surfaces); children of parents with school-only education had 1.9 times the average number of affected tooth surfaces than children who had a tertiary-educated parent (4.6 versus 2.4 surfaces) and 1.6 times that of children of vocationally educated parents (4.6 versus 2.8 surfaces).

Among all children, those from low income households had 2.1 times the number of affected tooth surfaces than children from high income households (4.4 versus 2.1 surfaces) and 1.6 times children from medium income households (4.4 versus 2.7 surfaces). Children from Remote/Very remote areas had 1.5 times the number of decayed, missing and filled tooth surfaces compared to children in Major cities (4.4 versus 2.9 surfaces). Differences were also seen between children aged 5–6 years (2.7 surfaces) and those aged 7–8 years (3.6 surfaces).

In the 5–6-year age group, larger relative differences were observed. There was a 2.7-fold relative difference between Indigenous and non-Indigenous children (5.9 versus 2.5 surfaces); a 2.6-fold difference between children of parents with school-level education compared to children of tertiary-educated parents (4.5 versus 1.7 surfaces); a 3.3-fold difference between children from low income households relative to children from households with a high income; and a 3.9-fold relative difference between children who last visited for a problem compared to children whose reason for their last dental visit was for a check-up (7.5 versus 1.9 surfaces).

Differences were also observed for the 7–8-year and 9–10-year age groups for Indigenous identity, parental education, household income and reason for last dental visit.

In summary, the average number of decayed, missing and filled tooth surfaces was related to age group, Indigenous identity, parental education, household income, residential location and reason for last dental visit. The largest relative differences were seen in the 5–6-years age group.

Table 5-8: Average number of decayed, missing or filled tooth surfaces (dmfs) in the primary dentition in the Australian child population

| | Population: children aged 5–10 years | | | |
	All ages	5—6	7—8	9—10
All	3.1	2.7	3.6	3.2
	2.9–3.4	*2.4–3.0*	*3.3–3.9*	*2.9–3.5*
Sex				
Male	3.3	2.6	3.8	3.3
	3.0–3.5	*2.2–3.1*	*3.4–4.2*	*3.0–3.7*
Female	3.0	2.8	3.4	3.0
	2.8–3.3	*2.3–3.2*	*2.9–3.8*	*2.6–3.4*
Indigenous identity				
Non-Indigenous	2.9	2.5	3.3	3.0
	2.7–3.1	*2.2–2.8*	*3.0–3.6*	*2.8–3.3*
Indigenous	6.3	5.9	7.2	5.9
	5.2–7.4	*3.7–8.0*	*5.7–8.6*	*4.4–7.3*
Parents' country of birth				
Australian born	3.0	2.4	3.3	3.2
	2.7–3.2	*2.0–2.7*	*3.0–3.7*	*2.8–3.6*
Overseas born	3.5	3.3	4.0	3.1
	3.2–3.8	*2.7–3.9*	*3.5–4.5*	*2.8–3.5*
Parental education				
School	4.6	4.5	5.1	4.1
	4.1–5.0	*3.7–5.2*	*4.5–5.7*	*3.5–4.7*
Vocational training	2.8	2.2	3.3	3.0
	2.5–3.2	*1.7–2.7*	*2.6–3.9*	*2.5–3.6*
Tertiary education	2.4	1.7	2.7	2.7
	2.2–2.5	*1.4–2.0*	*2.4–3.0*	*2.4–3.0*
Household income				
Low	4.4	4.3	5.0	4.0
	4.1–4.8	*3.7–4.9*	*4.4–5.6*	*3.5–4.6*
Medium	2.7	2.2	2.9	3.0
	2.5–2.9	*1.8–2.6*	*2.6–3.2*	*2.6–3.3*
High	2.1	1.3	2.5	2.4
	1.8–2.3	*1.0–1.7*	*2.1–3.0*	*2.0–2.9*
Residential location				
Major city	2.9	2.5	3.3	2.8
	2.6–3.1	*2.1–2.9*	*2.9–3.7*	*2.5–3.1*
Inner regional	3.6	2.7	4.3	3.9
	3.2–4.1	*2.1–3.3*	*3.5–5.0*	*3.2–4.6*
Outer regional	3.8	3.5	4.1	3.7
	3.1–4.5	*2.4–4.6*	*3.4–4.8*	*2.9–4.4*
Remote/Very remote	4.4	4.5	4.2	4.6
	3.2–5.7	*2.7–6.2*	*2.9–5.5*	*2.4–6.8*
Reason for last dental visit				
Check-up	2.4	1.9	2.6	2.6
	2.2–2.6	*1.5–2.2*	*2.3–2.9*	*2.3–2.9*
Dental problem	6.7	7.5	7.4	5.4
	6.2–7.2	*6.3–8.7*	*6.6–8.2*	*4.8–6.0*

Row 1: Means were computed using weighted data.
Row 2: 95% CI: Confidence intervals for estimates were computed using weighted data.
Columns are arranged by age at time of Survey.

Permanent dentition

Permanent teeth (sometimes referred to as adult teeth or secondary teeth) start erupting from around the age of 6 years. There are usually 28 permanent teeth erupted by age 15 years, and a further 4 wisdom teeth (third molars) that usually erupt later.

Untreated dental caries

The percentage of Australian children with at least one untreated decayed tooth in their mouth is shown in Table 5-9. The highest percentage of children with at least one untreated decayed tooth in their mouth was among Indigenous children (22.9%) and the lowest percentage was among children from high income households (6.6%).

Approximately one child in ten has a permanent tooth with untreated decay (10.9%) with the percentages increasing across younger to older children; 6–8 years (5.7%), 9–11 years (11.5%), and 12–14 years (15.4%).

Indigenous children overall had more than a two-fold difference in the percentage of children with untreated decay compared with non-Indigenous children (22.9% versus 10.1%). Among ages 6–8 years there were 13.1% of Indigenous children compared with 5.1% of non-Indigenous children with untreated decayed teeth. The prevalence in those aged 9–11 years was 25.6% versus 10.5%; and 31.8% versus 14.6% in those aged 11–14 years among Indigenous and non-Indigenous children, respectively.

Overall, children of vocational education parents or tertiary-education parents had a lower percentage of untreated decay compared with children whose parents had school-level education (9.7% and 8.1% versus 14.9%. This pattern was observed across children aged 6–8 years, 9–11 years and 12–14 years.

A higher percentage of children from low income households (15.3%) had untreated permanent tooth decay compared with children from medium (9.2%) or high (6.6%) income households. The same pattern was observed among all age groups.

Overall, a higher percentage of children from Remote/Very remote (21.6%) and Outer regional residential locations (12.3%) had permanent teeth with untreated decay compared with children from Major cities (9.9%). Differences were also observed among children aged 9–11 years and 12–14 years from Remote/Very remote and Major city locations (21.5% versus 10.4%) and (35.9% versus 13.8%), respectively.

The prevalence of untreated permanent tooth dental decay was higher (15.4%) among children who last attended for a dental problem compared with children who attended for a check-up (9.3%). The same pattern was observed across all age groups.

The prevalence of untreated decayed permanent teeth among children was related to age, Indigenous identity, parent education level, household income, residential location and reason for last dental visit.

Table 5-9: Percentage of children with untreated dental caries in the permanent dentition in the Australian child population

	Population: children aged 6–14 years			
	All ages	6–8	9–11	12–14
All	10.9	5.7	11.5	15.4
	10.0–11.8	*4.9–6.5*	*10.1–13.0*	*13.9–17.0*
Sex				
Male	10.8	5.3	11.2	15.9
	9.7–11.8	*4.4–6.4*	*9.5–13.1*	*13.9–18.1*
Female	11.0	6.0	11.8	14.9
	9.9–12.1	*4.9–7.3*	*10.1–13.7*	*12.9–17.1*
Indigenous identity				
Non-Indigenous	10.1	5.1	10.5	14.6
	9.3–11.0	*4.4–6.0*	*9.1–11.9*	*13.1–16.1*
Indigenous	22.9	13.1	25.6	31.8
	18.8–27.7	*9.4–18.0*	*20.2–31.9*	*22.9–42.1*
Parents' country of birth				
Australian born	10.7	5.7	11.1	15.1
	9.7–11.7	*4.8–6.7*	*9.5–12.8*	*13.3–17.1*
Overseas born	11.0	5.6	11.6	15.7
	9.8–12.2	*4.2–7.2*	*9.5–14.0*	*13.6–17.9*
Parental education				
School	14.9	7.7	16.8	19.7
	13.3–16.6	*6.1–9.6*	*14.1–19.9*	*16.7–23.0*
Vocational training	9.7	6.2	8.8	13.8
	8.5–11.2	*4.7–8.2*	*6.9–11.2*	*11.2–16.7*
Tertiary education	8.1	4.2	8.2	12.1
	7.2–9.0	*3.4–5.2*	*6.9–9.6*	*10.4–14.0*
Household income				
Low	15.3	8.0	17.4	20.0
	13.8–16.9	*6.3–10.1*	*14.7–20.3*	*17.4–22.9*
Medium	9.2	5.2	8.8	13.5
	8.2–10.2	*4.2–6.3*	*7.4–10.4*	*11.6–15.6*
High	6.6	3.1	5.7	11.2
	5.5–7.8	*2.1–4.4*	*4.3–7.4*	*8.7–14.1*
Residential location				
Major city	9.9	5.6	10.4	13.8
	8.8–11.0	*4.6–6.8*	*8.7–12.3*	*11.9–16.0*
Inner regional	12.1	5.8	13.5	16.7
	10.6–13.7	*4.4–7.6*	*10.9–16.4*	*13.9–19.8*
Outer regional	12.3	5.0	12.5	18.6
	9.8–15.2	*3.5–7.0*	*9.7–16.0*	*14.4–23.7*
Remote/Very remote	21.6	9.0	21.5	35.9
	15.1–29.9	*4.8–16.0*	*11.8–36.0*	*25.8–47.4*
Reason for last dental visit				
Check-up	9.3	4.0	9.3	13.3
	8.4–10.2	*3.3–4.8*	*7.9–10.9*	*11.9–14.9*
Dental problem	15.4	9.7	16.2	21.1
	13.6–17.4	*7.3–12.7*	*13.5–19.2*	*17.3–25.3*

Row 1: Proportions were computed using weighted data.
Row 2: 95% CI: Confidence intervals for estimates were computed using weighted data.
Columns are arranged by age at time of Survey.

The average number of untreated decayed permanent tooth surfaces among Australian children aged 6–14 years is shown in Table 5-10. The average overall was 0.2 untreated decayed permanent tooth surfaces, which increased across the age groups from 0.1 untreated decayed surfaces among children aged 6–8 years to 0.2 surfaces among those aged 9–11 years and 0.4 surfaces among those aged 12–14 years.

Overall, Indigenous children had 3.5 times more untreated decayed permanent tooth surfaces than non-Indigenous children (0.2 versus 0.7). A similar pattern was observed among children aged 9–11 years and 12–14 years.

Children whose parents had school-level education had a higher number of untreated decayed permanent tooth surfaces (0.4) compared with children whose parents had vocational or tertiary-level education (0.2 surfaces and 0.1 surfaces, respectively). The same pattern was observed in children aged 9–11 years and 12–14 years.

Overall, children from low income households had more untreated decayed permanent tooth surfaces (0.4) than children from medium and high income households (0.2 and 0.1 surfaces, respectively). A similar pattern was observed among children aged 9–11 years and 12–14 years.

Children from Remote/Very remote residential locations had 2 to 3 more untreated decayed permanent tooth surfaces than children in Outer regional, Inner regional and Major city residential locations. The pattern was most pronounced among children aged 9–11 years and 12–14 years.

Children who last attended for a dental problem (0.4) had twice the number of untreated decayed permanent tooth surfaces than children who last attended for a check-up (0.2). Similar differences were observed among those aged 9–11 years and 12–14 years.

In summary, the number of untreated decayed permanent tooth surfaces was related to Indigenous identity, parent level of education, household income, residential location and reason for last dental visit.

Table 5-10: Average number of untreated decayed permanent tooth surfaces in the Australian child population

	Population: children aged 6–14 years			
	All ages	6–8	9–11	12–14
All	0.2	0.1	0.2	0.4
	0.2–0.3	0.1–0.1	0.2–0.3	0.3–0.5
Sex				
Male	0.2	0.1	0.2	0.4
	0.2–0.3	0.1–0.1	0.2–0.3	0.3–0.5
Female	0.3	0.1	0.2	0.4
	0.2–0.3	0.1–0.1	0.2–0.3	0.3–0.5
Indigenous identity				
Non-Indigenous	0.2	0.1	0.2	0.3
	0.2–0.2	0.1–0.1	0.2–0.2	0.3–0.4
Indigenous	0.7	0.2	0.7	1.2
	0.4–0.9	0.1–0.3	0.4–1.0	0.7–1.8
Parents' country of birth				
Australian born	0.2	0.1	0.2	0.4
	0.2–0.3	0.1–0.1	0.2–0.3	0.3–0.5
Overseas born	0.2	0.1	0.2	0.4
	0.2–0.3	0.1–0.1	0.2–0.3	0.3–0.5
Parental education				
School	0.4	0.1	0.4	0.6
	0.3–0.5	0.1–0.2	0.3–0.5	0.5–0.8
Vocational training	0.2	0.1	0.2	0.3
	0.2–0.2	0.1–0.1	0.1–0.2	0.2–0.4
Tertiary education	0.1	0.1	0.1	0.2
	0.1–0.2	0.1–0.1	0.1–0.2	0.2–0.3
Household income				
Low	0.4	0.1	0.4	0.6
	0.3–0.4	0.1–0.2	0.3–0.5	0.5–0.7
Medium	0.2	0.1	0.2	0.3
	0.2–0.2	0.1–0.1	0.1–0.2	0.2–0.4
High	0.1	0.1	0.1	0.2
	0.1–0.1	0.0–0.1	0.1–0.1	0.1–0.3
Residential location				
Major city	0.2	0.1	0.2	0.3
	0.2–0.2	0.1–0.1	0.2–0.3	0.3–0.4
Inner regional	0.3	0.1	0.3	0.4
	0.2–0.3	0.1–0.1	0.2–0.3	0.3–0.6
Outer regional	0.3	0.1	0.3	0.5
	0.2–0.4	0.1–0.1	0.1–0.5	0.3–0.7
Remote/Very remote	0.6	0.2	0.5	1.1
	0.3–0.9	0.1–0.3	0.3–0.8	0.5–1.8
Reason for last dental visit				
Check-up	0.2	0.1	0.2	0.3
	0.2–0.2	0.1–0.1	0.1–0.2	0.2–0.3
Dental problem	0.4	0.2	0.3	0.7
	0.3–0.5	0.1–0.2	0.3–0.4	0.5–0.9

Row 1: Means were computed using weighted data.
Row 2: 95% CI: Confidence intervals for estimates were computed using weighted data.
Columns are arranged by age at time of Survey.

Tooth loss due to dental caries

The percentage of Australian children with missing permanent teeth due to dental decay is shown in Table 5-11. Overall, 0.8% of Australian children had at least one permanent tooth missing due to dental decay with a pattern of increasing percentage of children across the age groups. The oldest age group (12–14 years), had four times the percentage of children with missing permanent teeth compared with children aged 9–11 years (1.6% versus 0.4%).

The highest percentage of children with any missing permanent teeth due to dental decay overall was among Indigenous children and children who attended for a problem at their last dental visit (1.4%). The highest percentage of children with missing permanent teeth due to dental decay among the various age groups was among those aged 12–14 years whose last dental visit was for a problem (3.5%).

In summary, the percentage of children with any missing permanent teeth because of dental decay was related to the age of the child and reason for last dental visit.

Table 5-11: Percentage of children with missing teeth due to caries in the permanent dentition in the Australian child population

	Population: children aged 6–14 years			
	All ages	6–8	9–11	12–14
All	0.8	0.2	0.4	1.6
	0.6–0.9	*0.1–0.4*	*0.3–0.6*	*1.2–2.1*
Sex				
Male	0.5	0.1	0.4	1.0
	0.3–0.7	*0.0–0.6*	*0.2–0.7*	*0.6–1.6*
Female	1.0	0.3	0.4	2.3
	0.8–1.4	*0.2–0.7*	*0.3–0.7*	*1.5–3.2*
Indigenous identity				
Non-Indigenous	0.7	0.2	0.4	1.6
	0.6–0.9	*0.1–0.4*	*0.2–0.6*	*1.1–2.1*
Indigenous	1.4	0.2	0.9	3.4
	0.8–2.5	*0.0–1.1*	*0.3–2.5*	*1.7–6.9*
Parents' country of birth				
Australian born	0.7	0.2	0.3	1.6
	0.5–1.0	*0.1–0.5*	*0.2–0.5*	*1.1–2.4*
Overseas born	0.9	0.3	0.6	1.7
	0.6–1.2	*0.1–0.8*	*0.3–1.2*	*1.0–2.6*
Parental education				
School	1.0	0.2	0.5	2.1
	0.6–1.5	*0.1–0.6*	*0.2–1.0*	*1.2–3.7*
Vocational training	0.9	0.5	0.7	1.5
	0.5–1.6	*0.2–1.8*	*0.3–1.7*	*0.7–3.1*
Tertiary education	0.5	0.1	0.2	1.2
	0.4–0.6	*0.0–0.3*	*0.1–0.4*	*0.8–1.7*
Household income				
Low	1.1	0.3	0.8	2.1
	0.7–1.6	*0.1–1.1*	*0.5–1.4*	*1.2–3.4*
Medium	0.7	0.1	0.3	1.7
	0.5–1.0	*0.0–0.2*	*0.1–0.6*	*1.1–2.7*
High	0.6	0.4	0.2	1.2
	0.3–1.0	*0.1–1.0*	*0.0–1.3*	*0.6–2.3*
Residential location				
Major city	0.7	0.2	0.4	1.5
	0.5–1.0	*0.1–0.6*	*0.2–0.7*	*1.0–2.3*
Inner regional	0.6	0.1	0.4	1.3
	0.4–0.9	*0.0–0.7*	*0.2–0.9*	*0.8–2.2*
Outer regional	1.3	0.3	0.8	2.7
	0.8–2.0	*0.1–0.6*	*0.3–1.7*	*1.6–4.7*
Remote/Very remote	1.0	0.4	0.2	2.5
	0.3–2.9	*0.1–2.7*	*0.1–0.6*	*0.7–8.5*
Reason for last dental visit				
Check-up	0.6	0.1	0.4	1.2
	0.4–0.8	*0.0–0.4*	*0.2–0.6*	*0.8–1.8*
Dental problem	1.4	0.5	0.7	3.5
	1.0–2.0	*0.2–1.2*	*0.3–1.5*	*2.3–5.3*

Row 1: Proportions were computed using weighted data.
Row 2: 95% CI: Confidence intervals for estimates were computed using weighted data.
Columns are arranged by age at time of Survey.

Filled teeth due to dental caries

The percentage of Australian children with at least one permanent tooth that has been filled because of dental decay is shown in Table 5-12. Overall, 15.6% of Australian children had at least one permanent tooth filled because of dental decay, which increased across age groups from 3.8% among ages 6–8 years to 14.5% among ages 9–11 years, and 28.3% among ages 12–14 years. The highest percentage overall of children with filled permanent teeth (22.3%) was among children whose last dental visit was for a dental problem, and it was the highest among children aged 12–14 years who last attended because of a dental problem (39.2%).

Indigenous children had a higher percentage of children with a filled permanent tooth due to dental decay (20.0%) compared with non-Indigenous children (15.4%). Among the specific age groups, Indigenous children aged 9–11 years had 1.7 times higher percentage of children with a permanent tooth with a filling due to dental decay than non-Indigenous children (24.3% versus 13.9%).

A higher percentage of children whose parents had school-level education (17.5%) had filled permanent teeth due to dental decay compared with children whose parents had tertiary level education (14.0%).

Children from low income households had a higher percentage of filled permanent teeth (17.3%) compared with children from high income households (13.7%).

Children from Outer regional residential locations had a higher percentage of filled permanent teeth (17.8%) compared with children from Major cities (14.8%), and the difference was reflected also among ages 9–11 years (18.2% versus 13.1%) and 12–14 years (31.2% versus 27.0%).

Children who last attended for a dental problem also had a higher percentage (22.3%) of children with filled permanent teeth because of dental decay when compared with children who last attended for a check-up (15.8%). The same pattern was observed across all age groups with the relative difference among the age groups being 2.3 times, 1.6 times and 1.5 times among children aged 6–8 years, 9–11 years and 12–14 years, respectively.

In summary, the percentage of children with at least one filled permanent tooth because of dental decay was related to Indigenous identity, parental education, household income, residential location and reason for last dental visit.

Oral health of Australian children

Table 5-12: Percentage of children with filled teeth due to caries in permanent dentition in Australian child population

	Population: children aged 6–14 years			
	All ages	**6–8**	**9–11**	**12–14**
All	**15.6**	**3.8**	**14.5**	**28.3**
	14.7–16.5	*3.2–4.5*	*13.3–15.6*	*26.6–30.0*
Sex				
Male	14.5	3.3	13.2	27.2
	13.4–15.6	*2.5–4.2*	*11.8–14.7*	*24.9–29.7*
Female	16.8	4.4	15.8	29.5
	15.5–18.0	*3.5–5.5*	*14.0–17.6*	*27.2–31.8*
Indigenous identity				
Non-Indigenous	15.4	3.8	13.9	28.0
	14.4–16.3	*3.2–4.5*	*12.7–15.1*	*26.3–29.8*
Indigenous	20.0	4.8	24.3	33.4
	16.9–23.4	*2.8–8.1*	*19.1–30.3*	*26.1–41.5*
Parents' country of birth				
Australian born	16.0	3.6	14.7	29.5
	14.9–17.1	*2.9–4.4*	*13.2–16.2*	*27.5–31.6*
Overseas born	14.9	4.3	14.0	26.1
	13.5–16.2	*3.2–5.7*	*12.2–16.0*	*23.4–29.0*
Parental education				
School	17.5	4.6	16.3	30.3
	15.9–19.2	*3.2–6.5*	*14.0–18.9*	*27.1–33.7*
Vocational training	16.7	3.6	15.2	30.1
	14.9–18.7	*2.5–5.1*	*12.7–18.0*	*26.3–34.2*
Tertiary education	14.0	3.5	13.3	25.9
	12.9–15.1	*2.8–4.4*	*11.9–14.9*	*24.0–27.9*
Household income				
Low	17.3	4.3	16.4	30.1
	15.8–18.9	*3.1–5.8*	*14.3–18.6*	*27.0–33.3*
Medium	15.8	3.7	14.6	28.7
	14.5–17.1	*2.8–4.9*	*12.8–16.4*	*26.2–31.3*
High	13.7	3.5	12.9	25.7
	12.3–15.2	*2.5–4.8*	*10.7–15.3*	*23.0–28.7*
Residential location				
Major city	14.8	3.7	13.8	27.0
	13.7–16.0	*3.0–4.6*	*12.3–15.3*	*24.8–29.3*
Inner regional	17.7	4.3	16.9	31.2
	15.8–19.8	*2.9–6.2*	*14.5–19.5*	*28.0–34.5*
Outer regional	17.8	4.4	16.2	31.2
	15.8–19.9	*3.2–6.1*	*13.5–19.2*	*27.6–35.0*
Remote/Very remote	11.9	1.5	7.2	28.6
	8.0–17.3	*0.5–4.3*	*3.6–14.1*	*21.1–37.6*
Reason for last dental visit				
Check-up	15.8	3.6	13.5	27.1
	14.8–16.8	*2.9–4.5*	*12.2–14.9*	*25.3–29.0*
Dental problem	22.3	7.8	22.2	39.2
	20.2–24.3	*5.9–10.1*	*19.4–25.1*	*34.8–43.7*

Row 1: Proportions were computed using weighted data.
Row 2: 95% CI: Confidence intervals for estimates were computed using weighted data.
Columns are arranged by age at time of Survey.

Table 5-13 shows the average number of filled permanent tooth surfaces due to dental decay among Australian children. On average, there were 0.4 permanent tooth surfaces filled because of dental decay and a pattern of increasing number of filled surfaces is seen across the age groups.

The highest average number of permanent tooth surfaces with a filling was seen among children whose last dental visit was for a dental problem (0.7 surfaces). A similar pattern was observed among all age groups and was highest among children aged 12–14 years (1.4 surfaces). The relative difference in the average number of filled permanent tooth surfaces was 1.8 times greater among children who last visited for a dental problem than those who visited for a check-up, and ranged from 1.8 times among children aged 12–14 years to twice the average among those aged 6–8 and 9–11 years.

In summary, the average number of permanent tooth surfaces filled because of dental decay was related to reason for last dental visit.

Table 5-13: Average number of filled tooth surfaces due to caries in the permanent dentition in the Australian child population

	Population: children aged 6–14 years			
	All ages	6–8	9–11	12–14
All	0.4	0.1	0.4	0.9
	0.4–0.5	0.1–0.1	0.3–0.4	0.8–1.0
Sex				
Male	0.4	0.1	0.3	0.8
	0.4–0.5	0.1–0.1	0.3–0.4	0.7–0.9
Female	0.5	0.1	0.4	0.9
	0.4–0.5	0.1–0.2	0.3–0.4	0.8–1.1
Indigenous identity				
Non-Indigenous	0.4	0.1	0.3	0.9
	0.4–0.5	0.1–0.1	0.3–0.4	0.8–1.0
Indigenous	0.6	0.1	0.6	1.0
	0.4–0.7	0.0–0.2	0.4–0.8	0.7–1.4
Parents' country of birth				
Australian born	0.5	0.1	0.4	0.9
	0.4–0.5	0.1–0.1	0.3–0.4	0.8–1.0
Overseas born	0.4	0.1	0.3	0.8
	0.4–0.5	0.1–0.2	0.3–0.4	0.7–0.9
Parental education				
School	0.5	0.1	0.4	1.0
	0.5–0.6	0.1–0.2	0.3–0.5	0.8–1.2
Vocational training	0.4	0.1	0.3	0.9
	0.4–0.5	0.0–0.1	0.3–0.4	0.7–1.0
Tertiary education	0.4	0.1	0.3	0.8
	0.4–0.4	0.1–0.1	0.3–0.4	0.7–0.9
Household income				
Low	0.5	0.1	0.4	0.9
	0.4–0.6	0.1–0.1	0.3–0.5	0.8–1.1
Medium	0.4	0.1	0.3	0.9
	0.4–0.5	0.1–0.2	0.3–0.4	0.8–1.0
High	0.4	0.1	0.3	0.8
	0.3–0.5	0.0–0.1	0.3–0.4	0.7–1.0
Residential location				
Major city	0.4	0.1	0.3	0.8
	0.4–0.5	0.1–0.1	0.3–0.4	0.7–0.9
Inner regional	0.6	0.1	0.5	1.1
	0.5–0.6	0.1–0.1	0.3–0.6	0.9–1.3
Outer regional	0.5	0.1	0.4	0.9
	0.4–0.6	0.1–0.1	0.3–0.4	0.7–1.1
Remote/Very remote	0.4	0.0	0.2	1.1
	0.2–0.6	0.0–0.0	0.0–0.4	0.5–1.6
Reason for last dental visit				
Check-up	0.4	0.1	0.3	0.8
	0.4–0.5	0.1–0.1	0.3–0.3	0.7–0.9
Dental problem	0.7	0.2	0.6	1.5
	0.6–0.9	0.1–0.3	0.5–0.8	1.3–1.8

Row 1: Means were computed using weighted data.
Row 2: 95% CI: Confidence intervals for estimates were computed using weighted data.
Columns are arranged by age at time of Survey.

Total caries experience in the permanent dentition

The percentage of Australian children with any dental decay experience is shown in Table 5-14. Overall, 23.5% of Australian children had any dental decay experience with the highest percentage found among children whose last dental visit was because of a dental problem (32.3%). More than one in three Australian children aged 12–14 years have experienced dental decay in their permanent teeth (38.2%).

A higher percentage (36.0%) of Indigenous children had any permanent tooth decay experience compared with non-Indigenous children (22.7%). The pattern was similar across all the age groups.

A higher percentage of children whose parents had school-level education (28.2%) had experienced permanent tooth decay compared with children whose parents had either vocational or tertiary-level education, 23.6% and 20.0%, respectively. The pattern was observed among children aged 6–8 years and 9–11 years, and in the children aged 12–14 years, the difference was between children whose parents had school-level education (42.9%) and those whose parents had tertiary-level education (33.8%).

Overall, a gradient of higher percentage of children with permanent tooth dental decay experience with the level of household income was observed. A higher percentage of children from low income households (28.1%) experienced permanent tooth dental decay than children from medium income households (22.4%), and a higher percentage of children from medium income households experienced permanent tooth dental decay than children from high income households (18.9%).

A higher percentage of children from Remote/Very remote residential locations (28.3%) had permanent tooth decay experience compared with children from Major cities (22.2%). The pattern was observed across all age groups.

A higher percentage of children who last attended for a dental problem (32.3%) had experienced permanent tooth decay compared with children who last attended for a check-up (22.3%). This pattern was seen among all age groups with nearly 51% of children aged 12–14 years who last attended for a dental problem having experienced dental decay in their permanent teeth.

In summary, the percentage of Australian children who had permanent tooth decay experience was related to age, Indigenous identity, parental education level, household income, residential location and reason for last dental visit.

Table 5-14: Percentage of children with overall caries experience in the permanent dentition in the Australian child population

	Population: children aged 6–14 years			
	All ages	6–8	9–11	12–14
All	23.5	9.2	22.8	38.2
	22.3–24.6	*8.2–10.3*	*21.2–24.5*	*36.3–40.0*
Sex				
Male	22.4	8.4	21.7	37.5
	21.0–23.9	*7.2–9.7*	*19.7–23.9*	*35.0–40.1*
Female	24.6	10.2	24.0	38.8
	23.1–26.1	*8.6–11.9*	*21.8–26.3*	*36.2–41.4*
Indigenous identity				
Non-Indigenous	22.7	8.8	21.7	37.4
	21.6–23.9	*7.8–9.8*	*20.0–23.4*	*35.5–39.2*
Indigenous	36.0	16.4	41.3	53.7
	31.8–40.4	*12.2–21.7*	*34.9–47.9*	*44.6–62.5*
Parents' country of birth				
Australian born	23.6	9.0	22.9	38.7
	22.2–25.0	*7.9–10.2*	*20.8–25.0*	*36.4–41.0*
Overseas born	23.1	9.7	22.5	37.1
	21.5–24.8	*7.8–11.8*	*20.0–25.2*	*34.1–40.1*
Parental education				
School	28.2	12.0	28.2	42.9
	26.2–30.2	*9.8–14.5*	*24.9–31.7*	*39.2–46.5*
Vocational training	23.6	9.5	21.3	38.7
	21.6–25.7	*7.6–11.8*	*18.4–24.5*	*34.7–42.8*
Tertiary education	20.0	7.5	19.6	33.8
	18.7–21.3	*6.5–8.7*	*17.8–21.4*	*31.5–36.1*
Household income				
Low	28.1	11.7	29.3	41.9
	26.3–30.0	*9.8–13.8*	*26.3–32.5*	*38.7–45.1*
Medium	22.4	8.6	20.7	37.5
	20.9–23.9	*7.3–10.1*	*18.8–22.8*	*34.8–40.2*
High	18.9	6.9	17.0	33.9
	17.1–20.8	*5.4–8.6*	*14.6–19.7*	*30.7–37.3*
Residential location				
Major city	22.2	9.1	21.3	36.3
	20.7–23.7	*7.8–10.5*	*19.2–23.4*	*33.8–38.7*
Inner regional	25.9	9.7	26.6	40.4
	23.7–28.2	*7.8–12.0*	*23.4–30.0*	*37.1–43.8*
Outer regional	26.3	8.8	25.0	43.3
	23.5–29.3	*7.0–11.0*	*21.6–28.8*	*38.9–47.8*
Remote/Very remote	28.3	10.6	26.7	50.0
	20.4–37.8	*5.5–19.5*	*16.2–40.8*	*37.3–62.5*
Reason for last dental visit				
Check-up	22.3	7.4	20.5	35.5
	21.1–23.6	*6.4–8.4*	*18.6–22.4*	*33.5–37.4*
Dental problem	32.3	16.7	32.1	50.9
	30.0–34.8	*13.6–20.3*	*28.8–35.6*	*46.2–55.5*

Row 1: Proportions were computed using weighted data.
Row 2: 95% CI: Confidence intervals for estimates were computed using weighted data.
Columns are arranged by age at time of Survey.

Table 5-15 shows the average number of decayed, missing or filled permanent tooth surfaces among Australian children. On average, there were 0.7 permanent tooth surfaces affected by decay experience among Australian children with the averages being higher among older children. The highest average number of permanent tooth surfaces affected by dental decay experience was among Indigenous children (1.3 surfaces).

Indigenous children had a higher number of permanent tooth surfaces decayed, missing or filled due to dental decay (1.3) than non-Indigenous children (0.7) and the pattern was repeated for children aged 9–11 years and 12–14 years.

Children whose parents had school-level education had a higher average number of permanent tooth surfaces that were decayed, missing or filled (1.0 surfaces) than children whose parents had vocational training (0.7 surfaces) or tertiary-level education (0.6 surfaces). A difference in the average number of similarly affected permanent tooth surfaces was observed among those aged 9–11 years and 12–14 years between children whose parents had school-level education and children whose parents had tertiary-level education.

Children from low income households had a higher number of permanent tooth surfaces that were decayed, missing, or filled (0.9 surfaces) than among children from medium (0.7 surfaces) or high income (0.6 surfaces) households. A similar pattern was observed among children aged 9–11 years, and between children from low (1.6 surfaces) and high income (1.1 surfaces) households among those aged 12–14 years.

Children whose last dental visit was for a dental problem had higher numbers of permanent tooth surfaces that were decayed, filled or missing because of dental decay (1.2 surfaces) than children whose last dental visit was for a check-up (0.6 surfaces). The pattern was reflected across all age groups with the average number of decayed, filled or missing permanent tooth surfaces among children whose last dental visit was for a dental problem was twice the average of those children who last attended for a check-up.

In summary, the average number of permanent tooth surfaces that were decayed, filled or missing because of dental decay was related to Indigenous identity, parent education level, household income and reason for last visit.

Table 5-15: Average number of decayed, missing or filled tooth surfaces (DMFS) due to caries in the permanent dentition in the Australian child population

| | Population: children aged 6–14 years | | | |
	All ages	6–8	9–11	12–14
All	0.7	0.2	0.6	1.3
	0.7–0.8	0.2–0.2	0.6–0.7	1.2–1.5
Sex				
Male	0.7	0.2	0.6	1.3
	0.6–0.7	0.1–0.2	0.5–0.7	1.1–1.4
Female	0.8	0.2	0.6	1.4
	0.7–0.9	0.2–0.3	0.6–0.7	1.3–1.6
Indigenous identity				
Non-Indigenous	0.7	0.2	0.6	1.3
	0.6–0.7	0.2–0.2	0.5–0.6	1.2–1.4
Indigenous	1.3	0.3	1.4	2.4
	1.0–1.6	0.2–0.5	1.0–1.7	1.6–3.2
Parents' country of birth				
Australian born	0.7	0.2	0.6	1.4
	0.7–0.8	0.2–0.2	0.5–0.7	1.2–1.5
Overseas born	0.7	0.2	0.6	1.3
	0.6–0.8	0.2–0.3	0.5–0.7	1.1–1.4
Parental education				
School	1.0	0.3	0.8	1.7
	0.8–1.1	0.2–0.3	0.7–0.9	1.5–2.0
Vocational training	0.7	0.2	0.6	1.2
	0.6–0.8	0.1–0.3	0.4–0.7	1.0–1.4
Tertiary education	0.6	0.2	0.5	1.1
	0.5–0.6	0.1–0.2	0.4–0.5	1.0–1.2
Household income				
Low	0.9	0.3	0.8	1.6
	0.8–1.0	0.2–0.3	0.7–1.0	1.4–1.8
Medium	0.7	0.2	0.5	1.3
	0.6–0.7	0.1–0.2	0.4–0.6	1.1–1.4
High	0.6	0.2	0.4	1.1
	0.5–0.6	0.1–0.2	0.3–0.5	0.9–1.3
Residential location				
Major city	0.7	0.2	0.6	1.2
	0.6–0.7	0.2–0.2	0.5–0.6	1.1–1.3
Inner regional	0.9	0.2	0.7	1.6
	0.7–1.0	0.2–0.3	0.6–0.9	1.3–1.8
Outer regional	0.8	0.2	0.7	1.5
	0.6–1.0	0.1–0.3	0.5–0.9	1.1–1.9
Remote/Very remote	1.0	0.2	0.7	2.3
	0.6–1.5	0.1–0.4	0.4–1.1	1.5–3.1
Reason for last dental visit				
Check-up	0.6	0.2	0.5	1.1
	0.6–0.7	0.1–0.2	0.4–0.6	1.0–1.2
Dental problem	1.2	0.4	1.0	2.3
	1.0–1.3	0.3–0.5	0.9–1.2	1.9–2.7

Row 1: Means were computed using weighted data.
Row 2: 95% CI: Confidence intervals for estimates were computed using weighted data.
Columns are arranged by age at time of Survey.

Prevalence of non-cavitated carious lesions

Table 5-16 shows the percentage of children with at least one permanent tooth with a white spot lesion. A white spot lesion (or can be called non-cavitated carious lesions) is an early stage of dental decay, before it has progressed to a cavity, where the lesion can be stopped from progressing to the cavity stage through appropriate preventive care. Overall, 17.3% of Australian children presented with a white spot lesion. There was a pattern of a higher percentage of children with a spot lesion among older children. The highest percentage of children with white spot lesions was among children from Remote/Very remote residential locations (26.3%) and the lowest percentage (14.0%) was among children whose parents had tertiary-level education.

A higher percentage of Indigenous children (26.4%) presented with white spot lesions than non-Indigenous children (16.7%). A similar pattern of difference between Indigenous and non-Indigenous children was observed across all age groups.

A higher percentage of children whose parents had school-level education (20.7%) had a white spot lesion in their permanent teeth compared with children whose parents had vocational training (17.9%) or tertiary-level education (13.9%). Across all age groups, a higher percentage of children affected with white spot lesions in their permanent teeth was observed among children whose parents had school-level education compared with children whose parents had tertiary level education.

There was a gradient in the percentage of children affected with white spot lesions in their permanent teeth among the income groups with a higher percentage observed among children from low income households (21.1%) compared with children from medium income households (16.7%) and children from high income households (12.0%).

A higher percentage of children from Remote/Very remote residential locations were affected with white spot lesions in their permanent teeth (27.6%) compared with children from Major cities (15.5%). A similar pattern of the differences was observed among children aged 6–8 years and 9–11 years.

A higher percentage of children whose last dental visit was for a dental problem were affected with white spot lesions in their permanent teeth (19.7%) compared with children who last attended for a check-up (16.7%). The difference was reflected similarly among children aged 12–14 years.

In summary, the percentage of children affected with white spot lesions in their permanent teeth was related to age group, Indigenous identity, parent education level, household income, residential location and reason for last dental visit.

Oral health of Australian children

Table 5-16: Percentage of children with non-cavitated carious lesions in the permanent dentition in the Australian child population

| | Population: children aged 6–14 years | | | |
	All ages	6–8	9–11	12–14
All	17.3	6.9	17.1	27.6
	16.0–18.5	*5.9–8.1*	*15.5–18.8*	*25.4–29.8*
Sex				
Male	18.7	7.0	17.7	31.6
	17.2–20.2	*5.7–8.4*	*15.8–19.8*	*28.9–34.4*
Female	15.8	6.8	16.5	23.5
	14.4–17.2	*5.5–8.3*	*14.5–18.8*	*20.9–26.2*
Indigenous identity				
Non-Indigenous	16.7	6.4	16.5	27.0
	15.5–18.0	*5.3–7.5*	*14.9–18.1*	*24.8–29.3*
Indigenous	26.4	15.7	27.1	38.9
	21.7–31.7	*11.4–21.1*	*19.7–36.0*	*30.2–48.2*
Parents' country of birth				
Australian born	17.5	6.9	17.6	27.8
	16.1–18.9	*5.8–8.1*	*15.7–19.7*	*25.4–30.4*
Overseas born	16.7	6.8	16.2	27.1
	14.9–18.7	*5.3–8.8*	*13.9–18.7*	*23.6–30.8*
Parental education				
School	20.7	9.2	21.2	30.8
	18.7–22.9	*7.3–11.7*	*18.2–24.5*	*27.3–34.5*
Vocational training	17.9	6.4	16.7	29.4
	15.8–20.1	*4.8–8.4*	*14.0–19.7*	*25.0–34.2*
Tertiary education	13.9	5.1	13.7	23.4
	12.6–15.1	*4.2–6.2*	*12.1–15.4*	*20.7–26.2*
Household income				
Low	21.1	8.5	20.7	32.9
	19.3–23.0	*6.7–10.5*	*18.2–23.4*	*29.5–36.4*
Medium	16.7	6.4	16.4	27.2
	15.2–18.3	*5.1–7.9*	*14.2–18.8*	*24.3–30.2*
High	12.0	4.5	11.5	20.7
	10.5–13.6	*3.4–6.0*	*9.5–13.8*	*17.5–24.2*
Residential location				
Major city	15.5	5.7	15.1	25.8
	14.0–17.1	*4.5–7.2*	*13.3–17.1*	*23.1–28.6*
Inner regional	19.5	7.8	18.9	31.0
	17.1–22.0	*6.0–10.0*	*15.8–22.4*	*26.4–35.9*
Outer regional	22.1	10.9	23.2	31.2
	18.5–26.2	*7.6–15.3*	*18.2–29.1*	*25.9–37.0*
Remote/Very remote	27.6	16.4	33.8	33.4
	18.7–38.7	*8.7–28.9*	*18.8–52.9*	*22.7–46.0*
Reason for last dental visit				
Check-up	16.7	6.3	15.7	25.5
	15.4–18.0	*5.3–7.3*	*14.0–17.4*	*23.3–27.8*
Dental problem	19.7	7.9	18.5	34.9
	17.6–21.9	*5.7–10.8*	*15.7–21.7*	*30.3–39.7*

Row 1: Proportions were computed using weighted data.
Row 2: 95% CI: Confidence intervals for estimates were computed using weighted data.
Columns are arranged by age at time of Survey.

5.4 Fissure sealant use

The back (molar) teeth account for most of the caries experience in the permanent teeth of children and adolescents. The molar teeth have many grooves (fissures) and pits on the chewing (occlusal) surface and on the buccal and palatal surfaces, which can be difficult to keep clean. These are the sites most susceptible for developing caries.

Fissure sealants are materials that are applied to the pits and fissure surfaces of teeth to create a thin barrier, which protect the sealed surfaces from caries. Fissure sealant materials fall into two categories: resin–based sealants or glass–ionomer (cement) sealants. Fissure sealants are applied to the pit and fissure surfaces by dental professionals. Fissure sealant use may reflect the access to dental care for prevention or level of perceived risk of having future dental caries. Table 5-17 describes the proportion of children who had at least one tooth with a fissure sealant.

Nearly 27% of Australian children aged 6–14 years had at least one tooth with a fissure sealant, i.e. one in every four children aged 6–14 years had fissure-sealed teeth. As expected, this proportion increased across older age groups. Some 40% of Australian children aged 12–14 years had at least one fissure sealed tooth, which was nearly four times higher than that of the youngest age group (11.7%).

Across all ages combined, there was little variation between population subgroups. The proportion with a fissure sealant was highest among children living in Outer regional (30.2%) and lowest among Indigenous children (23.9%).

There were some statistically significant differences between population subgroups among children aged 12–14 years. Children whose parents had school-only education had a significantly lower proportion of fissure sealed (36.1%) teeth than children whose parents had some tertiary education (42.5%). The proportion of fissure-sealed teeth was significantly lower among males compared to females.

In summary, the proportion of children with at least one fissure sealed tooth was related to sex and parental education in the oldest age group (12–14 years) only.

Table 5-17: Percentage of children with at least one fissure sealant in the permanent dentition in the Australian child population

	Population: children aged 6–14 years			
	All ages	6–8	9–11	12–14
All	26.8	11.7	28.3	40.4
	25.5–28.1	*10.6–12.8*	*26.3–30.3*	*38.1–42.6*
Sex				
Male	25.1	10.9	27.3	37.5
	23.6–26.6	*9.6–12.4*	*24.8–29.8*	*34.7–40.3*
Female	28.6	12.5	29.3	43.3
	26.9–30.3	*11.1–14.0*	*27.0–31.7*	*40.3–46.2*
Indigenous identity				
Non-Indigenous	27.0	11.8	28.4	40.5
	25.6–28.4	*10.7–13.0*	*26.4–30.5*	*38.1–42.8*
Indigenous	23.9	10.5	27.9	35.6
	20.6–27.5	*6.8–15.7*	*22.1–34.5*	*28.5–43.3*
Parents' country of birth				
Australian born	27.1	12.2	28.7	40.3
	25.6–28.6	*10.9–13.5*	*26.2–31.3*	*37.6–43.0*
Overseas born	26.3	10.9	27.6	40.2
	24.4–28.3	*9.3–12.7*	*25.2–30.1*	*36.7–43.8*
Parental education				
School	24.9	10.6	27.0	36.1
	23.0–27.0	*8.8–12.6*	*23.7–30.5*	*32.6–39.7*
Vocational training	27.1	10.2	28.4	41.2
	24.9–29.3	*8.3–12.4*	*24.9–32.1*	*37.4–45.0*
Tertiary education	28.2	12.9	29.6	43.0
	26.4–29.9	*11.4–14.6*	*26.9–32.4*	*40.1–45.9*
Household income				
Low	25.8	11.9	25.9	38.4
	23.9–27.9	*10.0–14.2*	*23.2–28.7*	*34.8–42.1*
Medium	26.6	10.7	28.1	40.6
	24.9–28.3	*9.2–12.2*	*25.2–31.2*	*37.7–43.6*
High	28.6	13.1	31.6	42.5
	26.5–30.8	*11.0–15.6*	*28.5–34.9*	*38.5–46.6*
Residential location				
Major city	26.0	10.8	27.4	40.0
	24.3–27.8	*9.5–12.2*	*24.8–30.1*	*37.1–42.9*
Inner regional	28.1	13.5	29.2	40.6
	25.3–30.9	*11.1–16.3*	*25.3–33.4*	*36.1–45.4*
Outer regional	30.2	14.3	32.2	42.7
	26.9–33.7	*11.3–17.8*	*27.5–37.3*	*38.3–47.2*
Remote/Very remote	25.9	13.3	28.3	37.4
	21.2–31.1	*9.3–18.6*	*21.5–36.2*	*26.2–50.1*
Reason for last dental visit				
Check-up	29.8	12.5	30.6	42.4
	28.2–31.3	*11.1–14.0*	*28.2–33.0*	*40.0–44.8*
Dental problem	27.1	17.8	27.2	37.8
	25.0–29.3	*15.2–20.7*	*24.0–30.6*	*33.4–42.3*

Row 1: Proportions were computed using weighted data.
Row 2: 95% CI: Confidence intervals for estimates were computed using weighted data.
Columns are arranged by age at time of Survey.

5.5 Oral hygiene status

Prevalence of dental plaque

Plaque index includes the presence of moderate or abundant soft deposit within the gingival pocket, or the tooth and gingival margin visible to the naked eye (score of 2 or over of the Loe and Silness plaque index) (1963).

Table 5-18 shows the percentage of children who presented with plaque. The lowest percentage was among children aged 5–6 years from households with a high income (25.7%) while the highest percentage was among Indigenous children aged 7–8 years (69.7%).

Overall, 42.6% of children had at least one tooth index with plaque, varying across age groups from 32.4% (5–6 years) to 49.5% (9–10 years).

More Indigenous children had plaque than non-Indigenous children among all children (60.1% versus 41.5). Males had a higher percentage (47.9%) of dental plaque than females (37.0 %).

A higher proportion of children whose parents had school-only education had plaque compared to children of parents who had a tertiary education (47.3% versus 38.2%). This pattern was seen across all age groups with a relative ratio varying from 1.2 (7–8 years and 9–10 years) to 1.4 (5–6 years).

There was a gradient in the percentage of children with plaque across household income groups with 48.8% of children from low income households having plaque compared to 35.1% of children from high income households, a 1.4 relative ratio. The percentage ratio of dental plaque between children from low and medium income households and between children from medium and high income households was 1.2. In each specific two-year age group, there were more children with plaque in low income households relative to the medium and high income households.

The highest percentage of children with plaque was among those who had made their last dental visit for a problem. Among all children who last visited for a problem, there were 1.2 times more children with plaque compared to children who last visited for a check-up. This difference was 1.4 in the 5–6-year age group, 1.2-fold in the 7–8-year group, 1.1 times in the 9–10-year age group, 1.2 in the 11–12-year age group and 1.3 in the 13–14-year age group.

In summary, the prevalence of plaque among children was related to sex, Indigenous status, parental education, household income and reason for last dental visit.

Table 5-18: Percentage of children with a plaque index score of two or more (visible plaque accumulation) in the Australian child population

	Population: children aged 5–14 years					
	All ages	5–6	7–8	9–10	11–12	13–14
All	42.6	32.4	48.6	49.5	47.8	35.1
	40.6–44.6	*29.5–35.5*	*45.4–51.8*	*46.6–52.3*	*45.1–50.6*	*32.1–38.2*
Sex						
Male	47.9	34.3	51.6	56.0	54.8	43.3
	45.7–50.1	*30.9–37.8*	*47.8–55.4*	*52.3–59.6*	*51.3–58.3*	*39.6–47.1*
Female	37.0	30.5	45.3	42.8	40.3	26.9
	34.7–39.4	*27.0–34.2*	*41.6–49.1*	*39.2–46.6*	*37.0–43.8*	*23.4–30.7*
Indigenous identity						
Non-Indigenous	41.5	31.2	47.3	48.6	46.8	34.2
	39.5–43.5	*28.3–34.3*	*44.1–50.5*	*45.6–51.5*	*44.0–49.6*	*31.2–37.4*
Indigenous	60.1	49.6	69.7	64.5	62.0	53.7
	54.3–65.8	*39.3–59.8*	*60.3–77.7*	*55.3–72.7*	*52.5–70.7*	*41.4–65.5*
Parents' country of birth						
Australian born	42.9	32.1	48.8	50.9	48.2	35.0
	40.7–45.1	*28.7–35.7*	*45.2–52.4*	*47.4–54.4*	*45.0–51.3*	*31.5–38.7*
Overseas born	41.9	32.6	48.3	47.1	46.8	35.1
	39.4–44.5	*28.6–36.8*	*43.6–52.9*	*43.2–51.1*	*42.8–50.8*	*31.0–39.5*
Parental education						
School	47.3	38.6	52.0	52.5	54.8	39.3
	44.3–50.3	*33.4–44.0*	*46.6–57.4*	*47.3–57.7*	*50.2–59.2*	*34.7–44.1*
Vocational training	43.4	30.7	53.9	52.2	45.2	36.1
	40.6–46.2	*26.2–35.5*	*48.4–59.3*	*47.2–57.1*	*40.2–50.3*	*31.1–41.4*
Tertiary education	38.2	27.9	43.6	45.4	43.4	31.1
	36.0–40.5	*24.9–31.2*	*40.3–47.0*	*41.9–48.9*	*40.2–46.8*	*27.3–35.1*
Household income						
Low	48.8	36.0	53.7	58.5	54.9	41.9
	46.0–51.6	*31.3–41.0*	*49.2–58.2*	*54.0–62.8*	*50.5–59.3*	*37.1–46.8*
Medium	41.0	30.3	48.8	45.9	46.6	33.6
	38.6–43.4	*26.8–34.1*	*45.0–52.6*	*41.9–50.0*	*42.7–50.5*	*29.5–38.1*
High	35.1	25.7	39.6	42.8	39.9	28.1
	32.4–37.8	*21.6–30.3*	*34.9–44.5*	*37.9–47.8*	*35.7–44.2*	*23.3–33.5*
Residential location						
Major city	38.8	28.2	44.2	45.2	44.9	31.9
	36.2–41.4	*24.7–32.1*	*40.1–48.3*	*41.6–48.8*	*41.4–48.5*	*28.2–36.0*
Inner regional	49.6	39.6	56.0	58.7	52.3	41.7
	45.6–53.6	*33.5–46.0*	*49.5–62.3*	*53.3–64.0*	*47.1–57.5*	*36.0–47.5*
Outer regional	49.8	42.4	58.4	55.6	55.7	37.9
	44.9–54.7	*36.1–48.8*	*51.7–64.8*	*48.3–62.8*	*48.5–62.7*	*31.6–44.8*
Remote/Very remote	62.8	58.4	73.1	65.5	58.6	56.9
	53.8–70.9	*47.0–69.0*	*60.1–83.1*	*50.6–77.8*	*47.5–68.9*	*36.5–75.2*
Reason for last dental visit						
Check-up	39.8	29.5	44.9	46.3	44.9	32.8
	37.7–41.8	*26.4–32.8*	*41.3–48.6*	*42.9–49.8*	*42.0–47.9*	*29.7–35.9*
Dental problem	49.6	41.4	53.0	53.0	54.4	41.7
	46.6–52.6	*35.2–47.9*	*48.1–57.8*	*48.3–57.6*	*48.9–59.7*	*35.3–48.4*

Row 1: Proportions were computed using weighted data.
Row 2: 95% CI: Confidence intervals for estimates were computed using weighted data.
Columns are arranged by age at time of Survey.

Prevalence of gingival inflammation

Gingival index includes the presence of redness, hypertrophy, oedema and glazing with bleeding on swiping with probe or ulceration with spontaneous bleeding, or bleeding after drying with air (score of 2 or over of the Loe and Silness gingival index). (Silness J and Loe H 1964).

Table 5–19 describes the percentage of children who presented gingivitis. Overall, nearly one-fifth of the children (21.8%) had gingivitis with children aged 5–6 years presenting the lowest percentage (12.5%). Lower percentages of gingivitis were found among children from high income households when compared to those from low income households in all age groups. This difference was 1.8 times higher in the 5–6-year age group, 1.3 in the 7–8-year age group, 1.4 in the 9–10-year age group, 1.6 in the 11–12-year age group and 1.7 times in 13–14-year age group.

More Indigenous children had gingivitis than non-Indigenous children (34.4% versus 21.1%) and it was seen in all age groups. The highest difference was observed among children aged 7–8 years (41.2% versus 21.5%). Overall, a lower percentage of gingivitis was found among females, however, this pattern was not consistent across the age groups.

The percentage of gingivitis was 1.3 times higher in children whose parents had school-level education (24.7%) when compared to children of parents who had tertiary education (18.4%). A similar pattern was seen across all age groups with the highest ratio observed among children aged 5–6 years.

There was a gradient in the percentage of children with gingivitis across household income groups and its pattern remains the same across the age groups. The ratio between children from low and medium income households varied from 1.1 (7–8-year age group) to 1.3 (5–6-year and 13–14-year age groups) and between children from medium and high income households was from 1.2 in the 9–10-year age group to 1.4 in the 5–6-year age group. In each specific two-year age group, there were more children with plaque in low income households relative to medium and high income households.

Higher percentage of children with gingivitis was found among those who had made their last dental visit for a problem. Among all children who last visited for a problem, there were 1.2 times more children with gingivitis compared to children who last visited for a check-up. The highest relative ratio was 1.6 in the 5–6-year age group and the lowest (1.1) was found in the 7–8 and 9–10-year age groups.

In summary, the prevalence of gingivitis among children's dentition was related to Indigenous status, parental education, household income, residential location and reason for last dental visit.

Oral health of Australian children

Table 5-19: Percentage of children with gingivitis (gingival index score of 2+) in the Australian child population

	Population: children aged 5–14 years					
	All ages	5–6	7–8	9–10	11–12	13–14
All	21.8	12.5	22.6	25.8	25.4	23.1
	20.3–23.5	*10.6–14.6*	*20.3–25.2*	*23.3–28.4*	*23.2–27.8*	*20.4–26.0*
Sex						
Male	23.9	12.9	23.3	28.3	28.4	27.2
	22.1–25.8	*10.5–15.8*	*20.3–26.5*	*25.1–31.7*	*25.5–31.5*	*23.7–31.0*
Female	19.6	12.0	21.9	23.2	22.2	18.9
	17.9–21.4	*9.9–14.4*	*19.1–25.1*	*20.4–26.4*	*19.6–25.1*	*15.8–22.6*
Indigenous identity						
Non-Indigenous	21.1	12.0	21.5	25.2	24.4	22.5
	19.5–22.7	*10.2–14.2*	*19.2–24.0*	*22.7–27.8*	*22.2–26.7*	*19.8–25.5*
Indigenous	34.4	17.6	41.2	35.7	41.1	37.5
	28.4–40.9	*12.0–25.2*	*31.7–51.4*	*26.9–45.7*	*30.2–53.1*	*26.4–50.0*
Parents' country of birth						
Australian born	22.2	11.5	21.9	27.4	26.4	24.2
	20.5–23.9	*9.6–13.8*	*19.4–24.6*	*24.5–30.4*	*23.8–29.2*	*20.9–27.9*
Overseas born	21.0	13.7	23.8	22.7	23.4	21.6
	18.9–23.3	*10.8–17.3*	*20.2–27.8*	*19.4–26.5*	*20.3–26.7*	*18.0–25.7*
Parental education						
School	24.7	16.1	26.0	24.8	29.4	27.2
	22.3–27.3	*13.0–19.8*	*21.7–30.8*	*20.6–29.6*	*25.7–33.4*	*22.6–32.3*
Vocational training	23.0	11.0	22.2	29.2	25.6	26.2
	20.8–25.3	*8.2–14.5*	*18.4–26.7*	*25.1–33.6*	*21.6–30.1*	*21.2–31.8*
Tertiary education	18.4	9.8	20.1	23.2	21.0	18.3
	16.7–20.2	*7.9–12.3*	*17.4–23.1*	*20.6–26.1*	*18.5–23.7*	*15.5–21.4*
Household income						
Low	25.8	15.3	25.4	28.8	30.8	28.7
	23.4–28.3	*12.0–19.3*	*21.7–29.5*	*24.9–33.1*	*26.9–35.1*	*24.3–33.4*
Medium	20.4	11.2	20.3	24.9	23.3	22.3
	18.6–22.3	*9.3–13.3*	*17.6–23.1*	*21.5–28.6*	*20.4–26.4*	*18.8–26.3*
High	16.7	8.7	19.1	20.1	19.2	17.1
	14.8–18.8	*6.5–11.7*	*15.6–23.3*	*16.7–24.0*	*16.2–22.6*	*13.6–21.4*
Residential location						
Major city	19.6	10.8	20.1	22.6	23.6	21.3
	17.7–21.6	*8.5–13.6*	*17.2–23.3*	*19.6–25.9*	*21.0–26.5*	*18.2–24.8*
Inner regional	26.8	17.1	27.8	33.0	28.2	27.8
	23.7–30.1	*13.6–21.2*	*22.8–33.4*	*28.3–38.1*	*23.6–33.2*	*21.0–35.7*
Outer regional	23.2	12.6	24.7	27.0	27.0	24.0
	18.9–28.2	*9.0–17.4*	*18.6–32.1*	*20.9–34.2*	*20.6–34.5*	*18.6–30.3*
Remote/Very remote	38.1	23.7	43.6	47.1	45.7	29.6
	30.6–46.3	*12.3–40.8*	*36.7–50.7*	*29.8–65.1*	*35.7–56.0*	*17.1–46.1*
Reason for last dental visit						
Check-up	20.6	10.6	21.1	23.9	23.9	21.5
	19.1–22.3	*8.4–13.2*	*18.5–23.8*	*21.3–26.8*	*21.5–26.3*	*18.8–24.6*
Dental problem	24.8	17.0	23.6	26.7	27.3	27.9
	22.3–27.5	*12.9–22.1*	*19.6–28.2*	*22.4–31.4*	*23.0–32.1*	*22.3–34.3*

Row 1: Proportions were computed using weighted data.
Row 2: 95% CI: Confidence intervals for estimates were computed using weighted data.
Columns are arranged by age at time of Survey.

5.6 Other oral conditions

Prevalence of dental trauma

Children whose dental examination revealed the presence of any trauma in their permanent dentition were classified as having dental trauma. Trauma was examined based on worst condition observed among six anterior permanent teeth in the upper jaw. Visual assessment of trauma was confirmed by interview. This report describes the proportion of children who had any trauma in their upper anterior teeth.

Table 5-20 presents the percentage of children who had dental trauma. Overall, the percentage of dental trauma was 9.9%, varying from 3.1% among children aged 5–6 years to 14.1% in 13–14-year age group. Percentage of dental trauma was lower in females in all age groups with the exemption of children aged 7–8 years.

More Indigenous children had dental trauma than non-Indigenous children (14.3% versus 9.6%), however, this difference was not consistent in all age groups.

Overall, percentages of dental trauma did not vary much across parental education levels and a similar pattern was observed across age groups. No significant variation was observed in percentages of dental trauma across levels of household income.

Higher percentage of children with dental trauma was among those who had last made a dental visit for a problem. In all children, those who last visited for a problem had 38% (13.2%) higher percentage of dental trauma compared with children who last visited for a check-up (9.6%). This ratio was 2.3 in the 5–6-year age group, two-fold in the 7–8-year group, 1.3 times in the 9–10-year age group, 1.6 in the 11–12-year group and 1.3 in the 13–14-year age group.

In summary, the prevalence of dental trauma among children's dentition was related to sex, Indigenous status and reason for last dental visit.

Table 5-20: Percentage of children with any dental trauma in the Australian child population

	Population: children aged 5–14 years					
	All ages	**5–6**	**7–8**	**9–10**	**11–12**	**13–14**
All	9.9	3.1	3.9	9.3	13.9	14.1
	9.2–10.6	*2.0–4.8*	*3.1–4.9*	*8.2–10.5*	*12.5–15.4*	*12.5–15.9*
Sex						
Male	12.1	4.2	3.9	10.7	17.2	18.5
	11.1–13.2	*2.4–7.3*	*2.9–5.2*	*9.1–12.5*	*15.1–19.4*	*16.2–21.0*
Female	7.6	2.0	3.9	7.8	10.4	9.8
	6.9–8.4	*1.1–3.6*	*2.8–5.2*	*6.5–9.4*	*8.9–12.0*	*8.0–11.9*
Indigenous identity						
Non-Indigenous	9.6	3.1	3.8	8.9	13.3	14.0
	8.9–10.4	*1.9–4.9*	*3.0–4.8*	*7.8–10.1*	*11.9–14.7*	*12.3–15.8*
Indigenous	14.3	3.2	5.0	13.3	24.5	19.2
	11.4–17.8	*0.6–15.0*	*2.6–9.4*	*8.0–21.3*	*17.8–32.8*	*11.8–29.8*
Parents' country of birth						
Australian born	10.4	2.4	3.9	10.4	14.7	14.9
	9.7–11.3	*1.4–4.1*	*3.0–5.2*	*8.9–12.0*	*13.0–16.4*	*13.0–17.1*
Overseas born	8.8	4.3	3.8	7.2	12.4	12.9
	7.7–10.1	*2.2–8.3*	*2.5–5.5*	*5.8–8.9*	*9.9–15.3*	*10.4–15.9*
Parental education						
School	10.5	1.9	5.0	9.1	13.9	15.8
	9.1–12.1	*0.7–5.4*	*3.5–7.1*	*7.1–11.6*	*11.2–17.0*	*12.4–19.8*
Vocational training	10.5	1.7	4.2	9.6	13.1	16.7
	9.2–12.0	*0.8–3.9*	*2.5–7.2*	*7.4–12.2*	*10.6–16.0*	*13.6–20.4*
Tertiary education	9.1	4.3	2.9	9.3	13.7	11.9
	8.2–10.0	*2.5–7.2*	*2.0–4.3*	*7.6–11.3*	*11.9–15.8*	*10.0–14.0*
Household income						
Low	10.9	2.0	5.5	9.6	15.4	14.7
	9.7–12.2	*0.7–5.6*	*3.9–7.8*	*7.8–11.7*	*12.7–18.6*	*12.2–17.7*
Medium	9.5	3.1	3.0	9.2	14.1	13.4
	8.5–10.6	*1.7–5.6*	*2.1–4.3*	*7.6–11.2*	*11.9–16.5*	*11.0–16.3*
High	9.5	4.2	3.4	9.7	12.1	14.5
	8.3–10.7	*2.0–8.5*	*2.1–5.3*	*7.3–12.7*	*9.9–14.6*	*11.5–18.1*
Residential location						
Major city	9.2	2.4	3.7	9.0	13.3	12.4
	8.3–10.2	*1.2–4.5*	*2.7–5.1*	*7.7–10.6*	*11.6–15.2*	*10.4–14.7*
Inner regional	10.9	5.1	4.4	9.8	13.4	17.0
	9.5–12.4	*2.5–10.1*	*2.9–6.5*	*7.6–12.5*	*11.0–16.2*	*13.7–20.7*
Outer regional	12.5	4.1	3.9	11.5	17.5	19.1
	11.1–14.1	*1.9–8.6*	*2.7–5.7*	*8.6–15.1*	*14.3–21.4*	*15.3–23.5*
Remote/Very remote	10.3	0.2	4.5	4.0	19.1	18.2
	7.1–14.6	*0.0–1.5*	*1.5–12.7*	*1.2–12.5*	*10.7–31.7*	*9.3–32.6*
Reason for last dental visit						
Check-up	9.6	2.6	3.5	8.8	12.1	13.7
	8.8–10.4	*1.5–4.4*	*2.6–4.5*	*7.5–10.5*	*10.7–13.5*	*12.0–15.6*
Dental problem	13.2	5.9	6.9	11.3	19.4	17.9
	11.6–14.9	*2.3–14.6*	*4.7–10.1*	*8.9–14.4*	*15.8–23.6*	*13.9–22.7*

Row 1: Proportions were computed using weighted data.
Row 2: 95% CI: Confidence intervals for estimates were computed using weighted data.
Columns are arranged by age at time of Survey.

Prevalence of oral mucosal condition

Children whose examination revealed ulcers or other non-ulcerated mucosal conditions were classified as having mucosal lesions. Odontogenic abscesses were not included in this classification. Table 5-21 describes the proportion of children who had any of those conditions observed at the time of examination.

The overall percentage of oral mucosal conditions was 8.4% and the lowest percentage was among children aged 5–6 years (6.3%). Other age groups had similar percentages varying from 8.7% (9–10 years) to 9.2 (13–14 years). No significant differences were found in the percentages of oral mucosal lesions according to sex.

Among all age groups, the percentage of non-Indigenous children with oral mucosal lesions was lower (7.5%) than in Indigenous children (8.5%). However, the difference was not statistical significant.

A similar proportion of all children with oral mucosal lesions was observed across levels of parental education.

Children residing in outer regional areas had a higher proportion of oral mucosal lesions when compared with children from Major cities (11.9% versus 7.9%).

Overall, there was no variation in the percentage of oral mucosal lesions according to reason for last dental visit and it was seen across age groups.

In summary, the prevalence of oral mucosal lesions among children in the primary dentition was related to age group.

Table 5-21: Percentage of children with oral mucosal lesions in the Australian child population

	Population: children aged 5–14 years					
	All ages	5–6	7–8	9–10	11–12	13–14
All	8.4	6.3	8.9	8.7	8.9	9.2
	7.8–9.1	5.3–7.5	7.8–10.3	7.5–10.0	7.8–10.2	8.0–10.6
Sex						
Male	8.4	6.2	9.1	9.1	8.0	9.7
	7.6–9.3	4.7–8.1	7.6–11.0	7.6–10.8	6.7–9.6	8.0–11.6
Female	8.4	6.5	8.7	8.3	9.9	8.8
	7.7–9.3	5.3–7.9	7.2–10.6	6.8–10.1	8.2–11.9	7.3–10.7
Indigenous identity						
Non-Indigenous	8.5	6.4	9.1	8.8	9.0	9.2
	7.8–9.2	5.3–7.7	7.8–10.5	7.6–10.1	7.8–10.4	7.9–10.6
Indigenous	7.5	5.1	7.9	8.2	6.4	10.8
	5.7–9.7	2.8–9.0	4.3–14.1	4.7–14.1	3.6–11.1	6.0–18.7
Parents' country of birth						
Australian born	8.6	6.5	8.9	8.8	8.9	9.8
	7.8–9.4	5.4–7.9	7.4–10.7	7.4–10.4	7.6–10.4	8.3–11.7
Overseas born	8.2	6.0	9.1	8.6	9.0	8.3
	7.2–9.3	4.4–8.1	7.3–11.2	6.7–11.0	7.2–11.2	6.3–10.8
Parental education						
School	8.4	5.2	8.9	9.2	8.4	10.1
	7.4–9.4	3.8–7.1	6.8–11.5	6.9–12.2	6.5–10.8	7.8–13.0
Vocational training	8.8	6.5	9.7	8.4	8.9	10.3
	7.5–10.3	4.7–8.8	7.4–12.6	6.1–11.5	6.7–11.7	7.7–13.6
Tertiary education	8.6	7.1	9.0	8.7	9.7	8.3
	7.7–9.5	5.5–9.1	7.4–10.9	7.4–10.3	8.2–11.5	6.8–10.2
Household income						
Low	8.3	6.1	8.6	9.4	8.3	9.0
	7.4–9.2	4.5–8.1	6.9–10.7	7.3–11.9	6.6–10.4	7.1–11.5
Medium	8.4	6.9	9.0	6.7	8.7	10.8
	7.5–9.4	5.5–8.7	7.2–11.1	5.4–8.3	7.1–10.7	8.5–13.5
High	8.8	6.0	9.7	10.2	10.1	8.3
	7.6–10.2	4.3–8.5	7.3–12.7	8.0–13.0	7.8–12.9	6.4–10.8
Residential location						
Major city	7.9	5.6	8.5	8.1	8.5	8.7
	7.1–8.7	4.4–7.2	7.1–10.2	6.7–9.6	7.1–10.2	7.1–10.5
Inner regional	8.6	7.5	7.8	8.8	9.3	9.2
	7.5–9.8	5.5–10.1	5.9–10.2	6.6–11.7	7.4–11.7	6.9–12.2
Outer regional	11.9	9.6	12.8	11.8	12.2	12.7
	9.3–15.1	6.3–14.5	9.2–17.6	8.0–17.2	8.5–17.3	10.0–16.0
Remote/Very remote	9.0	5.1	13.5	11.6	4.4	9.9
	6.6–12.3	2.5–10.2	6.4–26.2	5.5–23.1	1.7–11.0	4.5–20.4
Reason for last dental visit						
Check-up	8.5	6.5	8.6	8.6	8.9	9.5
	7.8–9.4	5.2–8.2	7.1–10.2	7.4–10.1	7.6–10.4	8.1–11.0
Dental problem	8.3	5.3	9.4	8.4	9.8	7.4
	7.2–9.6	3.6–7.8	7.0–12.6	6.3–11.1	7.2–13.1	5.2–10.6

Row 1: Proportions were computed using weighted data.
Row 2: 95% CI: Confidence intervals for estimates were computed using weighted data.
Columns are arranged by age at time of Survey.

Prevalence of odontogenic abscess

An odontogenic abscess is a localised infection around the tooth apex and submucosa due to gross caries or trauma. If an odontogenic abscess was observed in the examination, attempts were made to link the abscess with the tooth or teeth for its origin in that child. This section describes the proportion of children who were observed with an odontogenic abscess at the time of the examination.

Table 5-22 describes the proportion of children who had odontogenic abscess. Overall, the proportion of odontogenic abscess was low (1.8%). The lowest prevalence across age groups was found in children aged 13–14 years (0.4%) and the highest percentage was in 7–8-year age group (3.4%). Males had greater percentage of odontogenic abscess (4.1%) than females (2.5%) in children aged 7–8 years only.

Percentages of odontogenic abscess were consistently higher among Indigenous children compared to that percentage among non-Indigenous children. However, no significant difference was observed.

A higher proportion of children whose parents had school-only education had odontogenic abscess compared to children of parents who had vocational and tertiary education (2.5% versus 1.3% and 1.5%, respectively). There was a 2.8 and 2.2-fold difference in the percentage of children with odontogenic abscess between children whose parents' highest education was school-level and children of tertiary-educated parents in the 5-6 year and 7–8-year age groups, respectively.

The percentage of children with odontogenic abscess varied from 0.5% (aged 11–12 years) to 3.9% (aged 5–6 years) in children from low income households. In children from medium income households the percentage of odontogenic abscess varied from 0.0% (aged 13–14 years) to 2.5% (aged 7–8 years) and from 0.6% (aged 13–14 years) to 2.7% (aged 7–8 years) among children from high income households. There was not a clear gradient across income household groups.

Higher percentage of children with odontogenic abscess was in those who had last made a dental visit for a problem. Among all children who last visited for a problem, there were 3.5 times more children with odontogenic abscess compared to children who last visited for a check-up. This ratio was 5.4-fold in the 5–6-year age group, 2.8-fold in the 7–8-year group, 2.6 times in the 9–10-year age group and 6.5-fold in the 13–14-year age group.

In summary, the prevalence of odontogenic abscess among children in the primary dentition was related to parental education and reason for last dental visit.

Table 5-22: Percentage of children with odontogenic abscesses in the Australian child population

	Population: children aged 5–14 years					
	All ages	5–6	7–8	9–10	11–12	13–14
All	1.8	2.6	3.4	1.9	0.7	0.4
	1.5–2.2	*2.0–3.5*	*2.6–4.3*	*1.4–2.6*	*0.4–1.2*	*0.1–0.9*
Sex						
Male	2.0	2.5	4.1	2.4	0.9	0.0
	1.6–2.5	*1.6–3.8*	*3.1–5.5*	*1.6–3.6*	*0.5–1.7*	*0.0–0.1*
Female	1.6	2.8	2.5	1.5	0.5	0.7
	1.2–2.0	*1.9–4.1*	*1.7–3.7*	*1.0–2.2*	*0.2–1.0*	*0.3–1.6*
Indigenous identity						
Non-Indigenous	1.8	2.5	3.3	1.9	0.7	0.4
	1.4–2.1	*1.8–3.4*	*2.5–4.2*	*1.4–2.6*	*0.4–1.2*	*0.2–0.9*
Indigenous	2.1	2.9	5.6	1.3	0.1	0.1
	1.2–3.8	*1.0–8.4*	*2.6–12.0*	*0.4–3.7*	*0.0–0.9*	*0.0–0.5*
Parents' country of birth						
Australian born	1.6	2.0	3.3	2.0	0.6	0.2
	1.3–2.0	*1.4–3.0*	*2.5–4.5*	*1.3–2.9*	*0.3–1.2*	*0.0–1.0*
Overseas born	2.0	3.3	3.5	1.9	0.8	0.7
	1.6–2.7	*2.1–5.3*	*2.4–5.1*	*1.2–2.9*	*0.4–1.6*	*0.2–1.9*
Parental education						
School	2.5	4.2	6.0	1.7	1.0	0.1
	1.9–3.5	*2.7–6.5*	*4.2–8.5*	*0.8–3.3*	*0.4–2.5*	*0.0–1.0*
Vocational training	1.3	2.4	1.7	2.2	0.3	0.0
	0.9–1.8	*1.3–4.4*	*1.0–3.1*	*1.3–3.8*	*0.1–1.4*	—
Tertiary education	1.5	1.5	2.7	2.0	0.7	0.7
	1.2–1.9	*0.9–2.5*	*1.8–3.9*	*1.3–3.0*	*0.3–1.3*	*0.3–1.8*
Household income						
Low	2.3	3.9	4.8	1.7	0.5	0.6
	1.7–3.1	*2.5–6.2*	*3.3–6.9*	*1.1–2.8*	*0.2–1.2*	*0.2–2.2*
Medium	1.5	1.4	2.5	2.4	0.9	0.0
	1.1–1.9	*0.9–2.3*	*1.6–3.9*	*1.5–3.7*	*0.4–2.0*	*0.0–0.1*
High	1.5	2.2	2.7	1.5	0.6	0.6
	1.1–2.1	*1.2–3.9*	*1.6–4.6*	*0.7–3.4*	*0.2–1.4*	*0.1–2.4*
Residential location						
Major city	1.8	2.6	3.0	1.9	0.7	0.5
	1.4–2.3	*1.8–3.8*	*2.2–4.3*	*1.3–2.8*	*0.4–1.3*	*0.2–1.3*
Inner regional	2.2	3.0	4.7	2.3	1.0	0.0
	1.6–3.0	*1.7–5.3*	*3.0–7.2*	*1.4–3.6*	*0.4–2.4*	—
Outer regional	1.4	2.0	3.4	1.6	0.1	0.1
	0.8–2.2	*1.0–3.9*	*1.5–7.6*	*1.0–2.6*	*0.0–0.5*	*0.0–0.4*
Remote/Very remote	1.3	2.5	2.4	1.4	0.0	0.1
	0.4–3.9	*0.7–8.1*	*0.9–5.9*	*0.3–6.6*	—	*0.0–0.9*
Reason for last dental visit						
Check-up	1.1	1.5	2.3	1.4	0.7	0.2
	0.9–1.5	*0.9–2.4*	*1.5–3.4*	*0.9–2.3*	*0.3–1.3*	*0.0–0.8*
Dental problem	3.9	8.1	6.4	3.6	0.7	1.3
	3.1–5.0	*5.3–12.2*	*4.6–8.9*	*2.4–5.6*	*0.2–2.0*	*0.4–4.3*

Row 1: Proportions were computed using weighted data.
Row 2: 95% CI: Confidence intervals for estimates were computed using weighted data.
Columns are arranged by age at time of Survey.

Prevalence of enamel hypoplasia

Enamel hypoplasia is the most common abnormality of development and mineralisation of human teeth. Enamel hypoplasia in this Survey was recorded when there was hypoplasia that produced detectable loss of enamel. The assessment was based on visual criteria. Enamel hypoplasia was recorded if observed on primary, permanent dentitions or both dentitions. Children whose examination revealed any hypoplasia on dentition was classified as having hypoplasia.

Table 5-23 describes percentages of enamel hypoplasia. Overall, the proportion of children with any enamel hypoplasia was 10.3%. The lowest percentage across age groups was seen in children aged 5–6 years (8.4%). No significant variation was identified across the other age groups.

More Indigenous children had enamel hypoplasia than non-Indigenous children among all children (13.3% versus 10.1%).

No clear gradient was seen across parental education levels and household income levels. Overall, a lower proportion of children living in Major cities (9.6%) had enamel hypoplasia compared to children from Outer regional areas (12.2%) and from Remote/Very remote areas (15.3%). This pattern was seen when children from Major cities (10.5%) were compared to those living in Remote/Very remote areas (25.2%) in the 7–8-year age group and when children from Major cities (10.2%) were compared to those living in Outer regional (14.8%) and in Remote/Very remote areas (18.5%) in the 9–10-year age group.

The highest percentage of children with enamel hypoplasia was among those who had made their last dental visit for a problem. Among all children who last visited for a problem, there were 1.2 times more children with enamel hypoplasia compared to children who last visited for a check-up. This ratio was 1.3 in the 5–6-year age group, 1.3 times in the 9–10-year age group, 1.4 in the 11–12-year age group and 1.2 in the 13–14-year age group.

In summary, the prevalence of enamel hypoplasia among children was related to Indigenous status, residential location and reason for last dental visit.

Table 5-23: Percentage of children with any enamel hypoplasia in the Australian child population

	Population: children aged 5–14 years					
	All ages	5–6	7–8	9–10	11–12	13–14
All	10.3	8.4	11.2	11.4	10.5	10.0
	9.6–11.0	*7.3–9.6*	*9.8–12.7*	*10.1–12.9*	*9.3–11.8*	*8.6–11.7*
Sex						
Male	10.1	8.1	10.9	11.3	9.9	10.3
	9.2–11.0	*6.6–9.8*	*9.1–13.1*	*9.6–13.2*	*8.3–11.7*	*8.3–12.7*
Female	10.5	8.7	11.5	11.5	11.2	9.7
	9.6–11.5	*7.1–10.5*	*9.8–13.3*	*9.7–13.7*	*9.6–13.1*	*7.8–12.0*
Indigenous identity						
Non-Indigenous	10.1	8.3	10.9	11.3	10.5	9.8
	9.5–10.9	*7.2–9.6*	*9.5–12.5*	*9.9–12.8*	*9.2–11.8*	*8.3–11.5*
Indigenous	13.3	10.6	16.8	12.7	11.3	15.5
	10.9–16.0	*6.7–16.4*	*11.6–23.9*	*8.0–19.6*	*7.2–17.3*	*9.2–25.1*
Parents' country of birth						
Australian born	10.6	8.5	11.5	12.1	10.6	10.4
	9.7–11.5	*7.1–10.0*	*9.8–13.4*	*10.3–14.0*	*9.2–12.2*	*8.6–12.5*
Overseas born	9.9	8.3	10.8	10.4	10.3	9.5
	8.9–10.9	*6.7–10.3*	*8.8–13.2*	*8.5–12.5*	*8.4–12.6*	*7.4–12.1*
Parental education						
School	9.2	6.5	9.1	11.5	8.6	10.7
	8.1–10.5	*4.6–9.0*	*6.9–11.9*	*9.1–14.5*	*6.6–11.1*	*8.0–14.2*
Vocational training	10.7	8.3	11.0	11.7	12.7	9.9
	9.4–12.1	*6.2–11.1*	*8.5–14.2*	*9.2–14.8*	*10.1–16.0*	*7.3–13.3*
Tertiary education	10.5	9.5	11.7	10.7	10.8	9.7
	9.6–11.5	*8.1–11.2*	*9.8–14.1*	*9.1–12.5*	*9.1–12.7*	*7.7–12.0*
Household income						
Low	9.7	7.3	9.4	13.4	8.7	9.9
	8.6–10.9	*5.7–9.4*	*7.5–11.6*	*10.9–16.4*	*6.9–10.9*	*7.3–13.2*
Medium	10.3	8.8	10.5	10.2	11.0	11.1
	9.4–11.3	*7.0–10.9*	*8.8–12.5*	*8.5–12.2*	*9.0–13.3*	*8.9–13.7*
High	10.7	9.4	12.6	10.7	12.3	8.3
	9.5–11.9	*7.3–12.0*	*9.6–16.4*	*8.4–13.5*	*9.7–15.4*	*6.4–10.8*
Residential location						
Major city	9.6	8.0	10.5	10.2	9.9	9.6
	8.8–10.5	*6.7–9.6*	*8.7–12.5*	*8.7–12.0*	*8.4–11.6*	*7.8–11.8*
Inner regional	10.9	9.7	10.8	12.8	11.2	10.0
	9.5–12.4	*7.6–12.3*	*8.6–13.4*	*10.0–16.2*	*9.0–13.8*	*7.3–13.5*
Outer regional	12.2	7.3	12.9	14.8	13.5	12.4
	10.4–14.3	*5.4–9.9*	*10.1–16.2*	*11.2–19.4*	*10.0–17.9*	*8.9–17.1*
Remote/Very remote	15.3	10.8	25.2	18.5	10.7	9.9
	10.5–21.7	*3.0–31.9*	*15.9–37.3*	*10.5–30.7*	*5.7–19.1*	*4.0–22.8*
Reason for last dental visit						
Check-up	10.2	8.7	11.4	10.6	10.2	9.9
	9.4–11.0	*7.4–10.3*	*9.7–13.3*	*9.2–12.2*	*8.8–11.8*	*8.3–11.7*
Dental problem	12.4	11.7	11.0	13.6	14.0	11.5
	11.0–14.0	*8.6–15.7*	*8.6–13.9*	*10.6–17.3*	*10.7–18.2*	*8.4–15.5*

Row 1: Proportions were computed using weighted data.
Row 2: 95% CI: Confidence intervals for estimates were computed using weighted data.
Columns are arranged by age at time of Survey.

Prevalence of non-fluorotic enamel opacity

Non-fluorotic enamel opacities were considered when a non-fluorotic discoloration (enamel hypoplasia or other opacities of non-fluorotic origin) was observed on the buccal surfaces of the upper permanent incisors. Table 5-24 describes the proportion of children who had non-fluorotic enamel opacities. Overall, the proportion of non-fluorotic enamel opacities was 8.8%.

Percentages of non-fluorotic enamel opacities varied from 7.6% (5–6-year age group) to 10.2% (13–14-year age group).

Non-significant variation in the percentage of non-fluorotic enamel opacities was seen across parental education and household income levels. Overall, a higher proportion of children living in Major cities (9.5%) had non-fluorotic enamel opacities compared to children from Inner regional (8.1%), Outer regional (6.1%) and from Remote/Very remote areas (5.7%). There was a 7.8-fold difference in the percentage of children with non-fluorotic enamel opacities between children living in Major cities and those living in Remote and Very remote areas in the 5–6-year age group. The same pattern was seen in 7–8, 9–10, 11–12 and 13–14-year age groups with relative ratios of 1.3, 1.4, 1.7 and 2.1, respectively.

Among children aged 5–6 years who last visited for a problem, there were two times more children with non-fluorotic enamel opacities compared to children who last visited for a check-up. This ratio was 1.2-fold in the 7–8-year and 13–14-year age groups. However, the difference was not statistically significant.

In summary, the prevalence of non-fluorotic enamel opacities among children aged 5–14 years was related to residential location.

Table 5-24: Percentage of children with any non-fluorotic enamel opacities in the Australian child population

	Population: children aged 5–14 years					
	All ages	5–6	7–8	9–10	11–12	13–14
All	8.8	7.6	7.8	8.7	8.5	10.2
	8.0–9.6	*5.3–11.0*	*6.5–9.3*	*7.6–10.0*	*7.4–9.7*	*8.6–12.2*
Sex						
Male	8.4	8.5	7.2	8.5	8.3	9.6
	7.5–9.5	*4.9–14.4*	*5.5–9.4*	*7.1–10.2*	*6.9–10.0*	*7.3–12.5*
Female	9.2	7.0	8.4	9.0	8.7	10.9
	8.2–10.2	*4.5–10.7*	*6.8–10.3*	*7.5–10.8*	*7.2–10.4*	*8.7–13.5*
Indigenous identity						
Non-Indigenous	8.9	7.9	7.9	8.8	8.7	10.3
	8.2–9.8	*5.4–11.4*	*6.6–9.6*	*7.6–10.1*	*7.6–9.9*	*8.6–12.3*
Indigenous	6.8	5.3	5.3	7.6	5.1	10.3
	4.7–9.5	*1.1–21.8*	*2.2–12.1*	*4.2–13.3*	*2.9–9.0*	*5.3–18.9*
Parents' country of birth						
Australian born	9.0	8.8	8.2	8.8	8.6	10.6
	8.2–10.0	*5.6–13.5*	*6.6–10.2*	*7.5–10.3*	*7.3–10.1*	*8.7–13.0*
Overseas born	8.4	6.1	7.2	8.9	8.2	9.7
	7.4–9.6	*3.7–10.0*	*5.5–9.4*	*7.2–11.0*	*6.5–10.2*	*7.3–12.8*
Parental education						
School	7.9	6.0	6.5	8.5	7.1	9.5
	6.8–9.2	*2.8–12.3*	*4.5–9.3*	*6.5–11.2*	*5.3–9.5*	*7.0–12.8*
Vocational training	10.0	6.9	9.4	7.9	9.1	13.7
	8.6–11.6	*3.3–13.8*	*6.7–13.0*	*5.9–10.5*	*7.0–11.9*	*10.4–17.8*
Tertiary education	9.1	9.2	8.3	9.6	8.9	9.3
	8.1–10.1	*5.4–15.2*	*6.6–10.3*	*8.2–11.3*	*7.4–10.6*	*7.4–11.8*
Household income						
Low	8.8	11.4	6.4	9.5	8.0	10.5
	7.6–10.1	*5.7–21.7*	*4.7–8.7*	*7.6–11.8*	*6.5–9.9*	*7.8–13.9*
Medium	8.7	7.2	8.0	8.2	8.8	9.7
	7.6–9.8	*4.3–11.8*	*6.3–10.2*	*6.6–10.1*	*7.2–10.8*	*7.4–12.8*
High	9.3	4.6	9.8	9.5	8.4	10.4
	8.0–10.8	*2.2–9.3*	*7.0–13.5*	*7.4–12.1*	*6.5–10.7*	*7.5–14.3*
Residential location						
Major city	9.5	9.3	8.1	9.4	9.1	11.6
	8.5–10.6	*6.0–14.0*	*6.4–10.2*	*7.9–11.0*	*7.7–10.7*	*9.4–14.3*
Inner regional	8.1	4.7	7.8	7.9	8.0	8.9
	6.8–9.5	*1.7–12.4*	*5.7–10.6*	*5.8–10.7*	*6.0–10.5*	*6.3–12.5*
Outer regional	6.1	4.7	6.1	6.8	6.3	5.4
	4.8–7.7	*1.8–11.9*	*3.8–9.6*	*4.5–10.0*	*4.4–8.9*	*3.6–8.0*
Remote/Very remote	5.7	1.2	6.4	6.6	5.4	5.4
	2.3–13.5	*0.2–8.3*	*1.9–19.3*	*1.8–20.8*	*1.4–18.7*	*1.3–19.7*
Reason for last dental visit						
Check-up	9.1	7.9	8.2	9.0	8.6	10.3
	8.2–10.0	*5.3–11.7*	*6.5–10.3*	*7.8–10.5*	*7.3–10.0*	*8.5–12.3*
Dental problem	9.8	15.8	9.5	9.7	7.9	12.0
	8.4–11.5	*7.3–30.8*	*6.8–13.2*	*7.5–12.5*	*5.8–10.8*	*8.3–17.1*

Row 1: Proportions were computed using weighted data.
Row 2: 95% CI: Confidence intervals for estimates were computed using weighted data.
Columns are arranged by age at time of Survey.

Prevalence of dental fluorosis (TF score of 1+ and TF score of 3+)

In this study, dental fluorosis was measured among children aged 8–14 years with the Thylstrup & Fejerskov Index (TF) (Fejerskov et al. 1988). Buccal surfaces of two permanent maxillary central incisors were assessed for presence and severity of dental fluorosis. The TF Index is a 'dry' index, i.e. teeth are assessed when they are dry. In this study, buccal surfaces of the two maxillary central incisors were dried with compressed air for 30 seconds and then assessed for presence of enamel opacities. The Russell differential diagnostic criteria (Russell 1961) were used to differentiate fluorotic from non-fluorotic opacities. Confirmed dental fluorosis was then assessed for severity using the TF Index.

This section reports the prevalence of any dental fluorosis, TF score of 1 or higher (TF1+) and the prevalence of more definite dental fluorosis representing those children with a TF score of 3 or higher (TF3+).

Table 5-25 shows the percentage of children who presented TF1+ and TF3+ scores. Overall, 16.8% and 0.9% of children had scores TF1+ and TF3+, respectively.

Indigenous children had lower TF1+ and TF3+ scores than non-Indigenous children; however, the difference was not statistically significant. No significant variation was seen across parental education and household income.

Children living in outer regional areas had lower TF1+ scores than children living in Major cities.

In summary, the prevalence of TF1+ among children aged 8–14 years was related to residential location.

Table 5-25: Percentage of children with dental fluorosis in the Australian child population

	Population: children aged 8–14 years	
	TF 1+	TF 3+
All	16.8	0.9
	15.5–18.1	*0.7–1.1*
Sex		
Male	16.7	0.7
	15.3–18.3	*0.5–0.9*
Female	16.8	1.1
	15.3–18.4	*0.8–1.5*
Indigenous identity		
Non-Indigenous	17.0	0.9
	15.7–18.3	*0.7–1.1*
Indigenous	13.6	0.3
	10.2–18.0	*0.1–0.6*
Parents' country of birth		
Australian born	17.0	0.8
	15.6–18.5	*0.6–1.1*
Overseas born	16.3	1.0
	14.6–18.1	*0.7–1.3*
Parental education		
School	17.1	0.9
	15.0–19.6	*0.6–1.4*
Vocational training	16.0	1.1
	14.0–18.2	*0.7–1.7*
Tertiary education	16.8	0.8
	15.3–18.5	*0.6–1.0*
Household income		
Low	16.5	0.9
	14.6–18.5	*0.6–1.5*
Medium	15.8	1.1
	14.0–17.8	*0.8–1.5*
High	17.9	0.6
	15.9–20.1	*0.4–0.9*
Residential location		
Major city	17.6	0.9
	15.9–19.4	*0.7–1.2*
Inner regional	15.5	0.9
	13.2–18.0	*0.6–1.3*
Outer regional	12.5	0.9
	10.5–14.8	*0.5–1.4*
Remote/Very remote	23.3	1.3
	13.6–36.9	*0.6–2.5*
Reason for last dental visit		
Check-up	16.4	1.0
	15.1–17.8	*0.8–1.2*
Dental problem	16.3	0.6
	14.2–18.7	*0.4–1.0*

Row 1: Proportions were computed using weighted data.
Row 2: 95% CI: Confidence intervals for estimates were computed using weighted data.
Columns are arranged by age at time of Survey.

Prevalence of children with severe/handicapping malocclusions

To estimate malocclusion in children aged 12–14 years, the Dental Aesthetic Index (Cons et al. 1986) was used. This index takes into account ten specific occlusal traits including missing visible teeth in the anterior segment. The DAI index provides a guide for treatment indications, which vary from no, or slight need for, mandatory treatment. Children with a DAI score equal between 31 and 35 are considered as having severe malocclusion and those with a score of 36 or over are considered as having severe or handicapping malocclusion. Table 5-26 shows the percentage of children who present severe and handicapping malocclusion. Variations between subgroups were observed. However, most variations, except for the difference between the low and high income groups in the prevalence of severe malocclusion, have overlapping confidence intervals.

A similar percentage was seen for severe (14.2%) and handicapping malocclusion (14.0%), with males having 1.2 times more of both conditions than females. Handicapping malocclusion was 1.5 times higher in Indigenous children than non-Indigenous children.

A higher proportion of children whose parents had school-level education had severe (14.9%) and handicapping (14.8%) malocclusion compared to children of parents who had tertiary education (12.9% and 12.6%, respectively). There was a 1.2-fold difference in the percentage of children with severe and handicapping malocclusion between children whose parents' highest education level was vocational training and children of tertiary-educated parents.

There was a gradient in the percentage of children with severe and handicapping malocclusion across household income groups with 16.2% of children from low income households having severe malocclusion compared to 13.3% of those from medium income households and 10.7% of those from high income households. The gradient for handicapping malocclusion across income household levels was 16.0%, 13.9% and 12.2% from low, medium and high income groups, respectively.

The highest percentage of children with severe and handicapping malocclusion was in those who had last made a dental visit for a problem. Among all children who last visited for a problem, there were 1.1 and 1.7 times more children with severe and handicapping malocclusion, respectively, compared to children who last visited for a check-up.

In summary, the prevalence of severe malocclusion in children aged 12–14 years was related to household income. There were variations by parental education and reason for last dental visit. Handicapping malocclusion follows the same pattern. However, the observed variations were not statistically significant.

Oral health of Australian children

Table 5-26: Percentage of children with severe malocclusion or handicapping malocclusion in the Australian child population

| | Population: children aged 12–14 years | |
	Severe malocclusion (DAI: 31–<36)	Handicapping (DAI≥36)
All	14.2	14.0
	12.9–15.7	*12.5–15.7*
Sex		
Male	15.7	15.2
	13.6–18.0	*13.3–17.2*
Female	12.7	12.8
	11.0–14.7	*10.8–15.2*
Indigenous identity		
Non-Indigenous	14.0	13.9
	12.7–15.4	*12.4–15.5*
Indigenous	14.5	20.7
	7.9–25.1	*11.7–33.7*
Parents' country of birth		
Australian born	14.0	14.1
	12.5–15.8	*12.3–16.0*
Overseas born	14.0	14.1
	12.0–16.4	*11.8–16.8*
Parental education		
School	14.9	14.8
	12.4–17.8	*12.0–18.1*
Vocational training	15.1	15.7
	12.2–18.5	*12.2–20.0*
Tertiary education	12.9	12.6
	11.2–14.8	*11.0–14.5*
Household income		
Low	16.2	16.0
	13.6–19.1	*13.5–19.0*
Medium	13.3	13.9
	11.3–15.6	*11.5–16.6*
High	10.7	12.2
	8.8–13.0	*9.9–14.9*
Residential location		
Major city	14.5	14.8
	12.9–16.4	*12.8–17.0*
Inner regional	13.6	12.4
	11.5–16.1	*10.3–14.9*
Outer regional	13.0	11.2
	10.5–16.0	*8.9–13.9*
Remote/Very remote	15.2	15.4
	7.2–29.2	*7.2–29.9*
Reason for last dental visit		
Check-up	11.9	12.6
	10.4–13.5	*11.0–14.4*
Dental problem	13.4	21.7
	10.1–17.6	*17.8–26.3*

Row 1: Proportions were computed using weighted data.
Row 2: 95% CI: Confidence intervals for estimates were computed using weighted data.

5.7 Caries experience by state/territory

Australian states and territories have different sociodemographic and socioeconomic profiles. More importantly, states and territories have different population preventive programs and policies in dental service provision. For example, Queensland (Qld) had only under 5% of the state population covered by water fluoridation until 2010–12. New South Wales (NSW) and Victoria (Vic) do not have universal school dental programs. The differences can lead to varying levels of dental caries experience and treatment for dental caries.

Tables 5-27 to 5-32 present prevalence and severity of dental caries and its components across states and territories. Each of these tables presents data for all ages combined and three age groups for Australia and states and territories in alphabetical order. Table 5-33 presents state/territory breakdowns of provision of fissure sealants for children.

Across states and territories, children in the Northern Territory (NT) had the highest average number of untreated decayed primary tooth surfaces (2.6), followed by children in Qld (1.6) (Table 5-27). Children in South Australia (SA), Australian Capital Territory (ACT) and Tasmania (Tas) had their average number of decayed primary tooth surfaces lower than the national average. Average number of filled primary tooth surfaces was highest in Qld (2.3) and lowest in ACT and NSW.

Total dental caries experience in the primary dentition measured at surface and tooth levels was highest in NT children, followed by that in Qld children (Table 5-28). Children in ACT had lowest average total caries experience. For all states and territories, total caries experience in the primary dentition peaked at ages 7–8 years.

The prevalence of untreated dental caries and overall caries experience in the primary dentition was highest among NT children (39.5% and 53.1%, respectively), followed by children in Qld (29.9% and 50.2%) (Table 5-29). The prevalence of untreated dental caries in ACT, SA, WA and Tas was lower than the national average. The prevalence of overall dental caries experience was lowest in ACT.

Table 5-27: Average number of untreated decayed (ds) or filled tooth surfaces (fs) in the primary dentition by state/territory

	Population: children aged 5–10 years			
	All ages	5–6	7–8	9–10
Australia				
ds	1.3	1.5	1.4	1.0
	1.2–1.4	*1.3–1.7*	*1.2–1.6*	*0.9–1.1*
fs	1.5	0.9	1.8	1.8
	1.4–1.6	*0.8–1.1*	*1.6–1.9*	*1.6–2.0*
ACT				
ds	0.8	1.0	0.9	0.6
	0.6–1.1	*0.6–1.3*	*0.6–1.2*	*0.4–0.8*
fs	1.0	0.7	1.2	1.3
	0.9–1.2	*0.5–0.9*	*0.8–1.5*	*1.0–1.5*
NSW				
ds	1.5	1.5	1.7	1.2
	1.2–1.8	*1.1–2.0*	*1.3–2.1*	*0.9–1.5*
fs	1.0	0.6	1.3	1.1
	0.8–1.2	*0.4–0.8*	*1.0–1.6*	*0.9–1.4*
NT				
ds	2.6	3.5	2.3	2.1
	1.2–4.0	*0.8–6.1*	*1.3–3.3*	*0.3–3.9*
fs	1.6	0.7	2.0	2.1
	1.1–2.1	*0.2–1.1*	*1.2–2.9*	*1.2–3.0*
Qld				
ds	1.6	2.0	1.5	1.1
	1.2–1.9	*1.5–2.6*	*1.1–2.0*	*0.8–1.5*
fs	2.3	1.5	2.8	2.7
	2.1–2.6	*1.2–1.9*	*2.4–3.3*	*2.2–3.2*
SA				
ds	0.6	0.4	0.7	0.6
	0.4–0.7	*0.2–0.5*	*0.4–1.0*	*0.2–1.0*
fs	1.6	0.8	1.9	2.1
	1.4–1.8	*0.5–1.1*	*1.5–2.4*	*1.7–2.4*
Tas				
ds	0.9	0.8	1.1	0.7
	0.6–1.1	*0.5–1.1*	*0.6–1.5*	*0.4–1.1*
fs	1.4	0.8	1.4	1.9
	1.1–1.7	*0.5–1.1*	*1.0–1.9*	*1.4–2.4*
Vic				
ds	1.2	1.5	1.2	0.9
	0.9–1.4	*1.0–1.9*	*0.8–1.5*	*0.7–1.1*
fs	1.3	0.9	1.4	1.7
	1.1–1.5	*0.6–1.1*	*1.2–1.6*	*1.4–2.1*
WA				
ds	1.0	1.2	1.1	0.5
	0.7–1.2	*0.8–1.7*	*0.6–1.6*	*0.3–0.7*
fs	1.8	1.1	2.1	2.4
	1.5–2.2	*0.3–1.8*	*1.5–2.7*	*1.8–3.0*

Row 1: Means were computed using weighted data.
Row 2: 95% CI: Confidence intervals for estimates were computed using weighted data.
Columns are arranged by age at time of Survey.

Table 5-28: Average number of dmfs and dmft in the primary dentition by state/territory

| | Population: children aged 5–10 years | | | |
	All ages	5–6	7–8	9–10
Australia				
dmfs	3.1	2.7	3.6	3.2
	2.9–3.4	*2.4–3.0*	*3.3–3.9*	*2.9–3.5*
dmft	1.5	1.3	1.7	1.5
	1.4–1.6	*1.2–1.4*	*1.6–1.8*	*1.4–1.6*
ACT				
dmfs	2.1	1.8	2.3	2.2
	1.7–2.5	*1.4–2.3*	*1.7–2.9*	*1.7–2.7*
dmft	1.0	0.9	1.1	1.1
	0.8–1.2	*0.7–1.1*	*0.8–1.4*	*0.8–1.3*
NSW				
dmfs	2.8	2.4	3.4	2.7
	2.4–3.3	*1.8–2.9*	*2.7–4.1*	*2.1–3.3*
dmft	1.2	1.1	1.4	1.2
	1.1–1.4	*0.8–1.3*	*1.2–1.7*	*1.0–1.5*
NT				
dmfs	4.7	4.5	5.0	4.7
	3.1–6.4	*1.9–7.2*	*3.3–6.6*	*2.5–6.9*
dmft	2.4	2.5	2.3	2.3
	1.7–3.1	*1.2–3.8*	*1.7–3.0*	*1.4–3.1*
Qld				
dmfs	4.3	4.0	4.8	4.2
	3.8–4.8	*3.2–4.8*	*4.1–5.5*	*3.5–4.9*
dmft	2.1	2.0	2.3	2.0
	1.9–2.3	*1.6–2.3*	*2.0–2.6*	*1.7–2.3*
SA				
dmfs	2.5	1.4	3.2	3.1
	2.2–2.9	*1.0–1.8*	*2.5–3.9*	*2.5–3.7*
dmft	1.2	0.7	1.5	1.5
	1.1–1.4	*0.5–0.9*	*1.2–1.8*	*1.2–1.8*
Tas				
dmfs	2.7	1.8	3.4	2.9
	2.3–3.2	*1.3–2.3*	*2.5–4.3*	*2.1–3.7*
dmft	1.4	1.0	1.6	1.5
	1.1–1.6	*0.7–1.3*	*1.2–2.0*	*1.2–1.8*
Vic				
dmfs	2.8	2.6	3.0	2.9
	2.4–3.2	*1.9–3.2*	*2.5–3.4*	*2.5–3.3*
dmft	1.5	1.3	1.6	1.5
	1.3–1.6	*1.0–1.6*	*1.4–1.8*	*1.3–1.7*
WA				
dmfs	3.1	2.5	3.6	3.2
	2.6–3.6	*1.6–3.4*	*2.7–4.4*	*2.5–3.8*
dmft	1.4	1.2	1.6	1.5
	1.2–1.6	*0.8–1.5*	*1.3–2.0*	*1.2–1.7*

Row 1: Means were computed using weighted data.
Row 2: 95% CI: Confidence intervals for estimates were computed using weighted data.
Columns are arranged by age at time of Survey.

Oral health of Australian children

Table 5-29: Prevalence of untreated decay and overall caries experience in the primary dentition by state/territory

	Population: children aged 5–10 years			
	All ages	5–6	7–8	9–10
Australia				
Untreated decay	27.1	26.1	28.4	27.0
	25.6–28.6	*23.9–28.3*	*26.0–30.8*	*24.9–29.1*
Overall caries experience	41.7	34.3	45.1	46.2
	40.1–43.3	*31.9–36.6*	*42.6–47.4*	*43.7–48.6*
ACT				
Untreated decay	21.1	19.2	23.1	21.2
	17.3–25.5	*15.9–23.0*	*18.0–29.2*	*15.3–28.5*
Overall caries experience	31.9	25.3	33.6	37.4
	27.8–36.3	*21.7–29.2*	*28.0–39.8*	*30.9–44.3*
NSW				
Untreated decay	27.6	26.3	29.1	27.5
	24.5–30.9	*22.3–30.8*	*24.4–34.3*	*23.2–32.1*
Overall caries experience	36.7	31.1	40.7	38.5
	33.4–40.1	*26.9–35.7*	*35.7–45.9*	*33.6–43.7*
NT				
Untreated decay	39.5	44.5	39.5	34.5
	29.3–50.7	*29.8–60.2*	*29.1–50.9*	*21.7–50.0*
Overall caries experience	53.1	50.7	52.2	56.5
	43.9–62.1	*36.6–64.8*	*41.2–62.9*	*43.9–68.2*
Qld				
Untreated decay	29.9	30.2	31.2	28.2
	26.8–33.1	*25.5–35.5*	*26.6–36.1*	*25.0–31.6*
Overall caries experience	50.2	42.4	53.6	54.9
	47.2–53.2	*37.3–47.5*	*48.6–58.4*	*50.8–58.9*
SA				
Untreated decay	16.6	15.2	18.0	16.7
	13.7–20.0	*10.7–21.1*	*13.2–24.2*	*12.3–22.2*
Overall caries experience	37.6	25.3	42.5	45.1
	33.8–41.4	*20.5–30.8*	*35.9–49.4*	*38.8–51.5*
Tas				
Untreated decay	22.7	22.0	23.4	22.9
	18.4–27.7	*15.5–30.3*	*16.6–31.9*	*16.9–30.2*
Overall caries experience	39.2	31.2	42.9	43.7
	34.8–43.8	*23.9–39.5*	*35.1–51.1*	*36.7–50.9*
Vic				
Untreated decay	29.3	26.6	29.7	31.8
	26.1–32.7	*21.6–32.2*	*24.7–35.0*	*27.2–36.8*
Overall caries experience	43.2	35.2	45.2	49.5
	39.7–46.7	*29.9–40.9*	*40.4–50.0*	*44.7–54.2*
WA				
Untreated decay	22.4	22.4	25.1	19.7
	19.0–26.1	*18.1–27.3*	*19.8–31.2*	*15.6–24.4*
Overall caries experience	40.3	31.6	44.2	45.5
	37.5–43.2	*26.8–36.8*	*39.4–49.1*	*40.6–50.5*

Row 1: Proportions were computed using weighted data.
Row 2: 95% CI: Confidence intervals for estimates were computed using weighted data.
Columns are arranged by age at time of Survey.

The prevalence and severity of untreated dental caries and overall dental caries experience in the permanent dentition by state/territory are presented in Tables 5-30 to 5-32.

The average number of untreated decayed tooth surfaces in the permanent dentition among children aged 6–14 years was relatively low (Table 5-30). Number of children with untreated dental caries increased sharply with age, especially among NT and Qld children. NT children aged 12–14 years had the highest average number of untreated dental caries (1.0), followed by Qld children of the same age (0.6). Children aged 12–14 years in ACT and SA had average number of untreated dental caries in the permanent dentition, lower than the national average. Average number of filled permanent tooth surfaces (FS) followed a similar age pattern. At age 12–14 years, children in Qld had the highest average number of filled tooth surfaces (1.5), followed by children of the same age group in WA (1.0).

The overall dental caries experience of the permanent dentition measured at surface and tooth levels also increased with age (Table 5-31). At age 12–14 years, children in Qld had the highest overall dental caries experience in the permanent dentition at both surface and tooth levels (2.2 and 1.6, respectively), closely followed by children of the same age in NT. Children aged 12–14 years in ACT and SA had, overall, lower dental caries experience than the national average.

Children in NT had the highest prevalence of untreated decay in the permanent dentition (20.3%) while children in SA had the lowest (3.5%) (Table 5-32). At age 12–14 years, children in NT also were most likely to have untreated decay in the permanent dentition, followed by children in Qld. The prevalence of overall dental caries experience in the permanent dentition was highest in NT children (32.9%), followed by Qld children (30.7%). However, for the 12–14-year age group, children in Qld had the highest prevalence of dental caries in the permanent dentition, followed by children from NT. The prevalence of dental caries in the permanent dentition of children from ACT, SA, Tas and NSW were lower than the national prevalence.

Table 5-30: Average number of untreated decayed (DS) and filled surfaces (FS) in the permanent dentition by state/territory

| | Population: children aged 6–14 years | | | |
	All ages	6–8	9–11	12–14
Australia				
DS	0.2	0.1	0.2	0.4
	0.2–0.3	*0.1–0.1*	*0.2–0.3*	*0.3–0.5*
FS	0.4	0.1	0.4	0.9
	0.4–0.5	*0.1–0.1*	*0.3–0.4*	*0.8–1.0*
ACT				
DS	0.1	0.1	0.2	0.1
	0.1–0.2	*0.0–0.1*	*0.1–0.2*	*0.0–0.2*
FS	0.2	0.1	0.2	0.2
	0.1–0.2	*0.1–0.1*	*0.1–0.3*	*0.1–0.4*
NSW				
DS	0.2	0.1	0.2	0.4
	0.2–0.3	*0.1–0.1*	*0.2–0.3*	*0.3–0.5*
FS	0.4	0.1	0.3	0.7
	0.3–0.4	*0.0–0.1*	*0.2–0.4*	*0.5–0.8*
NT				
DS	0.6	0.2	0.6	1.0
	0.1–1.1	*0.1–0.3*	*0.2–1.0*	*0.1–2.2*
FS	0.4	0.0	0.4	0.7
	0.2–0.5	*0.0–0.1*	*0.1–0.7*	*0.4–1.0*
Qld				
DS	0.3	0.1	0.3	0.6
	0.2–0.4	*0.1–0.1*	*0.2–0.3*	*0.4–0.8*
FS	0.8	0.1	0.6	1.5
	0.7–0.9	*0.1–0.2*	*0.5–0.7*	*1.3–1.7*
SA				
DS	0.1	0.0	0.0	0.1
	0.0–0.1	*0.0–0.1*	*0.0–0.1*	*0.0–0.1*
FS	0.3	0.1	0.2	0.5
	0.2–0.3	*0.0–0.1*	*0.2–0.3*	*0.4–0.7*
Tas				
DS	0.1	0.1	0.1	0.2
	0.1–0.2	*0.0–0.1*	*0.1–0.2*	*0.1–0.4*
FS	0.3	0.0	0.3	0.6
	0.2–0.4	*0.0–0.1*	*0.2–0.4*	*0.4–0.8*
Vic				
DS	0.2	0.1	0.2	0.3
	0.2–0.3	*0.1–0.1*	*0.1–0.4*	*0.2–0.4*
FS	0.4	0.1	0.2	0.8
	0.3–0.4	*0.1–0.1*	*0.2–0.3*	*0.6–0.9*
WA				
DS	0.2	0.1	0.2	0.4
	0.2–0.3	*0.1–0.2*	*0.2–0.3*	*0.2–0.5*
FS	0.5	0.1	0.3	1.0
	0.4–0.6	*0.0–0.2*	*0.2–0.4*	*0.8–1.1*

Row 1: Means were computed using weighted data.
Row 2: 95% CI: Confidence intervals for estimates were computed using weighted data.
Columns are arranged by age at time of Survey.

Table 5-31: Average number of DMFS and DMFT in the permanent dentition by state/territory

	Population: children aged 6–14 years			
	All ages	6–8	9–11	12–14
Australia				
DMFS	0.7	0.2	0.6	1.3
	0.7–0.7	*0.2–0.2*	*0.6–0.7*	*1.2–1.5*
DMFT	0.5	0.1	0.4	0.9
	0.5–0.5	*0.1–0.2*	*0.4–0.5*	*0.8–1.0*
ACT				
DMFS	0.3	0.2	0.4	0.4
	0.2–0.4	*0.1–0.2*	*0.2–0.5*	*0.2–0.6*
DMFT	0.2	0.1	0.2	0.3
	0.2–0.3	*0.1–0.1*	*0.2–0.3*	*0.2–0.5*
NSW				
DMFS	0.6	0.2	0.6	1.1
	0.5–0.7	*0.1–0.3*	*0.5–0.7*	*0.9–1.3*
DMFT	0.4	0.1	0.4	0.7
	0.4–0.5	*0.1–0.2*	*0.3–0.5*	*0.6–0.8*
NT				
DMFS	1.2	0.4	1.1	2.1
	0.5–1.8	*0.1–0.6*	*0.5–1.7*	*0.8–3.4*
DMFT	0.8	0.3	0.7	1.4
	0.4–1.1	*0.1–0.4*	*0.3–1.2*	*0.5–2.2*
Qld				
DMFS	1.1	0.2	0.9	2.2
	1.0–1.3	*0.2–0.3*	*0.8–1.1*	*1.9–2.5*
DMFT	0.8	0.2	0.7	1.6
	0.7–0.9	*0.1–0.2*	*0.6–0.8*	*1.4–1.8*
SA				
DMFS	0.4	0.1	0.3	0.7
	0.3–0.4	*0.1–0.2*	*0.2–0.4*	*0.5–0.8*
DMFT	0.3	0.1	0.2	0.5
	0.2–0.3	*0.0–0.1*	*0.2–0.3*	*0.4–0.6*
Tas				
DMFS	0.5	0.1	0.4	0.9
	0.4–0.6	*0.0–0.2*	*0.3–0.5*	*0.6–1.2*
DMFT	0.4	0.1	0.3	0.7
	0.3–0.5	*0.0–0.1*	*0.2–0.3*	*0.5–0.9*
Vic				
DMFS	0.6	0.2	0.5	1.2
	0.5–0.7	*0.2–0.3*	*0.4–0.6*	*0.9–1.4*
DMFT	0.5	0.2	0.4	0.8
	0.4–0.5	*0.1–0.2*	*0.3–0.5*	*0.7–1.0*
WA				
DMFS	0.7	0.2	0.5	1.3
	0.6–0.8	*0.2–0.3*	*0.4–0.6*	*1.1–1.6*
DMFT	0.5	0.1	0.4	0.9
	0.4–0.6	*0.1–0.2*	*0.3–0.5*	*0.8–1.1*

Row 1: Means were computed using weighted data.
Row 2: 95% CI: Confidence intervals for estimates were computed using weighted data.
Columns are arranged by age at time of Survey.

Oral health of Australian children

Table 5-32: Prevalence of untreated decay and overall caries experience in the permanent dentition by state/territory

	Population: children aged 6–14 years			
	All ages	6–8	9–11	12–14
Australia				
Untreated decay	**10.9**	**5.7**	**11.5**	**15.4**
	10.0–11.8	*4.9–6.5*	*10.1–13.0*	*13.9–17.0*
Overall caries experience	**23.5**	**9.2**	**22.8**	**38.2**
	22.3–24.6	*8.2–10.3*	*21.2–24.5*	*36.3–40.0*
ACT				
Untreated decay	5.5	2.9	6.4	7.1
	3.8–7.8	*1.8–4.7*	*4.2–9.8*	*3.9–12.5*
Overall caries experience	12.9	6.0	14.5	18.3
	10.7–15.5	*4.6–7.9*	*11.5–18.1*	*13.4–24.3*
NSW				
Untreated decay	10.7	5.2	12.1	14.7
	9.0–12.5	*3.8–7.1*	*9.5–15.3*	*11.9–18.1*
Overall caries experience	20.6	7.9	21.8	32.4
	18.5–22.9	*6.1–10.2*	*18.8–25.0*	*29.4–35.5*
NT				
Untreated decay	20.3	10.1	23.9	27.4
	12.2–31.9	*5.4–18.1*	*14.0–37.6*	*13.6–47.4*
Overall caries experience	32.9	13.7	38.6	47.2
	23.2–44.3	*7.9–22.6*	*24.6–54.7*	*30.8–64.2*
Qld				
Untreated decay	12.9	5.0	12.7	20.8
	11.0–15.0	*3.6–6.8*	*10.3–15.6*	*17.1–25.0*
Overall caries experience	30.7	10.6	30.8	50.4
	28.1–33.5	*8.6–12.9*	*27.6–34.3*	*46.5–54.2*
SA				
Untreated decay	3.5	2.8	3.1	4.6
	2.5–5.0	*1.4–5.4*	*1.7–5.6*	*2.8–7.5*
Overall caries experience	15.3	4.8	13.6	26.7
	13.1–17.6	*3.2–7.3*	*10.5–17.5*	*22.2–31.7*
Tas				
Untreated decay	6.8	3.3	7.8	9.0
	5.0–9.1	*1.6–6.4*	*5.2–11.7*	*5.4–14.5*
Overall caries experience	18.7	5.6	17.8	31.6
	15.6–22.3	*3.1–9.7*	*14.3–21.9*	*24.6–39.5*
Vic				
Untreated decay	10.8	6.9	10.8	14.7
	9.0–12.9	*5.3–8.9*	*7.9–14.7*	*11.7–18.2*
Overall caries experience	22.7	11.1	19.5	37.3
	20.3–25.3	*9.2–13.2*	*16.1–23.4*	*33.2–41.5*
WA				
Untreated decay	13.1	7.8	14.2	17.1
	11.0–15.5	*5.4–11.2*	*10.4–19.0*	*13.7–21.0*
Overall caries experience	26.3	10.0	24.3	44.0
	23.3–29.5	*7.4–13.4*	*20.2–28.7*	*38.0–50.2*

Row 1: Proportions were computed using weighted data.
Row 2: 95% CI: Confidence intervals for estimates were computed using weighted data.
Columns are arranged by age at time of Survey.

The percentage of children with fissure sealants and average number of fissure sealants per child varied greatly across states and territories (Table 5-33). The percentage of children having fissure sealants was highest in Tasmania (Tas) (41.9%) and lowest in NSW (16.8%). The percentage of children with fissure sealants in Tas., SA and Victoria (Vic) were higher than the national average, while that in NSW, NT and Qld were lower than the national average. The average number of fissure sealants per child was highest in Tas. and lowest in NSW and Qld.

Table 5-33: Fissure sealant used by state/territory

	Population: children aged 6–14 years			
	Per cent of children with at least one fissure sealed tooth		Average number of fissure sealed tooth surfaces per child	
Australia	Per cent	26.8	mean	1.0
	95% CI	25.5–28.2	95% CI	0.9–1.1
ACT	Per cent	31.9	mean	1.4
	95% CI	28.1–36.1	95% CI	1.2–1.6
NSW	Per cent	16.8	mean	0.6
	95% CI	14.5–19.4	95% CI	0.5–0.7
NT	Per cent	19.9	mean	0.7
	95% CI	16.2–24.2	95% CI	0.5–0.8
Qld	Per cent	22.5	mean	0.6
	95% CI	20.5–24.5	95% CI	0.6–0.7
SA	Per cent	36.8	mean	1.4
	95% CI	33.8–39.8	95% CI	1.2–1.5
Tas	Per cent	41.9	mean	1.8
	95% CI	36.7–46.7	95% CI	1.5–2.1
Vic	Per cent	39.9	mean	1.7
	95% CI	36.7–43.3	95% CI	1.5–1.8
WA	Per cent	26.3	mean	0.8
	95% CI	23.8–28.8	95% CI	0.7–0.9

Row 1: Proportions or means were computed using weighted data.
Row 2: 95% CI: Confidence intervals for estimates were computed using weighted data.

Oral health of Australian children

5.8 Clustering of dental caries in the Australian child population

Distribution of dental caries in a child population is highly skewed (Spencer 1997). It has been suggested that the majority of the population burden of dental caries is disproportionately experienced by a minority of children. Those children are often from a low socioeconomic background. This chapter reports significantly higher prevalence and severity of untreated decay and total caries experience among children identified as Indigenous, from families where parents had school-level education, low household income and living in remote or very remote areas, and those whose last dental visit was for a dental problem.

Lorenz curve (Lorenz 1905) is a graph on which the cumulative percentage of total distribution of a condition is plotted against the cumulative percentage of the corresponding population. The extent to which the curve sags below a straight diagonal line indicates the degree of inequality of distribution of the condition of interest in the population.

Lorenz curves of the distribution of untreated dental caries (ds and DS) and overall caries experience (dmfs and DMFS) were generated for children aged 5–10 and 11–14 years, respectively (Figure 5-1 and Figure 5-2). Data for the age group 11–14 years was used for the permanent dentition to reduce age effect in examining the clustering of dental caries experience.

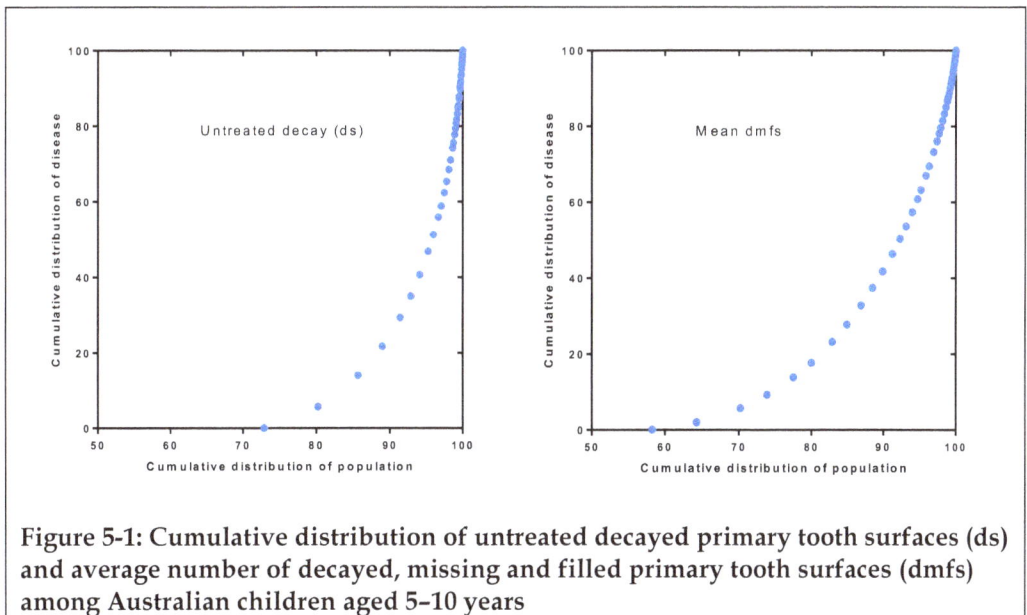

Figure 5-1: Cumulative distribution of untreated decayed primary tooth surfaces (ds) and average number of decayed, missing and filled primary tooth surfaces (dmfs) among Australian children aged 5–10 years

While 27% of children aged 5–10 years had untreated decay in the primary dentition, almost 80% of its total population burden was observed among 11% of the population (Figure 5-1). Likewise, 20% of the child population aged 5–10 years had over 80% of the total population burden of overall dental caries experience in the primary dentition.

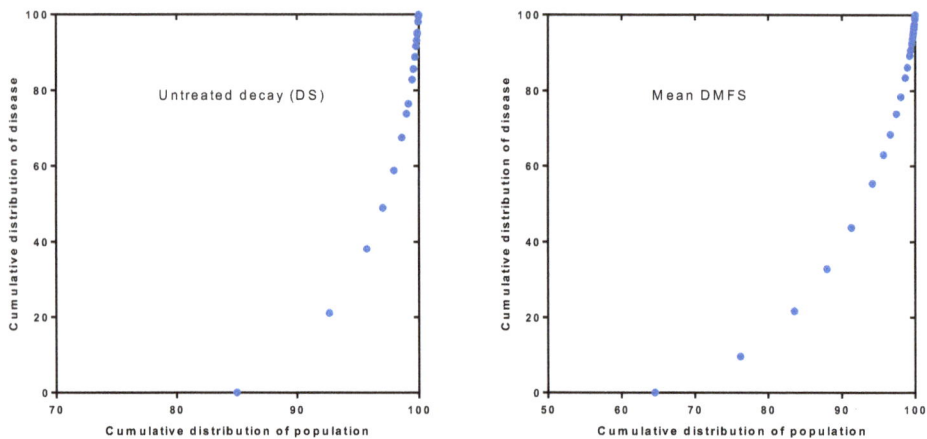

Figure 5-2: Cumulative distribution of untreated decayed permanent tooth surfaces (DS) and average number of decayed, missing and filled permanent tooth surfaces (DMFS) among Australian children aged 11–14 years

The distribution of dental caries in the permanent dentition was also highly skewed (Figure 5-2). Just over 7% of children aged 11–14 years carried almost 80% of the population burden of untreated decay in the permanent dentition. Likewise, around 17% of the child population aged 11–14 years had almost 80% of the population burden of overall dental caries experience in the permanent dentition. There is one caveat in interpreting this result; dental caries experience in the permanent dentition is strongly associated with increasing age. While this analysis was confined to children aged 11–14 years, the distribution was still influenced by age of children to some extent. However, the evidence of skewed distribution of dental caries was undeniable.

Summary

Dental caries experience

This chapter has provided a detailed description of the distribution of dental caries in the primary and permanent dentition of the Australian children. Different measures of the prevalence and severity of dental caries and its components were presented for different age groups and population sub-groups.

Untreated dental caries reflects both the population patterns of the disease and lack of the use of dental care. One in four and one in ten Australian children had untreated dental caries in their primary or permanent teeth, respectively. Children from a lower socioeconomic background were significantly more likely to have untreated dental caries. The severity of untreated decay was also higher among those children compared to their counterparts from higher socioeconomic backgrounds. A small group of children carried the majority of population burden of untreated dental caries. Untreated dental caries can have a significant impact on children's well-being.

Missing teeth due to dental caries was relatively low in the Australian child population. However, clear socioeconomic gradients were observed both in the prevalence and average number of missing teeth. Also, children whose last dental visit was for a dental problem had many times higher prevalence and average number of missing teeth due to dental caries.

Filled teeth due to dental caries is another indicator of the pattern of the disease and access to dental services. The socioeconomic gradients in prevalence and average number of filled teeth due to caries were less clear. However, those from lower socioeconomic backgrounds still had higher prevalence and average number of fillings due to dental caries. Those gradients mostly reflected higher patterns of dental caries in these socioeconomic groups.

Four in ten and almost one in four Australian children had experience of dental caries in their primary or permanent dentition, respectively. These figures confirm that dental caries is one of the most prevalent chronic health conditions in children. The prevalence and severity of dental caries in the permanent dentition quickly increased with age of children. Clear socioeconomic gradients were observed in the prevalence and severity of dental caries in Australian children. Those gradients were observed even in the youngest age group. Small groups of children carried the majority of the population burden of dental caries experience.

There were significant variations between Australian states and territories in the prevalence and severity of dental caries. These variations reflect differences in socioeconomic profiles of the population as well as presence or absence of population-based programs for caries prevention and dental service provision. Strong contrast was observed between states/territories by remoteness status, predominantly Major city status of ACT versus predominantly Remote/Very remote status of NT. Strong contrast was also observed between jurisdictions by population coverage of water fluoridation in the case of Qld versus other jurisdictions. States and territories with varying levels of school dental service coverage also differed in certain components of dental caries measurement.

Other oral conditions

Four in ten Australian children were observed with visible dental plaque at the time of the survey. Some one in five children had evidence of gingival inflammation. There were socioeconomic gradients in these indicators of oral hygiene status. Most notably, 60% of Indigenous children had visible dental plaque.

Any dental fluorosis (TF score of 1+) was observed on one in six children aged 8 years and older. However, the prevalence of moderate to severe dental fluorosis (TF score of 3+) was under 1%. There were very few children with a TF score of 4 or 5 even with the sample size of the Survey. Therefore, separate estimates of the prevalence of a TF score of 4 or 5 were not statistically reliable.

References

Casamassimo PS, Thikkurissy S, Edelstein BL & Maiorini E 2009. Beyond the dmft: the human and economic cost of early childhood caries. J Am Dent Assoc 140(6):650–7.

Cons, NC, Jenny J & Kohout F 1986. The Dental Aesthetic Index. Iowa: Iowa University Press.

Fejerskov O 2004. Changing paradigms in concepts on dental caries: consequences for oral health care. Caries Res 38(3):182-91.

Fejerskov O, Manji F & Baelum V 1988. Dental fluorosis: a handbook for health workers. Copenhagen: Munksgaard.

Fisher-Owens SA, Gansky SA, Platt LJ, Weintraub JA, Soobader MJ, Bramlett MD & Newacheck PW 2007. Influences on children's oral health: a conceptual model. Pediatrics 120(3):e510–520.

Harford J & Luzzi L 2013. Child and teenager oral health and dental visiting: results from the National Dental Telephone Interview Survey 2010. Dental statistics and research series 64. Canberra: Australian Institute of Health and Welfare.

Loe H & Silness J 1963. Periodontal disease in pregnancy. I. Prevalence and severity. Acta Odontol Scand 21:533-51.

Lorenz MO 1905. Methods of measuring the concentration of wealth. Publications of the American Statistical Association 9(70):209–19.

Mejia G, Amarasena N, Ha D, Roberts-Thomson K & Ellershaw A 2012. Child Dental Health Survey Australia 2007: 30-year trends in child oral health. Dental statistics and research series no. 60. Cat. no. DEN 217, Canberra: Australian Institute of Health and Welfare.

Mouradian WE, Wehr E & Crall JJ 2000. Disparities in children's oral health and access to dental care. J Am Dent Assoc 284:2625–31.

Russell AL 1961. The differential diagnosis of fluoride and nonfluoride enamel opacities. J Public Health Dent 21:143–6.

Spencer AJ 1997. Skewed distributions–new outcome measures. Community Dent Oral Epidemiol 25(1):52–9.

Silness J & Loe H 1964. Periodontal disease in pregnancy. II. Correlation between oral hygiene and periodontal condition. Acta Odontol Scand 22:121-35.

6 Patterns of dental services use by Australian children

DS Brennan, X Ju, N Amarasena, M Dooland, KG Peres, GC Mejia and AJ Spencer

Patterns of dental service use can be described using a range of approaches including measures related to first dental visit, usual dental visit pattern, and the most recent dental visit. First dental visit is considered important as it represents first contact with the dental system. The usual dental visit pattern of children is also of interest as it can reflect long-term attendance patterns. The most recent dental visit is considered important as it reflects current health behaviour.

In this chapter, measures related to first dental visit will be presented for: first making a dental visit before the age of 5 years, having a check-up as the reason for the first dental visit, and reporting having never made a dental visit. Information will also be presented related to usual dental visiting using the measure of irregular usual visit pattern. For the most recent dental visit: making a dental visit within the last 12 months, having a check-up as the reason for last dental visit, attending a private dental clinic at the last dental visit, whether parents or guardians attended with the child at their last dental visit, and rating of the last dental visit by the parent/guardian.

Frequency of dental visits and the reason for dental visits are key aspects related to access to dental care (Roberts-Thomson et al. 1995). Making a recent dental visit is indicative of access to the dental care system while visiting for the reason of a check-up is considered more likely to be associated with better health outcomes than visiting for a dental problem such as relief of pain (Crocombe et al. 2012). Hence, the dental profession tends to advocate a visit pattern of attending for annual dental check-ups to access preventive dental care or allow diagnosis of dental problems at an early stage, which can facilitate treatment before the disease progresses (Riley et al. 2013). For children, there are recommendations in relation to the desirability of making dental visits at an early age (Jones & Tomar 2005). While children who have not made a dental visit or report an irregular dental visit pattern could reflect a lack of perceived need, these measures could also reflect barriers to dental care that inhibit dental visiting or reflect problem-based attendance patterns.

Place of dental visiting and providers of dental care can also be important in establishing dental visit patterns and facilitating continuity of care. In Australia, the dental care system is predominantly based in private practice on a fee-for-service basis. However, school dental services provide dental care for children albeit with varying coverage between primary and secondary schools and across states and territories.

There are a range of outcomes to consider in evaluating dental health services. While clinical measures are of significance, it is also desirable to consider patient-based outcomes that measure the perceptions of those experiencing the health care, such as satisfaction with care and quality of life (Leplege & Hunt 1997; Tsakos et al. 2013).

Hence, it is important to consider the ratings of the dental care provided from the perspective of the child or the parent/guardian reporting on behalf of their child.

6.1 First dental visit

In this section, measures will be presented relating to first making a dental visit before the age of 5 years, having a check-up as the reason for the first dental visit, and reporting having never made a dental visit.

Table 6-1 presents the percentage of children who first visited a dental provider before the age of 5 years in the Australian child population. While the highest percentage was among children from households with a high income (69.4%) the lowest percentage was among Indigenous children (45.1%). Overall, 57.3% of children had made their first dental visit before the age of 5 years, but this did not vary across the age groups. The percentage of Australian children who first visited a dental provider before the age of 5 years was not related to sex.

Across all age groups, a lower percentage of Indigenous children had made their first dental visit before the age of 5 years than non-Indigenous children. The relative difference between Indigenous and non-Indigenous children was highest for children in the 11–12-year age group (1.4). There was no association between the percentage of children who first visited a dental provider before the age of 5 years and parents' country of birth.

A higher percentage of children whose parents had vocational training made their first dental visit before the age of 5 years (56.3%) compared to children of parents who had school-only education (45.4%). There was a 1.4-fold relative difference in the percentage of children with a first visit to a dental provider before the age of 5 years between children of tertiary-educated parents and children whose parents' highest education was at school. This pattern was consistent across all the age groups.

There was a gradient in the percentage of children who made their first dental visit before the age of 5 years across household income groups with 46.3% of children from low income households first making a dental visit before the age of 5 years compared to 58.2% of children from medium income households, a 1.3-fold relative difference. The relative differences between children from low and high income households as well as medium and high income households were 1.5 and 1.2, respectively. In each specific two-year age group, there were fewer children who made their first contact with a dental provider before the age of 5 years in low income households relative to the medium and high income households.

A higher percentage of children who last visited for a check-up had made their first dental visit before the age of 5 years (66.3%) compared to children who last visited for a problem (59.1%). This pattern was seen across all the age groups with children in 11–12-year age group having the highest relative difference (1.2).

In summary, the percentage of Australian children who first visited a dental provider before the age of 5 years was related to Indigenous identity, parental education, household income and reason for last dental visit.

Oral health of Australian children

Table 6-1: Percentage of children who first visited a dental provider before the age of 5 years in the Australian child population

	Population: children aged 5-14 years					
	All ages	5—6	7—8	9—10	11—12	13—14
All	57.3	55.8	57.5	58.3	57.3	57.4
	55.8–58.7	*53.2–58.3*	*55.1–59.9*	*55.6–60.9*	*55.0–59.5*	*54.7–60.1*
Sex						
Male	56.7	55.4	56.2	57.7	55.9	58.2
	54.9–58.4	*52.0–58.7*	*52.9–59.4*	*54.6–60.8*	*52.9–58.9*	*54.8–61.6*
Female	57.9	56.3	59.1	58.9	58.7	56.6
	56.1–59.7	*53.3–59.2*	*55.9–62.1*	*55.5–62.1*	*55.6–61.8*	*52.8–60.4*
Indigenous identity						
Non-Indigenous	57.9	56.4	58.3	59.0	58.3	57.7
	56.4–59.4	*53.8–58.9*	*55.8–60.7*	*56.3–61.6*	*55.9–60.6*	*54.9–60.5*
Indigenous	45.1	46.0	45.9	49.4	40.5	43.8
	40.2–50.0	*36.4–55.9*	*38.2–53.8*	*39.6–59.3*	*32.0–49.6*	*32.4–55.8*
Parents' country of birth						
Australian born	58.8	56.0	58.9	61.3	60.5	57.7
	57.2–60.5	*53.0–58.8*	*56.2–61.6*	*58.4–64.1*	*57.9–63.1*	*54.4–60.9*
Overseas born	54.2	55.3	54.7	53.3	51.5	56.1
	51.8–56.5	*51.0–59.5*	*50.5–58.8*	*49.2–57.3*	*47.7–55.2*	*52.1–60.1*
Parental education						
School	45.4	42.9	43.8	46.3	46.3	47.4
	43.1–47.7	*38.5–47.4*	*39.1–48.6*	*41.7–51.0*	*42.1–50.5*	*42.4–52.4*
Vocational training	56.3	52.6	55.3	58.2	60.1	55.3
	54.0–58.6	*47.8–57.5*	*50.3–60.1*	*53.7–62.5*	*55.7–64.4*	*50.4–60.2*
Tertiary education	65.3	65.1	65.8	65.8	63.8	65.7
	63.6–66.9	*62.1–68.1*	*63.0–68.5*	*62.6–68.9*	*61.0–66.6*	*62.4–68.9*
Household income						
Low	46.3	45.4	46.1	46.0	47.3	46.4
	44.1–48.4	*41.1–49.7*	*42.2–50.1*	*41.8–50.4*	*43.3–51.3*	*42.1–50.8*
Medium	58.2	58.9	57.6	59.3	57.8	57.4
	56.6–59.8	*55.9–61.9*	*54.4–60.8*	*56.0–62.5*	*54.5–61.0*	*53.7–61.0*
High	69.4	64.8	69.7	72.0	70.6	70.4
	67.2–71.5	*60.2–69.1*	*65.7–73.4*	*67.4–76.2*	*66.9–74.1*	*65.4–74.9*
Residential location						
Major city	57.0	56.2	57.1	58.0	56.5	57.0
	55.0–58.9	*52.8–59.6*	*53.9–60.3*	*54.5–61.5*	*53.5–59.5*	*53.4–60.6*
Inner regional	58.8	56.0	58.9	57.2	59.8	61.7
	56.3–61.2	*52.0–60.0*	*54.4–63.3*	*52.1–62.2*	*55.7–63.8*	*57.4–65.9*
Outer regional	57.5	53.2	58.6	63.2	58.0	54.8
	54.2–60.7	*47.3–59.0*	*52.6–64.3*	*57.9–68.1*	*53.3–62.6*	*49.2–60.2*
Remote/Very remote	52.1	51.9	54.8	55.0	53.4	45.0
	46.3–57.9	*42.6–61.0*	*43.7–65.5*	*45.9–63.7*	*42.5–64.0*	*31.5–59.3*
Reason for last dental visit						
Check-up	66.3	80.1	68.8	64.2	62.4	60.1
	64.9–67.7	*77.6–82.5*	*66.1–71.3*	*61.6–66.7*	*60.0–64.8*	*57.4–62.7*
Dental problem	59.1	74.3	62.1	57.2	52.3	52.8
	56.7–61.6	*69.0–79.0*	*57.7–66.2*	*52.3–62.0*	*47.5–57.0*	*46.7–58.8*

Row 1: Proportions were computed using weighted data.
Row 2: 95% CI: Confidence intervals for estimates were computed using weighted data.
Columns are arranged by age at time of Survey.

Table 6-2 presents the percentage of children who have never visited a dental provider in the Australian child population. The lowest and highest percentages were among children from households with a high income (6.9%) and low income (16.9%), respectively.

Overall, 11.3% of children have never visited a dental provider, but this varied across the age groups with the highest percentage (28.9%) among children aged 5–6 years.

The percentage of children who have never visited a dental provider was not related to sex, Indigenous identity and parents' country of birth.

A higher percentage of children whose parents had school-level education have never visited a dental provider (16.7%) compared to children of parents who had vocational training (11.4%). There was a 2.1-fold relative difference in the percentage of children who have never visited a dental provider between children whose parents had school-level education and children of tertiary-educated parents. This pattern was consistent across all the age groups with higher percentages of children whose parents only had school-level education have never visited a dental provider relative to the children of vocationally trained and tertiary-educated parents.

There was a gradient in the percentage of children who have never visited a dental provider across household income groups. Approximately 17% of children from low income households have never made a dental visit compared to 9.7% of children from medium income households, pointing to a 1.7-fold relative difference. The relative difference between children from low and high income households was 2.4 times and 1.4 times between medium and high income households. The relative differences between low and high income households increased from 2-fold in the 5–6-year age group to 8.6-fold in the 11–12-year age group, thereafter showing a sharp decline in the 13–14-year age group (1.5).

Across all age groups, there was no significant variation of the percentage of children who have never made a dental visit in regards to the residential location of the children.

In summary, the percentage of children who have never visited a dental provider in the Australian child population was associated with age group, parental education and household income.

Oral health of Australian children

Table 6-2: Percentage of children who have never visited a dental provider in the Australian child population

	Population: children aged 5—14 years					
	All ages	5—6	7—8	9—10	11—12	13—14
All	11.3	28.9	13.7	6.6	4.6	2.2
	10.2–12.5	*26.6–31.3*	*11.8–15.8*	*5.3–8.3*	*3.7–5.6*	*1.4–3.4*
Sex						
Male	12.0	29.2	15.3	7.8	4.7	2.3
	10.7–13.4	*26.1–32.5*	*12.6–18.4*	*5.9–10.2*	*3.6–6.2*	*1.2–4.2*
Female	10.6	28.5	11.9	5.5	4.5	2.1
	9.4–11.8	*25.8–31.4*	*10.0–14.1*	*4.0–7.5*	*3.3–6.0*	*1.2–3.6*
Indigenous identity						
Non-Indigenous	11.1	28.5	13.7	6.6	4.4	2.1
	10.0–12.3	*26.2–31.0*	*11.7–15.9*	*5.2–8.4*	*3.5–5.5*	*1.3–3.3*
Indigenous	13.6	34.0	12.0	5.6	6.7	6.3
	10.8–16.9	*25.8–43.4*	*7.4–19.0*	*2.8–11.2*	*3.3–12.9*	*2.0–18.3*
Parents' country of birth						
Australian born	10.6	29.0	12.1	5.8	3.3	2.4
	9.6–11.7	*26.3–31.8*	*10.3–14.2*	*4.4–7.5*	*2.5–4.3*	*1.4–3.8*
Overseas born	12.3	28.6	16.5	7.7	6.7	2.0
	10.5–14.4	*24.9–32.7*	*13.0–20.6*	*5.6–10.5*	*5.1–8.8*	*1.0–3.8*
Parental education						
School	16.7	40.1	20.2	11.6	7.5	4.3
	14.6–19.1	*35.5–44.9*	*15.9–25.4*	*8.5–15.6*	*5.6–10.0*	*2.3–8.1*
Vocational training	11.4	30.9	16.3	5.8	4.0	1.7
	10.0–13.1	*26.9–35.2*	*12.6–20.8*	*3.9–8.6*	*2.6–6.2*	*0.7–4.1*
Tertiary education	7.9	21.4	9.2	3.9	2.8	1.1
	7.0–9.0	*18.7–24.3*	*7.6–11.1*	*2.6–5.7*	*2.0–3.9*	*0.5–2.3*
Household income						
Low	16.9	40.5	21.0	11.2	8.6	3.0
	14.8–19.2	*36.1–45.0*	*17.4–25.2*	*8.5–14.6*	*6.6–11.0*	*1.7–5.3*
Medium	9.7	25.0	13.4	5.5	2.8	2.0
	8.7–10.9	*22.2–28.1*	*11.0–16.2*	*3.9–7.8*	*1.9–4.1*	*1.1–3.6*
High	6.9	20.6	7.1	1.9	1.0	2.1
	5.7–8.3	*16.9–24.9*	*5.1–9.8*	*1.1–3.6*	*0.5–2.0*	*0.8–5.6*
Residential location						
Major city	11.8	28.5	14.8	6.9	5.2	2.7
	10.4–13.4	*25.5–31.7*	*12.2–17.7*	*5.1–9.3*	*4.0–6.7*	*1.6–4.4*
Inner regional	11.1	29.5	13.2	7.9	3.5	1.7
	9.6–12.8	*25.6–33.7*	*10.3–16.7*	*5.5–11.2*	*2.3–5.4*	*0.8–3.4*
Outer regional	8.9	29.8	10.0	2.6	3.3	0.5
	7.3–10.8	*24.3–36.1*	*7.1–14.0*	*1.6–4.1*	*2.1–5.3*	*0.2–1.3*
Remote/Very remote	8.2	30.2	2.6	4.5	2.3	1.1
	5.1–12.9	*19.7–43.3*	*1.2–5.5*	*1.6–12.3*	*0.8–6.5*	*0.4–3.3*
Reason for last dental visit						
Check-up	0.0	0.0	0.0	0.0	0.0	0.0
	—	—	—	—	—	—
Dental problem	0.0	0.0	0.0	0.0	0.0	0.0
	—	—	—	—	—	—

Row 1: Proportions were computed using weighted data.
Row 2: 95% CI: Confidence intervals for estimates were computed using weighted data.
Columns are arranged by age at time of Survey.

Table 6-3 presents the percentage of children who first visited a dental provider for a check-up in the Australian child population. The highest percentage was among children who last visited for a check-up (92.4%) and the lowest percentage was among children whose last dental visit was for a problem (64.2%). Overall, there were 86.7% of children who first visited a dental provider for a check-up but this did not vary across the age groups. There was no variation in the percentage of children who first visited a dental provider for a check-up in relation to sex.

A higher percentage of non-Indigenous children first visited a dental provider for a check-up than Indigenous children (87.3% versus 77.3%). This was also seen among children in all age groups except the 7–8 year and 13–14-year age groups.

A higher proportion of children with Australian born parents had first visited a dental provider for a check-up (88.2%) compared to children with an overseas born parent (84.3%). However, this difference was not seen across the age groups and was limited to children aged 11–12 years (89.4% versus 83.8%).

A lower proportion of children whose parents only had school-only education visited a dental provider for a check-up in their first visit (81.2%) compared to children of tertiary-educated parents (89.6%). In each specific two-year age group, there were higher percentages of children whose parents had a tertiary education visiting for a check-up in their first visit relative to children whose parents had school-only education. There were higher percentages of children of vocationally trained parents making their first visit for a check-up compared to children whose parents had school-only education (87.7% versus 81.2%). However, this difference was seen only among children aged 7–8 and 11–12 years. Among all but 5–6-year-old children, there were no significant differences between children of tertiary-educated and vocationally trained parents in regards to the percentage of children who first visited a dental provider for a check-up.

Higher percentages of children from high income (92.4%) and medium income (89.1%) households had first visited a dental provider for a check-up relative to children from low income households (78.5%). This pattern was consistent across the age groups with the children aged 5–6 years showing the highest relative difference. Overall, a greater proportion of children from high income households made their first visit for a check-up compared to children from medium income households (92.4% versus 89.1%) but this difference was seen only among children aged 13–14 years.

Residential location was not related to the percentage of children who first visited a dental provider for a check-up in the Australian child population.

The percentage of children who first visited a dental provider for a check-up was 1.4 times more among children whose last visit was for a check-up than who last visited for a problem. This difference was consistent across the age groups.

In summary, the percentage of Australian children who first visited a dental provider for a check-up was related to Indigenous status, parents' country of birth, parental education, household income and reason for last dental visit.

Table 6-3: Percentage of children who first visited a dental provider for a check-up in the Australian child population

| | Population: children aged 5–14 years | | | | | |
	All ages	5–6	7–8	9–10	11–12	13–14
All	86.7	85.4	84.8	85.5	87.3	89.9
	85.8–87.7	*83.2–87.3*	*82.8–86.6*	*83.8–87.0*	*85.6–88.9*	*88.4–91.3*
Sex						
Male	85.7	84.0	83.2	85.7	86.2	88.7
	84.4–87.0	*80.9–86.7*	*80.1–85.8*	*83.5–87.7*	*83.6–88.4*	*86.4–90.7*
Female	87.8	86.7	86.5	85.3	88.5	91.1
	86.6–88.9	*84.2–89.0*	*84.0–88.6*	*82.8–87.5*	*86.5–90.3*	*88.9–92.9*
Indigenous identity						
Non-Indigenous	87.3	86.1	85.3	86.5	87.8	90.1
	86.3–88.2	*83.8–88.0*	*83.3–87.1*	*84.8–88.0*	*86.0–89.3*	*88.5–91.5*
Indigenous	77.3	72.2	79.2	68.9	79.4	87.4
	73.1–81.0	*60.7–81.4*	*70.2–86.0*	*59.3–77.1*	*71.4–85.6*	*78.0–93.2*
Parents' country of birth						
Australian born	88.2	86.6	86.8	86.6	89.4	91.1
	87.3–89.1	*84.2–88.6*	*84.6–88.7*	*84.7–88.3*	*87.6–90.9*	*89.2–92.6*
Overseas born	84.3	83.3	81.5	83.6	83.8	88.1
	82.4–85.9	*79.4–86.6*	*78.0–84.6*	*80.5–86.3*	*80.5–86.7*	*85.0–90.6*
Parental education						
School	81.2	78.5	76.6	81.2	81.4	85.8
	79.2–83.0	*73.3–82.9*	*72.0–80.6*	*77.3–84.7*	*77.4–84.8*	*81.9–88.9*
Vocational training	87.7	82.7	86.5	86.3	88.3	92.1
	86.0–89.1	*78.0–86.6*	*82.5–89.8*	*82.7–89.3*	*85.2–90.8*	*88.8–94.5*
Tertiary education	89.6	89.5	88.5	87.5	90.6	91.7
	88.5–90.5	*87.1–91.5*	*86.3–90.3*	*85.5–89.2*	*88.7–92.3*	*89.8–93.3*
Household income						
Low	78.5	73.7	77.4	75.2	78.3	85.1
	76.4–80.4	*68.4–78.4*	*73.2–81.0*	*71.1–78.9*	*74.5–81.6*	*81.3–88.2*
Medium	89.1	87.2	86.2	89.5	90.6	91.0
	88.1–90.0	*84.7–89.4*	*83.5–88.5*	*87.6–91.1*	*88.4–92.4*	*88.8–92.8*
High	92.4	92.3	90.8	90.8	93.2	95.0
	91.2–93.5	*89.3–94.5*	*87.7–93.2*	*88.2–92.8*	*90.8–95.0*	*92.9–96.5*
Residential location						
Major city	86.6	85.3	85.3	85.2	87.1	89.6
	85.3–87.8	*82.4–87.7*	*82.7–87.6*	*83.0–87.1*	*84.8–89.1*	*87.5–91.4*
Inner regional	87.4	87.5	82.5	86.9	88.3	90.9
	85.7–88.9	*83.8–90.5*	*77.7–86.4*	*83.6–89.6*	*85.2–90.8*	*88.3–93.0*
Outer regional	86.2	82.0	84.8	85.1	87.1	89.8
	84.0–88.1	*76.9–86.2*	*80.7–88.1*	*81.2–88.2*	*82.9–90.3*	*86.0–92.7*
Remote/Very remote	87.1	78.8	92.4	83.0	84.1	91.6
	79.6–92.1	*65.5–87.9*	*85.4–96.2*	*73.2–89.8*	*66.8–93.3*	*78.8–97.0*
Reason for last dental visit						
Check-up	92.4	93.8	91.7	91.5	92.3	92.6
	91.7–93.0	*92.5–95.0*	*90.2–93.0*	*90.2–92.7*	*90.9–93.4*	*91.1–93.9*
Dental problem	64.2	49.7	62.8	64.2	67.9	74.7
	61.3–67.1	*43.1–56.3*	*57.8–67.6*	*59.5–68.7*	*62.9–72.6*	*68.5–80.1*

Row 1: Proportions were computed using weighted data.
Row 2: 95% CI: Confidence intervals for estimates were computed using weighted data.
Columns are arranged by age at time of Survey.

6.2　Children's usual dental visit

Information is presented in this section related to usual dental visiting using the percentage of children with a usual visit pattern that was irregular.

Table 6-4 presents the percentage of children who usually have an irregular dental visiting pattern in the Australian child population. While the highest proportion was among children whose last dental visit was for a problem (33.9%) the lowest proportion was among children who last visited for a check-up (17.4%).

Overall, there were 20.9% of children who usually have an irregular dental visiting pattern but this did not vary across the age groups. There was no variation in the percentage of children who usually have an irregular dental visiting pattern in relation to sex.

There were higher percentages of Indigenous children with an irregular dental visiting pattern than non-Indigenous children (20.6% versus 20.4%) but this difference was confined only to the children aged 11–12 and 13–14 years.

Parents' country of birth was not related to the percentage of children who usually have an irregular dental visiting pattern.

There were higher percentages of children with an irregular dental visiting pattern in children whose parents had school-only education (29.9%) relative to the children of vocationally trained (20%) and tertiary-educated parents (16.3%). This difference was consistent across the age groups. Among all children of vocationally trained parents, a higher percentage of children had an irregular dental visiting pattern than children of tertiary-educated parents. However, this difference was not seen across the age groups.

There was a gradient in the percentage of children with an irregular dental visiting pattern across household income groups with 31.7% of children from low income households having an irregular dental visiting pattern compared to 19.1% of children from medium income households, a 1.7-fold relative difference. The relative differences between children from low and high income households as well as medium and high income households were 2.5 and 1.5, respectively. The relative difference between medium and high income groups was evident among all age groups except for the 5–6-year age group.

There was no association between the percentage of children with an irregular dental visiting pattern and their residential location.

The proportion of children with an irregular dental visiting pattern was nearly 2 times in children whose last visit was for a problem compared to children who last visited for a check-up. This pattern was consistent across the age groups.

In summary, the percentage of Australian children who usually have an irregular dental visiting pattern was related to Indigenous identity, parental education, household income and reason for last dental visit.

Table 6-4: Percentage of children who usually have an irregular dental visiting pattern in the Australian child population

	Population: children aged 5–14 years					
	All ages	5–6	7–8	9–10	11–12	13–14
All	20.9	27.8	23.1	19.7	18.7	17.1
	19.7–22.1	*25.3–30.5*	*21.0–25.4*	*17.8–21.7*	*17.0–20.7*	*15.2–19.3*
Sex						
Male	21.0	27.9	24.0	19.3	19.4	16.4
	19.6–22.5	*24.5–31.7*	*21.2–27.0*	*16.8–22.1*	*17.1–22.0*	*14.0–19.1*
Female	20.8	27.7	22.1	20.0	18.0	17.9
	19.2–22.4	*24.4–31.3*	*19.4–25.1*	*17.5–22.9*	*15.7–20.6*	*15.0–21.2*
Indigenous identity						
Non-Indigenous	20.4	27.3	22.8	19.3	18.1	16.7
	19.2–21.7	*24.8–29.9*	*20.7–25.0*	*17.4–21.4*	*16.3–20.0*	*14.7–19.0*
Indigenous	30.6	39.7	27.2	24.4	33.7	30.1
	26.0–35.7	*28.2–52.5*	*19.3–36.9*	*17.5–33.0*	*24.1–44.8*	*20.1–42.4*
Parents' country of birth						
Australian born	20.1	26.0	21.6	19.0	18.6	16.8
	18.8–21.4	*23.2–29.1*	*19.1–24.3*	*16.9–21.3*	*16.4–20.9*	*14.5–19.5*
Overseas born	22.4	30.9	25.5	20.9	19.2	18.0
	20.6–24.3	*27.0–35.2*	*22.3–29.1*	*17.7–24.5*	*16.5–22.3*	*14.7–21.8*
Parental education						
School	29.9	38.8	34.2	25.5	27.0	28.1
	27.7–32.2	*33.7–44.2*	*29.3–39.5*	*21.6–29.8*	*23.3–31.0*	*24.1–32.6*
Vocational training	20.0	27.3	22.6	20.6	18.4	14.3
	18.1–21.9	*22.6–32.5*	*18.7–27.0*	*17.1–24.7*	*15.2–22.2*	*11.1–18.3*
Tertiary education	16.3	23.5	18.0	15.9	13.7	11.3
	15.1–17.5	*20.6–26.7*	*15.9–20.4*	*13.6–18.4*	*11.7–16.0*	*9.4–13.6*
Household income						
Low	31.7	41.2	33.2	29.2	30.8	28.1
	29.6–33.9	*36.5–46.0*	*29.1–37.5*	*25.5–33.2*	*27.0–34.9*	*24.1–32.6*
Medium	19.1	25.8	22.7	19.0	16.2	14.1
	17.7–20.6	*22.8–29.2*	*19.9–25.8*	*16.4–21.9*	*13.8–18.8*	*11.7–17.0*
High	12.5	19.8	14.7	10.3	10.0	8.5
	11.1–14.0	*16.1–24.1*	*11.7–18.3*	*7.9–13.3*	*7.9–12.7*	*6.3–11.3*
Residential location						
Major city	19.9	27.0	21.9	18.7	17.5	16.4
	18.4–21.5	*23.9–30.3*	*19.3–24.7*	*16.3–21.3*	*15.2–20.0*	*13.8–19.3*
Inner regional	22.8	29.9	25.7	23.0	21.8	16.3
	20.6–25.2	*25.6–34.6*	*21.5–30.3*	*19.6–26.8*	*18.5–25.6*	*12.8–20.5*
Outer regional	22.6	28.5	25.2	19.0	20.0	22.5
	20.5–24.8	*23.0–34.7*	*21.1–29.8*	*15.2–23.4*	*15.9–24.9*	*18.5–27.0*
Remote/Very remote	29.3	42.5	32.6	29.2	27.4	22.8
	19.0–42.2	*34.6–50.8*	*16.1–54.9*	*18.0–43.8*	*11.4–52.6*	*9.4–45.9*
Reason for last dental visit						
Check-up	17.4	24.1	18.9	16.7	15.2	14.4
	16.3–18.6	*21.6–26.8*	*16.6–21.3*	*14.8–18.8*	*13.4–17.1*	*12.5–16.6*
Dental problem	33.9	41.8	35.8	29.3	32.9	31.9
	31.6–36.3	*35.7–48.2*	*31.5–40.4*	*25.3–33.6*	*28.5–37.5*	*26.2–38.2*

Row 1: Proportions were computed using weighted data.
Row 2: 95% CI: Confidence intervals for estimates were computed using weighted data.
Columns are arranged by age at time of Survey.

6.3   Children's most recent dental visit

In this section the following measures of the most recent dental visit are presented: making a dental visit within the last 12 months, having a check-up as the reason for last dental visit, attending a private dental clinic at the last dental visit, whether parents or guardians attended with the child at their last dental visit, and rating of the last dental visit by the parent/guardian.

Table 6-5 presents the percentage of children who last visited a dental provider within the last 12 months in the Australian child population. The highest percentage was among children from high income households (85.7%) while the lowest was among children from Remote/Very remote residential locations (71.3%).

Of all children, 81.1% visited a dental provider within the last 12 months but this did not vary across the age groups. Sex was not related to the percentage of children who last visited a dental provider within the last 12 months.

Higher percentages of non-Indigenous children (81.5%) than Indigenous children (74.9%) last visited a dental provider within the last 12 months. This difference was also seen among children aged 5–6 years and 9–10 years.

There was no association between the percentage of children who last visited a dental provider within the last 12 months and parents' country of birth.

Overall, a higher proportion of children with tertiary-educated parents had last visited a dental provider within the last 12 months (84.4%) compared to children whose parents had vocational training (80.9%) and school-only education (75.7%). Such a difference was seen between children of vocationally trained parents and school-only educated parents. However, this pattern was not seen across all age groups and evident only among children aged 13–14 years.

Children from high income households comprised the highest percentage of children who visited a dental provider within the last 12 months. Higher percentages of children from high income households had last visited a dental provider within the last 12 months (85.7%) relative to children from medium (81.5%) and low income households (76.4%). Although this difference existed between children from medium and low income groups, it was not seen across the age groups.

The percentage of children who last visited a dental provider within the last 12 months in the Australian child population was not associated with the residential location and reason for last dental visit.

In summary, the percentage of Australian children who visited a dental provider within the last 12 months was related to Indigenous status, parental education and household income.

Table 6-5: Percentage of children who last visited a dental provider at or less than 12 months in the Australian child population

	Population: children aged 5–14 years					
	All ages	5–6	7–8	9–10	11–12	13–14
All	81.1	81.6	81.4	81.2	81.5	80.1
	80.1–82.1	*79.4–83.7*	*79.4–83.2*	*79.3–83.0*	*79.9–83.1*	*77.8–82.2*
Sex						
Male	81.1	82.6	82.4	80.2	80.8	79.9
	79.8–82.3	*79.8–85.1*	*79.8–84.7*	*77.5–82.6*	*78.4–83.0*	*77.0–82.5*
Female	81.2	80.6	80.3	82.2	82.3	80.3
	79.7–82.5	*77.3–83.6*	*77.4–82.8*	*79.6–84.6*	*80.1–84.3*	*76.8–83.3*
Indigenous identity						
Non-Indigenous	81.5	81.7	81.8	81.8	82.1	80.3
	80.5–82.5	*79.5–83.8*	*79.9–83.7*	*79.8–83.6*	*80.4–83.7*	*78.0–82.5*
Indigenous	74.9	84.8	75.2	72.7	74.7	68.5
	70.7–78.7	*75.0–91.2*	*65.1–83.1*	*64.3–79.7*	*66.1–81.7*	*56.3–78.5*
Parents' country of birth						
Australian born	81.0	82.2	81.7	80.3	81.6	79.6
	79.8–82.2	*79.4–84.7*	*79.4–83.7*	*77.9–82.5*	*79.5–83.5*	*77.0–82.1*
Overseas born	81.5	81.4	80.9	83.0	81.9	80.4
	79.9–83.0	*77.5–84.7*	*77.2–84.2*	*80.1–85.5*	*79.0–84.5*	*76.4–83.9*
Parental education						
School	75.7	79.8	77.5	77.4	74.8	71.2
	73.5–77.8	*74.9–84.0*	*72.9–81.6*	*73.2–81.0*	*70.8–78.5*	*66.4–75.5*
Vocational training	80.9	82.8	78.9	77.5	83.3	82.0
	78.8–82.9	*78.5–86.3*	*74.3–82.9*	*72.9–81.5*	*79.5–86.6*	*77.9–85.5*
Tertiary education	84.4	82.7	84.3	85.6	84.8	84.5
	83.3–85.4	*80.0–85.2*	*82.1–86.2*	*83.3–87.6*	*82.8–86.6*	*81.8–86.9*
Household income						
Low	76.4	81.2	75.2	77.1	73.8	76.0
	74.5–78.2	*76.9–84.9*	*71.0–78.9*	*73.7–80.3*	*70.0–77.3*	*71.6–79.9*
Medium	81.5	79.1	82.9	80.0	83.6	81.8
	80.1–82.9	*75.3–82.4*	*79.7–85.6*	*77.1–82.6*	*81.1–85.8*	*78.6–84.6*
High	85.7	85.7	85.1	87.1	87.5	83.2
	84.2–87.2	*82.4–88.5*	*81.9–87.7*	*83.7–90.0*	*84.6–90.0*	*79.3–86.5*
Residential location						
Major city	82.1	81.6	82.1	82.8	82.8	81.1
	80.9–83.2	*78.8–84.0*	*79.7–84.3*	*80.5–84.9*	*80.6–84.7*	*78.0–83.8*
Inner regional	79.5	83.1	80.5	77.0	78.0	80.0
	77.4–81.5	*78.8–86.7*	*76.6–83.9*	*72.4–81.1*	*74.5–81.2*	*75.7–83.8*
Outer regional	80.3	84.3	80.9	81.3	80.5	76.3
	77.5–82.8	*79.3–88.3*	*75.3–85.4*	*76.8–85.1*	*75.7–84.6*	*70.9–80.9*
Remote/Very remote	71.3	62.6	70.8	70.5	81.1	69.4
	58.9–81.1	*38.9–81.4*	*50.8–85.0*	*50.0–85.1*	*72.0–87.8*	*52.1–82.6*
Reason for last dental visit						
Check-up	81.7	81.6	81.4	81.6	82.6	81.3
	80.6–82.7	*79.1–83.8*	*79.2–83.4*	*79.4–83.6*	*80.6–84.3*	*78.8–83.5*
Dental problem	80.2	83.1	82.8	80.9	78.3	75.3
	78.1–82.1	*78.0–87.2*	*78.5–86.4*	*76.8–84.4*	*73.9–82.1*	*69.4–80.3*

Row 1: Proportions were computed using weighted data.
Row 2: 95% CI: Confidence intervals for estimates were computed using weighted data.
Columns are arranged by age at time of Survey.

Table 6-6 presents the percentage of children who last visited a dental provider for a check-up in the Australian child population. The highest proportion was among children from high income households (87.5%) while the lowest was among Indigenous children (68.4%).

Overall, 80.2% of children last visited a dental provider for a check-up but this did not vary across the age groups. The percentage of children who last visited a dental provider for a check-up was not related to sex.

The proportion of non-Indigenous children who last visited a dental provider for a check-up was 1.2 times more than that of Indigenous children (80.8% versus 68.4%). This difference was also evident among children aged 9–10 and 11–12 years.

Parents' country of birth was not associated with the percentage of children who last visited a dental provider for a check-up.

A higher proportion of children whose parents had a tertiary education had last visited a dental provider for a check-up (83.6%) compared to children of vocationally trained parents (80.3%) as well as school-only educated parents (74.1%). Higher percentages of children of vocationally trained parents had last visited a dental provider for a check-up than children whose parents had school-level education. However, this pattern was not consistent across the age groups.

Children from high income households comprised the highest percentage of children who last visited a dental provider for a check-up. The relative difference between the children from high income households who last visited a dental provider for a check-up compared to low income households was 1.2 while that between children from medium and low as well as high and medium income households was 1.1. This difference was also seen among children aged 7–8, 9–10 and 11–12 years.

There was no relation between the percentage of children who last visited a dental provider for a check-up and their residential location.

In summary, Indigenous status, parental education and household income were related to the percentage of children who last visited a dental provider for a check-up in the Australian child population.

Oral health of Australian children

Table 6-6: Percentage of children who last visited a dental provider for a check-up in the Australian child population

	Population: children aged 5-14 years					
	All ages	5–6	7–8	9–10	11–12	13–14
All	**80.2**	**81.0**	**76.3**	**78.0**	**79.8**	**85.2**
	79.1–81.2	*78.5–83.4*	*74.1–78.4*	*76.1–79.7*	*78.0–81.5*	*83.4–86.8*
Sex						
Male	79.8	80.1	76.1	78.3	78.7	84.9
	78.3–81.1	*76.5–83.3*	*73.1–79.0*	*75.7–80.7*	*75.9–81.3*	*82.1–87.3*
Female	80.6	82.0	76.5	77.6	81.0	85.4
	79.2–81.9	*78.9–84.7*	*73.6–79.1*	*74.7–80.3*	*78.6–83.2*	*83.2–87.4*
Indigenous identity						
Non-Indigenous	80.8	81.5	76.9	78.6	80.7	85.4
	79.7–81.8	*78.9–83.9*	*74.7–79.1*	*76.7–80.4*	*79.0–82.4*	*83.6–87.0*
Indigenous	68.4	68.9	68.0	65.0	63.4	79.1
	62.9–73.4	*51.7–82.1*	*57.1–77.2*	*55.4–73.6*	*52.7–73.0*	*66.4–87.9*
Parents' country of birth						
Australian born	81.1	82.2	78.9	78.8	80.6	84.8
	80.0–82.2	*79.3–84.9*	*76.4–81.2*	*76.7–80.8*	*78.3–82.8*	*82.6–86.8*
Overseas born	78.6	78.8	72.1	76.5	78.5	85.9
	76.7–80.4	*74.6–82.5*	*68.3–75.6*	*72.9–79.7*	*75.4–81.4*	*83.2–88.2*
Parental education						
School	74.1	72.6	67.4	72.2	74.8	80.9
	72.2–76.0	*67.4–77.2*	*62.8–71.6*	*68.1–76.0*	*70.8–78.4*	*76.8–84.4*
Vocational training	80.3	76.6	77.6	79.2	78.0	87.4
	78.4–82.1	*71.4–81.1*	*72.8–81.8*	*75.4–82.5*	*74.1–81.5*	*83.9–90.2*
Tertiary education	83.6	86.2	80.4	80.5	84.1	86.9
	82.3–84.7	*83.1–88.9*	*77.9–82.7*	*78.1–82.8*	*82.0–85.9*	*84.6–88.9*
Household income						
Low	71.0	69.5	66.6	65.7	70.9	79.6
	68.9–73.0	*64.2–74.3*	*62.8–70.2*	*61.6–69.5*	*67.2–74.3*	*75.6–83.1*
Medium	81.3	82.1	77.4	78.4	81.4	86.5
	80.0–82.5	*79.0–84.8*	*74.4–80.2*	*75.9–80.7*	*78.7–83.8*	*83.9–88.8*
High	87.5	88.2	84.9	88.5	87.1	89.0
	86.0–88.8	*84.6–91.1*	*81.4–87.8*	*85.9–90.6*	*83.9–89.8*	*85.1–92.0*
Residential location						
Major city	81.1	81.2	77.5	79.0	81.1	86.2
	79.7–82.5	*77.8–84.2*	*74.5–80.2*	*76.5–81.2*	*78.8–83.2*	*83.9–88.3*
Inner regional	78.6	82.5	73.8	75.0	77.9	83.8
	76.8–80.3	*78.4–86.0*	*69.4–77.7*	*71.4–78.3*	*74.2–81.2*	*80.7–86.5*
Outer regional	76.4	77.2	71.8	75.2	77.2	79.8
	73.9–78.6	*72.1–81.5*	*66.3–76.8*	*70.8–79.2*	*72.3–81.5*	*74.3–84.4*
Remote/Very remote	83.2	73.5	86.4	92.4	63.2	91.3
	77.4–87.7	*56.0–85.8*	*79.8–91.1*	*77.0–97.8*	*41.2–80.8*	*81.6–96.1*
Reason for last dental visit						
Check-up	0.0	0.0	0.0	0.0	0.0	0.0
	—	—	—	—	—	—
Dental problem	0.0	0.0	0.0	0.0	0.0	0.0
	—	—	—	—	—	—

Row 1: Proportions were computed using weighted data.
Row 2: 95% CI: Confidence intervals for estimates were computed using weighted data.
Columns are arranged by age at time of Survey.

Table 6-7 presents the percentage of children whose most recent dental visit was at a private-practice location in the Australian child population. The highest proportion was among children from high income households (76.6%) and the lowest proportion was among Indigenous children (23.3%). Among all children there were 56.8% whose most recent dental visit was at a private-practice location but this did not vary across the age groups. The percentage of children whose most recent dental visit was at a private-practice location was not related to sex.

Overall, there were higher percentages of non-Indigenous children than Indigenous children whose most recent dental visit was at a private-practice location (58.4% versus 23.3%). This difference was evident across the age groups with the relative difference between non-Indigenous and Indigenous children being highest in children aged 11–12 years (3.31).

There was no association between the proportions of children whose most recent dental visit was at a private-practice location and parents' country of birth.

There was a gradient in the percentage of children whose most recent dental visit was at a private-practice location across parental education groups. Approximately 52.3% of children of vocationally trained parents had made their most recent dental visit at a private-practice location compared to 39.6% of children of school-only educated parents, pointing to a relative difference of 1.3. The relative differences between children of tertiary-educated parents and school-only educated parents as well as children of tertiary-educated parents and vocationally trained parents were 1.7 and 1.3, respectively. This pattern was consistent across the age groups.

The proportion of children from high income households whose most recent dental visit was at a private-practice location was 2.3 times compared to children from low income households and 1.3 times compared to children from medium income households. There were higher percentages of children from medium income households whose most recent dental visit was at a private-practice location (59.6%) compared to children from low income households (32.6%). This pattern was seen across the age groups with children aged 5–6 years showing the highest relative difference between low and high income households (2.7).

The percentage of children whose most recent dental visit was at a private-practice location was associated with their residential location with a higher proportion of children from Major cities visiting a private practice at their most recent visit (61.6%) compared to children from Inner regional (50.6%), Outer regional (39.3%) and Remote/Very remote (28.3%) locations. However, this difference was not seen across the age groups.

Among all children who last visited for a check-up, there were 1.3 times more children whose most recent dental visit was at a private-practice location compared to children who last visited for a problem. This pattern was consistent across the age groups.

In summary, the percentage of children whose most recent dental visit was at a private-practice location was related to Indigenous status, parental education, household income, residential location and reason for last dental visit.

Table 6-7: Percentage of children whose most recent dental visit was at a private practice in the Australian child population

	Population: children aged 5–14 years					
	All ages	5–6	7–8	9–10	11–12	13–14
All	56.8	57.9	54.6	52.4	55.5	63.0
	54.6–58.9	*54.2–61.5*	*51.1–58.0*	*49.3–55.6*	*52.8–58.1*	*59.6–66.3*
Sex						
Male	56.8	58.1	55.0	52.8	55.8	62.0
	54.4–59.2	*53.7–62.4*	*50.9–59.1*	*48.8–56.8*	*52.5–59.1*	*58.0–65.9*
Female	56.7	57.6	54.1	52.0	55.1	64.0
	54.1–59.4	*53.3–61.9*	*50.0–58.2*	*48.0–56.0*	*51.4–58.7*	*59.2–68.4*
Indigenous identity						
Non-Indigenous	58.4	59.4	56.3	54.1	57.7	64.1
	56.3–60.6	*55.7–62.9*	*52.8–59.7*	*50.9–57.3*	*55.0–60.4*	*60.7–67.4*
Indigenous	23.3	31.1	21.5	20.6	17.4	29.9
	18.4–29.0	*19.6–45.5*	*14.2–31.2*	*13.2–30.7*	*10.6–27.1*	*19.4–43.0*
Parents' country of birth						
Australian born	56.6	58.5	55.0	51.3	54.6	63.2
	54.2–58.9	*54.5–62.4*	*51.1–58.8*	*47.7–54.9*	*51.5–57.7*	*59.4–66.9*
Overseas born	57.3	57.3	53.9	54.3	57.6	62.4
	54.4–60.1	*51.6–62.8*	*49.3–58.5*	*49.6–58.9*	*53.7–61.4*	*57.5–67.1*
Parental education						
School	39.6	35.5	33.9	36.4	41.5	46.6
	36.8–42.4	*29.1–42.4*	*29.5–38.7*	*31.4–41.7*	*36.9–46.3*	*41.0–52.3*
Vocational training	52.3	50.0	50.2	47.6	51.9	59.4
	49.3–55.2	*44.5–55.6*	*44.6–55.9*	*42.3–53.0*	*46.9–56.8*	*54.2–64.4*
Tertiary education	68.3	70.9	65.9	63.4	66.1	75.4
	65.9–70.6	*67.0–74.5*	*62.0–69.6*	*59.8–66.9*	*62.9–69.1*	*72.0–78.5*
Household income						
Low	32.6	29.1	28.3	26.4	32.5	42.9
	30.3–35.0	*24.5–34.2*	*24.7–32.1*	*22.7–30.5*	*28.4–36.8*	*38.1–47.8*
Medium	59.6	60.2	57.6	55.6	57.6	66.8
	57.5–61.8	*56.2–64.0*	*53.6–61.5*	*51.7–59.5*	*54.0–61.0*	*62.9–70.5*
High	76.6	79.0	73.0	73.8	77.6	79.9
	74.0–79.0	*74.7–82.8*	*68.0–77.5*	*69.3–77.8*	*73.8–81.0*	*75.6–83.7*
Residential location						
Major city	61.6	62.8	59.7	58.5	59.8	67.0
	58.9–64.2	*58.3–67.1*	*55.5–63.9*	*54.7–62.3*	*56.3–63.1*	*62.7–71.1*
Inner regional	50.6	51.3	49.2	42.2	48.8	60.7
	46.6–54.6	*44.7–57.8*	*42.8–55.7*	*36.9–47.7*	*43.6–54.0*	*55.0–66.2*
Outer regional	39.3	34.6	35.4	34.6	41.9	46.8
	34.3–44.5	*27.1–42.9*	*29.8–41.3*	*27.9–41.9*	*33.9–50.4*	*40.3–53.3*
Remote/Very remote	28.3	33.2	11.2	21.7	38.0	35.0
	18.4–41.0	*15.0–58.3*	*3.3–31.4*	*16.2–28.4*	*19.9–60.1*	*16.6–59.2*
Reason for last dental visit						
Check-up	59.5	60.1	56.1	55.0	59.0	65.6
	57.2–61.7	*56.2–63.9*	*52.2–59.9*	*51.6–58.4*	*56.1–61.8*	*62.3–68.9*
Dental problem	46.1	48.0	49.6	43.5	42.0	48.1
	43.2–49.0	*41.7–54.4*	*44.8–54.4*	*38.6–48.5*	*37.1–47.1*	*40.8–55.5*

Row 1: Proportions were computed using weighted data.
Row 2: 95% CI: Confidence intervals for estimates were computed using weighted data.
Columns are arranged by age at time of Survey.

Table 6-8 presents the percentage of parents or guardians attending with their child at the most recent dental visit in the Australian child population. While the highest proportion was among parents with children who last visited for a dental problem, the lowest was among those who were from Remote/Very remote residential locations (87.7% versus 73.4%).

Overall, 84.1% of parents or guardians were attending with their child at the most recent dental visit but this did not vary across the age groups of children.

There was no association between the percentage of parents or guardians attending with their child at the most recent dental visit and child's sex.

Fewer Indigenous parents or guardians were attending with their child at the most recent dental visit (74.5%) compared to their non-Indigenous counterparts (84.5%). This difference was also evident among parents with children aged 11–12 years and 13–14 years who presented with almost identical relative differences (0.8).

Parents' country of birth, parental education and household income were not related to the percentage of parents or guardians attending with their child at the most recent dental visit in the Australian child population.

There was a mixed relationship between the percentage of parents or guardians attending with their child at the most recent dental visit and their residential location. Although there was no gradient in the percentage of parents or guardians attending with their child at the most recent dental visit across all residential groups, a higher proportion of parents or guardians from Major city (84.6%) and Inner regional areas (84.3%) were attending with their child at the most recent dental visit compared to their counterparts from Remote/Very remote locations (73.4%). This pattern was seen among parents whose children were in 5–6-year and 9–10-year age groups.

Among parents or guardians of all children who last made a dental visit for a problem, there were a higher percentage of parents or guardians attending with their child at the most recent dental visit compared to the parents or guardians of children who last visited for a check-up (87.7% versus 83.2%). However, this difference was seen only among parents with children aged 9–10 years.

In summary, the percentage of parents or guardians attending with their child at the most recent dental visit in the Australian child population was related to Indigenous status and reason for last dental visit.

Table 6-8: Percentage of guardians' attendance at child recent dental visit in the Australian child population

	Population: children aged 5-14 years					
	All ages	5–6	7–8	9–10	11–12	13–14
All	84.1	86.2	84.3	82.9	83.1	84.2
	83.0–85.1	*84.3–87.9*	*82.3–86.1*	*80.7–84.9*	*81.2–84.9*	*82.2–86.0*
Sex						
Male	84.1	85.7	84.0	82.6	84.8	83.9
	82.8–85.4	*83.0–88.0*	*81.5–86.3*	*79.8–85.0*	*82.4–86.9*	*81.1–86.3*
Female	84.0	86.8	84.6	83.2	81.4	84.5
	82.6–85.3	*84.2–89.0*	*82.0–87.0*	*80.6–85.6*	*78.7–83.9*	*81.8–86.9*
Indigenous identity						
Non-Indigenous	84.5	86.3	84.7	83.1	84.0	84.8
	83.4–85.5	*84.4–88.0*	*82.6–86.5*	*80.9–85.1*	*82.1–85.7*	*82.8–86.6*
Indigenous	74.5	84.2	77.3	77.0	66.5	70.5
	69.6–78.8	*73.5–91.1*	*67.8–84.6*	*67.8–84.2*	*56.0–75.6*	*57.0–81.2*
Parents' country of birth						
Australian born	84.1	86.7	84.6	82.7	83.6	83.6
	82.7–85.4	*84.1–88.9*	*82.2–86.6*	*80.0–85.0*	*81.3–85.8*	*80.9–86.0*
Overseas born	83.9	85.7	83.9	83.0	82.0	85.2
	82.5–85.3	*82.8–88.1*	*80.8–86.5*	*80.1–85.6*	*79.1–84.6*	*81.9–88.1*
Parental education						
School	81.4	84.6	82.1	83.4	79.1	79.9
	79.3–83.5	*80.3–88.0*	*78.1–85.4*	*79.3–86.8*	*75.2–82.5*	*75.2–84.0*
Vocational training	84.6	84.9	83.5	80.3	84.9	88.7
	82.7–86.4	*80.4–88.6*	*79.2–87.1*	*76.0–84.0*	*80.9–88.2*	*85.2–91.5*
Tertiary education	85.3	87.6	85.5	83.9	84.9	84.7
	84.1–86.4	*85.5–89.5*	*83.0–87.6*	*81.5–86.0*	*82.7–86.8*	*82.3–86.9*
Household income						
Low	81.5	83.3	82.2	79.7	80.9	81.8
	79.5–83.3	*79.3–86.6*	*78.8–85.2*	*75.2–83.5*	*77.4–84.0*	*77.9–85.2*
Medium	84.7	87.1	84.8	82.8	83.4	85.8
	83.2–86.0	*84.5–89.4*	*82.0–87.3*	*79.9–85.4*	*80.7–85.7*	*83.1–88.1*
High	85.8	87.0	85.8	85.0	85.6	85.6
	84.2–87.3	*83.7–89.8*	*82.5–88.7*	*81.6–87.8*	*82.4–88.3*	*81.9–88.6*
Residential location						
Major city	84.6	86.6	83.8	83.6	84.1	85.2
	83.3–85.8	*84.2–88.6*	*81.1–86.2*	*81.0–86.0*	*81.8–86.1*	*82.6–87.4*
Inner regional	84.3	87.6	87.3	82.0	81.5	84.5
	81.4–86.8	*82.7–91.3*	*83.4–90.4*	*75.8–86.9*	*77.4–85.0*	*80.3–87.9*
Outer regional	81.2	82.3	81.9	81.5	81.0	80.0
	78.1–84.0	*77.3–86.4*	*77.8–85.4*	*77.3–85.0*	*73.4–86.8*	*74.4–84.6*
Remote/Very remote	73.4	67.6	84.6	66.2	76.4	70.9
	64.5–80.7	*49.9–81.5*	*75.3–90.8*	*55.9–75.1*	*59.5–87.8*	*50.5–85.4*
Reason for last dental visit						
Check-up	83.2	85.6	83.1	81.5	82.4	83.8
	82.0–84.4	*83.4–87.6*	*80.7–85.3*	*79.0–83.8*	*80.3–84.3*	*81.7–85.8*
Dental problem	87.7	89.3	88.3	87.9	86.5	86.8
	86.1–89.2	*85.2–92.4*	*85.0–91.0*	*84.5–90.7*	*82.6–89.7*	*82.5–90.1*

Row 1: Proportions were computed using weighted data.
Row 2: 95% CI: Confidence intervals for estimates were computed using weighted data.
Columns are arranged by age at time of Survey.

Table 6-9 presents the percentage of parents reporting excellent or very good dental care for their child at the most recent dental visit in the Australian child population. The highest proportion was among parents from high income households (88.1%) while the lowest proportion was among parents from low income households (73.7%).

There was no relationship between the percentage of parents reporting excellent or very good dental care for their child at the most recent dental visit and child's sex.

A higher proportion of parents of non-Indigenous children had reported excellent or very good dental care for their child at the most recent dental visit compared to their Indigenous counterparts (82.2% versus 74.7%). This difference was also seen among parents whose children were in the 9–10, 11–12 and 13–14-year age groups.

Higher percentages of Australian born parents (84.8%) than overseas born parents (76.7%) had reported excellent or very good dental care for their child at the most recent dental visit. This pattern was consistent across the age groups with parents whose children were in the 11–12-year age group showing the highest relative difference (1.1).

The association between the percentage of parents reporting excellent or very good dental care for their child at the most recent dental visit and parental education showed a mixed pattern. Even though there was no gradient across the parental education groups, parents with vocational training (84.5%) and tertiary education (83.6%) backgrounds had reported excellent or very good dental care for their child at the most recent dental visit compared to the parents with school-level education (76.5%). This trend was also evident among parents with children aged 5–6, 11–12 and 13–14 years.

A higher proportion of parents from high income households (88.1%) had reported excellent or very good dental care for their child at the most recent dental visit compared to those from low income households (73.7%) pointing to a 1.2 relative difference. The relative differences between higher and medium as well as medium and low income households were 1.05 and 1.13, respectively. However, this difference was not seen across the age groups.

Residential location was not related to the percentage of parents reporting excellent or very good dental care for their child at the most recent dental visit.

The proportion of parents reporting excellent or very good dental care for their child at the most recent dental visit was greater among parents with children who last visited for a check-up (82.9%) compared to those who had last made a dental visit for a problem (77.5%). This difference was also seen among parents whose children were in the 7–8-year age group.

In summary, the percentage of parents reporting excellent or very good dental care for their child at the most recent dental visit in the Australian child population was related to Indigenous status, parents' country of birth, household income and reason for last dental visit.

Table 6-9: Percentage of parental reporting excellent or very good dental care at child's recent dental visit in the Australian child population

	Population: children aged 5–14 years					
	All ages	5–6	7–8	9–10	11–12	13–14
All	81.8	82.9	81.8	81.4	80.8	82.2
	80.8–82.8	*80.8–84.9*	*79.9–83.6*	*79.6–83.1*	*79.0–82.4*	*80.2–84.2*
Sex						
Male	81.0	83.0	79.8	80.3	80.3	81.8
	79.7–82.2	*80.3–85.5*	*77.0–82.4*	*77.9–82.6*	*77.9–82.6*	*78.8–84.5*
Female	82.6	82.8	83.9	82.5	81.2	82.7
	81.3–83.8	*79.8–85.5*	*81.6–86.0*	*79.8–84.8*	*78.9–83.4*	*79.9–85.2*
Indigenous identity						
Non-Indigenous	82.2	83.2	81.8	82.0	81.2	82.8
	81.2–83.1	*81.1–85.1*	*79.8–83.6*	*80.2–83.7*	*79.5–82.9*	*80.7–84.7*
Indigenous	74.7	82.2	84.4	69.1	70.6	69.7
	69.8–78.9	*69.9–90.3*	*76.5–89.9*	*59.3–77.4*	*61.7–78.2*	*55.9–80.7*
Parents' country of birth						
Australian born	84.8	86.4	84.7	83.9	84.3	85.0
	83.8–85.8	*84.2–88.4*	*82.5–86.7*	*81.7–85.9*	*82.3–86.0*	*82.7–87.1*
Overseas born	76.7	77.2	76.8	77.0	74.8	77.6
	74.9–78.4	*73.2–80.8*	*73.1–80.0*	*74.0–79.7*	*71.6–77.8*	*74.0–80.8*
Parental education						
School	76.5	76.4	78.8	77.3	75.1	75.8
	74.4–78.5	*71.2–80.9*	*74.6–82.4*	*73.2–81.0*	*71.2–78.5*	*70.9–80.0*
Vocational training	84.5	88.1	85.0	80.8	83.7	85.9
	82.8–86.1	*84.4–91.0*	*80.9–88.3*	*76.9–84.2*	*80.0–86.9*	*82.3–89.0*
Tertiary education	83.6	84.3	82.0	84.1	83.0	84.7
	82.4–84.7	*81.7–86.5*	*79.8–84.1*	*81.9–86.1*	*80.6–85.1*	*82.3–86.8*
Household income						
Low	73.7	75.4	75.2	74.3	70.4	74.3
	71.9–75.5	*70.2–80.0*	*71.1–78.9*	*70.8–77.5*	*66.7–73.9*	*70.2–78.0*
Medium	83.7	83.6	81.5	82.8	84.1	85.9
	82.5–84.8	*80.6–86.3*	*78.6–84.0*	*80.1–85.1*	*81.8–86.2*	*83.4–88.1*
High	88.1	89.4	89.0	87.2	88.5	86.8
	86.8–89.4	*86.3–91.8*	*86.4–91.2*	*84.0–89.8*	*85.8–90.7*	*83.3–89.6*
Residential location						
Major city	80.7	82.4	80.5	79.7	79.8	81.3
	79.4–82.0	*79.7–84.9*	*78.0–82.8*	*77.4–81.9*	*77.5–82.0*	*78.5–83.8*
Inner regional	84.8	85.5	83.7	86.0	82.0	87.0
	83.2–86.3	*81.7–88.6*	*80.0–86.8*	*82.6–88.7*	*78.5–85.1*	*83.9–89.6*
Outer regional	83.3	81.6	87.1	83.8	83.9	80.6
	80.8–85.6	*76.0–86.1*	*83.2–90.1*	*79.4–87.4*	*79.4–87.5*	*75.3–85.0*
Remote/Very remote	80.7	80.8	84.5	82.1	87.3	73.8
	70.7–87.9	*47.8–95.1*	*77.5–89.7*	*74.3–87.8*	*73.6–94.5*	*51.7–88.1*
Reason for the dental visit						
Check-up	82.9	83.8	83.5	82.7	81.9	82.8
	81.8–83.9	*81.6–85.7*	*81.5–85.4*	*80.8–84.5*	*80.0–83.6*	*80.5–84.9*
Dental problem	77.5	79.3	76.4	77.3	76.2	79.1
	75.3–79.5	*73.9–83.7*	*72.3–80.0*	*73.0–81.2*	*71.8–80.1*	*73.7–83.6*

Row 1: Proportions were computed using weighted data.
Row 2: 95% CI: Confidence intervals for estimates were computed using weighted data.
Columns are arranged by age at time of Survey.

6.4 Patterns of dental service use by state in the Australian child population

Table 6-10 presents patterns of dental service use by state in the Australian child population.

Overall, 57.3% of Australian children had made their first dental visit before the age of 5 years. The lowest proportion was among children from Queensland (49.8%) and the highest was among children from Tasmania (75.1%). In addition, higher proportions of children from South Australia (68.7%), Australian Capital Territory (67.4%) and Victoria (64.7%) had made their first dental visit before the age of 5 years compared to the Australian child population.

Nearly 11% of Australian children had never made a dental visit. While the lowest percentage was among children from Western Australia (7.3%) the highest was among children from New South Wales (15.6%). There were no differences between the proportions of children from other states/territories who had never made a dental visit and the corresponding national estimate.

Overall, 86.7% of Australian children had made their first dental visit for a check-up. The highest proportion was among Tasmanian children (92.9%) and the lowest was among children from Northern Territory (82.4%). A higher percentage of South Australian children (90.4%) had also made their first dental visit for a check-up compared to the Australian child population.

Among all Australian children, 20.9% had an irregular dental visiting pattern. The highest proportion was among children from Queensland (27.3%) while the lowest was among South Australian children (11.3%). Lower proportions of children from Tasmania (14%) and Western Australia (15.4%) had also shown an irregular dental visiting pattern compared to the corresponding national estimate.

Almost 81% of Australian children had visited a dental provider within the last 12 months. Despite the highest proportion being among Victorian and Western Australian children (83.8% each) and the lowest being among children from Northern Territory (74.6%), there were no differences between the national estimate and these proportions. However, higher proportions of South Australian children (83.4%) and a lower proportion of children from Queensland (76.4%) visited a dental provider within the last 12 months compared to the Australian child population.

Overall, 80.2% of Australian children had made their last dental visit for a check-up: the highest proportion was among South Australian children (85.1%) and the lowest was among children from Northern Territory (73.8%). Higher proportions of Western Australian children (84.8%) had also last visited for a check-up compared to the corresponding national estimate.

Nearly 57% of Australian children's most recent dental visit was at a private-practice location. The highest proportion was among children from New South Wales, which was about 3.4 times the proportion of Children from Northern Territory, who comprised the lowest proportion. A higher proportion of Victorian children (65.7%) and lower proportions of children from Tasmania (25.9%) and Western Australia (28.7%) had also

Oral health of Australian children

visited a private practice at their most recent dental visit compared to the Australian child population.

Overall, the percentage of guardians/parents attending with their child at the most recent dental visit was 84.1%: the highest was among South Australians (93.4%) while the lowest was among Queenslanders (67.8%). In addition, higher proportions of guardians/parents from Victoria (91.2%), Tasmania (90.5%), New South Wales (89.2%) and Australian Capital Territory (88.1%) were attending with their child at the most recent dental visit compared to the national estimate.

Almost 82% of parents/guardians of Australian children reported excellent/good dental care for their child at the most recent dental visit. While the highest proportion was among Tasmanians (87.4%) the lowest was among Queenslanders (77.6%). A higher proportion of South Australians also reported excellent/good dental care for their child at the most recent dental visit (86.3%) compared to the Australian child population.

In summary, the patterns of dental service use by Australian children varied across the states and territories. Most of the negative patterns were seen among children from Northern Territory.

Table 6-10: Patterns of dental service use by state/territory in the Australian child population

	Aus	ACT	NSW	NT	Qld	SA	Tas	Vic	WA
Population: children aged 5–14 years									
First dental visit <5 years old	57.3	67.4	53.7	55.0	49.8	68.7	75.1	64.7	54.0
	55.8-58.7	64.4-70.2	50.5-57.0	48.2-61.6	47.2-52.4	65.7-71.5	70.6-79.1	61.7-67.6	50.8-57.2
Never had a dental visit	11.3	10.3	15.6	8.1	9.3	8.7	8.1	10.3	7.3
	10.2-12.5	8.1-13.1	13.0-18.6	5.4-12.1	8.0-10.9	7.2-10.4	6.0-11.0	8.6-12.1	5.8-9.2
First dental visit for a check-up	86.7	88.5	84.5	82.4	85.7	90.4	92.9	87.9	89.4
	85.8-87.7	86.8-89.9	82.0-86.8	75.0-87.9	84.0-87.2	88.4-92.1	91.0-94.5	86.0-89.5	87.4-91.1
Irregular dental visiting pattern	20.9	19.4	22.3	25.9	27.3	11.3	14.0	18.6	15.4
	19.7-22.1	16.5-22.6	19.8-24.9	20.5-32.1	25.0-29.7	9.4-13.5	11.1-17.5	16.2-21.3	13.2-17.7
Last dental visit ≤12 months	81.1	78.5	81.0	74.6	76.4	83.4	82.9	83.8	83.8
	80.1-82.1	75.6-81.1	79.1-82.8	68.0-80.3	73.6-79.0	81.3-85.4	79.9-85.6	82.0-85.5	80.9-86.3
Last dental visit for a check	80.2	81.0	78.1	73.8	78.7	85.1	81.6	81.0	84.8
	79.1-81.2	78.0-83.6	75.4-80.5	66.5-80.1	76.7-80.6	83.3-86.8	78.9-84.1	78.9-83.0	82.6-86.7
Dental visiting in the private sector	56.8	50.8	72.7	21.7	43.9	51.7	25.9	65.7	28.7
	54.6-58.9	43.5-58.1	68.8-76.3	16.2-28.4	40.1-47.9	46.8-56.6	20.8-31.7	62.1-69.2	25.2-32.4
Guardians' attendance at child recent dental visit	84.1	88.1	89.2	76.0	67.8	93.4	90.5	91.2	79.5
	83.0-85.1	86.0-89.9	87.7-90.6	67.7-82.7	65.1-70.5	92.0-94.5	88.1-92.4	89.9-92.3	75.1-83.2
Parental reporting excellent/good dental care	81.8	83.1	80.8	79.4	77.6	86.3	87.4	84.5	82.9
	80.8-82.8	80.9-85.2	78.6-82.9	71.2-85.7	75.7-79.5	83.9-88.5	83.9-90.2	82.4-86.5	80.5-85.1

Row 1: Proportions were computed using weighted data.
Row 2: 95% CI: Confidence intervals for estimates were computed using weighted data.
Columns are arranged by age at time of Survey.

Oral health of Australian children

Summary

Patterns of dental service use were described using a range of measures related to first dental visit, usual dental visit pattern, and the most recent dental visit.

First dental visit

The percentage of Australian children who first visited a dental provider before the age of 5 years was related to Indigenous identity, parental education, household income and reason for last dental visit.

The percentage of children who have never visited a dental provider in the Australian child population was associated with age group, parental education and household income.

The percentage of Australian children who first visited a dental provider for a check-up was related to Indigenous status, parents' country of birth, parental education, household income and reason for the last dental visit.

Usual dental visit pattern

The percentage of Australian children who usually have an irregular dental visiting pattern was related to Indigenous identity, parental education, household income and reason for the last dental visit.

Most recent dental visit

The percentage of Australian children who visited a dental provider within the last 12 months was related to Indigenous status, parental education and household income.

Indigenous status, parental education and household income were related to the percentage of children who last visited a dental provider for a check-up in the Australian child population.

The percentage of children whose most recent dental visit was at a private-practice location was related to Indigenous status, parental education, household income, residential location and reason for last dental visit.

The percentage of parents or guardians attending with their child at the most recent dental visit in the Australian child population was related to Indigenous status and reason for last dental visit.

The percentage of parents reporting excellent or very good dental care for their child at the most recent dental visit in the Australian child population was related to Indigenous status, parents' country of birth, household income and reason for last dental visit.

The percentage of parents reporting excellent or very good dental care for their child at the most recent dental visit in the Australian child population was related to Indigenous status, parents' country of birth, household income and reason for last dental visit.

Conclusions

The majority of Australian children displayed a pattern of dental service use indicative of adequate access to dental care. Most children had accessed dental care recently, with 81.1% visiting within the last 12 months. The type of dental visit accessed at the last dental visit was favourable to prevention and early detection of dental problems, with 80.2% having a check-up visit. The dental care received by Australian children was rated as very good or excellent by 81.8% of parents or guardians.

However, despite the generally good levels of access to dental care by the majority of Australian children, there remained a substantial proportion of children (20.9%) that had an irregular pattern of dental visiting. Furthermore, many of the measures of dental service use were associated with lower socioeconomic status, particularly Indigenous status, parental education and household income.

References

Crocombe LA, Broadbent JM, Thomson WM, Brennan DS & Poulton R 2012. Impact of dental visiting trajectory patterns on clinical oral health and oral health-related quality of life. J Pub Health Dent 72:36-44.

Jones K & Tomar SL 2005. Estimated impact of competing policy recommendations for age of first dental visit. Pediatrics 115:906–14.

Leplege A & Hunt S 1997. The problem of quality of life in medicine. JAMA 278:45–50.

Riley P, Worthington HV, Clarkson JE & Beirne PV 2013. Recall intervals for oral health in primary care patients. Cochrane Database Syst Rev Dec;19(12): CD004346.

Roberts-Thomson K, Brennan DS & Spencer AJ 1995. Social inequality in the use and comprehensiveness of dental services. Aust J Pub Health 19:80–5.

Tsakos G, Allen PF & Steele JG 2013. What has oral health related quality of life ever done for us? Community Dent Health 30:66–7.

7 Australian children's oral health behaviours

JM Armfield, S Chrisopoulos, KG Peres, KF Roberts-Thomson and AJ Spencer

7.1 Patterns of toothbrushing practices

Brushing teeth with toothpaste is a widely adopted oral health behaviour in Australia (Slade et al. 2006). There is evidence that more than 90% of Australian children brush their teeth at least once a day (McLellan et al. 1999; Armfield & Spencer 2012) and that almost all children do so with a toothpaste containing fluoride (Armfield & Spencer 2012; Slade et al. 1995). Toothbrushes and fluoride toothpaste are readily available throughout the country and dental and other health authorities recommend brushing.

A great deal of evidence over a number of decades has found that regularly brushing children's teeth with fluoridated toothpaste reduces the risk of dental decay (Marinho et al. 2003a; Walsh et al. 2010). Toothbrushing not only removes plaque, which consists mostly of bacteria and is a risk factor for oral disease, but can be used to apply fluoride to the teeth via the application of toothpaste.

Australia's fluoride guidelines advise that brushing with fluoridated toothpaste commence from the age of 18 months (Australian Research Centre for Population Oral Health 2012). Table 7-1 shows the percentages of children who indicated that they had commenced brushing their teeth before the age of 18 months, by both the child's current age and various demographic and socioeconomic characteristics. The data are based on the recollection of the reporting parent, so parents of older children were having to recall the age of first brushing from further in their past than were parents of younger children. Overall, just over one-third of children commenced brushing with toothpaste before 18 months of age. There was little variation in reported early brushing commencement by child age at the time of the study.

Children were more likely to brush with toothpaste prior to 18 months if their parents were Australian born (36.0%) compared to those with an overseas-born parent (30.3%). In addition, the percentage of children brushing early was higher for those children whose parents had vocational (37.1%) or tertiary education (35.5%) than for those whose parents had no schooling beyond high school (29.2%). There was an income gradient in early-child toothbrushing. The lowest percentage was shown for children from the lowest household incomes (28.7%), followed by children from a medium household income (35.6%), with the highest percentage for children from families with a high household income (38.3%). Finally, those children who lived outside of a Major city, especially those from an Inner regional (38.0%) or Outer regional area (39.3%), were significantly more likely to have commenced toothbrushing early than were children who resided in a Major city (31.8%).

Table 7-1: Percentage of children who first brushed teeth with toothpaste before the age of 18 months in the Australian child population

	Population: children aged 5–14 years					
	All ages	5–6	7–8	9–10	11–12	13–14
All	33.8	35.7	34.7	33.0	33.3	32.3
	32.6–35.0	*33.7–37.8*	*32.5–37.1*	*31.0–35.0*	*31.4–35.2*	*30.0–34.6*
Sex						
Male	32.8	35.9	33.9	31.2	31.9	31.0
	31.4–34.3	*33.2–38.7*	*30.9–37.0*	*28.7–33.9*	*29.3–34.6*	*27.8–34.5*
Female	34.8	35.5	35.7	34.7	34.8	33.5
	33.3–36.4	*32.8–38.3*	*32.8–38.8*	*31.6–38.0*	*32.3–37.4*	*30.1–37.1*
Indigenous identity						
Non-Indigenous	34.1	36.1	34.8	33.6	33.4	32.3
	32.8–35.3	*34.1–38.2*	*32.4–37.3*	*31.6–35.8*	*31.5–35.5*	*29.9–34.7*
Indigenous	31.9	31.6	37.1	25.3	33.0	32.0
	27.2–37.0	*23.1–41.4*	*28.7–46.4*	*18.2–34.0*	*23.8–43.8*	*22.4–43.4*
Parents' country of birth						
Australian born	36.0	38.1	37.7	34.4	35.5	34.1
	34.7–37.3	*35.8–40.6*	*35.0–40.4*	*32.1–36.8*	*33.2–37.9*	*31.3–37.0*
Overseas born	30.3	31.8	29.9	30.8	29.7	29.0
	28.3–32.3	*28.6–35.3*	*26.3–33.8*	*27.4–34.4*	*26.5–33.1*	*25.4–32.9*
Parental education						
School	29.2	30.9	30.1	28.9	28.3	28.1
	27.2–31.3	*27.1–35.0*	*26.2–34.5*	*25.1–33.0*	*24.8–32.0*	*24.0–32.6*
Vocational training	37.1	41.5	39.2	35.4	37.1	33.1
	35.0–39.3	*36.8–46.2*	*34.2–44.4*	*31.2–39.8*	*33.0–41.5*	*28.3–38.3*
Tertiary education	35.5	36.8	35.9	34.8	35.5	34.5
	34.0–37.1	*34.1–39.6*	*33.0–39.0*	*31.7–37.9*	*33.1–38.1*	*31.6–37.5*
Household income						
Low	28.7	30.8	28.6	27.3	30.2	26.4
	26.8–30.5	*27.4–34.4*	*25.1–32.2*	*24.0–30.8*	*27.1–33.5*	*22.8–30.4*
Medium	35.6	39.4	35.6	35.9	32.9	34.0
	33.9–37.2	*36.4–42.6*	*32.3–39.0*	*32.9–38.9*	*29.9–36.1*	*30.3–37.8*
High	38.3	39.5	40.9	36.5	38.9	35.3
	36.3–40.3	*35.5–43.7*	*36.8–45.1*	*32.3–40.9*	*35.0–42.9*	*31.4–39.4*
Residential location						
Major city	31.8	34.2	31.8	30.8	32.0	30.1
	30.3–33.4	*31.6–36.8*	*28.9–34.8*	*28.3–33.3*	*29.5–34.5*	*27.2–33.2*
Inner regional	38.0	39.8	40.7	36.9	38.7	33.9
	35.9–40.1	*36.3–43.3*	*36.4–45.1*	*32.8–41.2*	*35.4–42.2*	*29.8–38.2*
Outer regional	39.3	41.6	42.3	39.9	33.3	39.4
	36.5–42.1	*36.8–46.7*	*37.6–47.2*	*34.8–45.1*	*28.2–38.9*	*33.9–45.2*
Remote/Very remote	35.0	26.5	41.1	35.4	23.0	48.8
	27.7–43.2	*19.7–34.6*	*26.0–58.1*	*25.5–46.7*	*13.9–35.5*	*32.9–64.9*
Reason for last dental visit						
Check-up	35.4	38.9	38.0	34.8	34.7	32.3
	34.1–36.8	*36.3–41.7*	*35.3–40.9*	*32.3–37.3*	*32.5–37.0*	*29.7–34.9*
Dental problem	33.4	33.3	32.5	32.9	33.3	35.3
	31.0–35.9	*28.3–38.7*	*28.2–37.2*	*28.8–37.4*	*28.8–38.1*	*29.8–41.2*

Row 1: Proportions were computed using weighted data.
Row 2: 95% CI: Confidence intervals for estimates were computed using weighted data.
Columns are arranged by age at time of Survey.

Because it is recommended that children commence brushing their teeth at approximately 2 years of age (Australian Research Centre for Population Oral Health 2012), it can be argued that fitting a 6-month window either side of this recommended age provides an approximate age range (vis-à-vis, 18–30 months) whereby brushing commencement could be considered to be consistent with the current recommendation.

Table 7-2 shows the percentages of children who were reported by their parents to have commenced toothbrushing between the age of 18 and 30 months. Overall, only about two in five children commenced brushing their teeth in this acceptable age range. There was little difference in recalled brushing commencement age by the age of the child at the time of the study.

Non-Indigenous children were significantly more likely to commence brushing between 18 and 30 months of age (40.6%) than were Indigenous children (31.6%). Also, a lower percentage of children with an overseas born parent commenced brushing between 18 and 30 months (36.0%) than did children of Australian born parents (42.4%). Children from both medium (42.5%) and high income families (42.0%) were more likely to commence brushing at the 'acceptable' age range than were children from low income families (36.4%).

There were no significant differences in the commencement of toothbrushing between 18 and 30 months of age by sex of the child, residential location or reason for last dental visit.

Table 7-2: Percentage of children who first brushed teeth with toothpaste between the age of 18 and 30 months in the Australian child population

	Population: children aged 5–14 years					
	All ages	5–6	7–8	9–10	11–12	13–14
All	40.1	41.6	40.3	41.3	38.0	39.3
	38.9–41.2	*39.4–43.8*	*38.2–42.4*	*39.2–43.4*	*36.0–40.0*	*37.1–41.6*
Sex						
Male	39.9	39.6	40.4	41.8	38.4	39.6
	38.5–41.5	*36.8–42.5*	*37.2–43.7*	*38.8–44.8*	*35.6–41.3*	*36.4–42.9*
Female	40.2	43.6	40.1	40.8	37.5	39.0
	38.8–41.7	*40.7–46.6*	*37.3–42.9*	*37.9–43.7*	*34.9–40.2*	*35.9–42.2*
Indigenous identity						
Non-Indigenous	40.6	42.1	40.8	41.9	38.7	39.6
	39.4–41.8	*39.9–44.3*	*38.6–43.1*	*39.8–44.0*	*36.6–40.9*	*37.3–42.0*
Indigenous	31.6	35.2	33.3	34.6	24.2	31.1
	27.1–36.6	*26.5–44.9*	*25.8–41.7*	*26.0–44.5*	*17.9–31.9*	*21.5–42.7*
Parents' country of birth						
Australian born	42.4	43.5	41.9	44.0	41.0	41.3
	41.0–43.7	*41.0–46.1*	*39.4–44.5*	*41.5–46.6*	*38.5–43.6*	*38.2–44.5*
Overseas born	36.0	37.9	37.4	36.8	32.8	35.4
	34.4–37.7	*34.2–41.7*	*34.1–40.9*	*33.5–40.2*	*29.7–36.0*	*32.1–38.8*
Parental education						
School	37.3	39.2	36.3	40.1	33.8	37.6
	35.2–39.6	*35.1–43.3*	*32.4–40.4*	*35.6–44.8*	*30.1–37.8*	*33.0–42.5*
Vocational training	40.6	39.7	39.5	42.4	40.6	40.8
	38.3–43.0	*35.2–44.4*	*34.7–44.4*	*37.9–46.9*	*36.0–45.3*	*35.3–46.5*
Tertiary education	41.8	43.5	42.8	42.0	40.1	40.2
	40.3–43.2	*40.6–46.5*	*39.9–45.8*	*39.3–44.8*	*37.5–42.8*	*37.6–42.9*
Household income						
Low	36.4	38.3	35.7	37.5	32.5	37.9
	34.4–38.3	*34.5–42.2*	*32.1–39.5*	*33.5–41.6*	*29.3–35.9*	*33.6–42.3*
Medium	42.5	42.9	44.2	43.5	42.4	39.7
	40.8–44.2	*39.8–46.0*	*41.1–47.3*	*40.4–46.6*	*39.2–45.7*	*35.8–43.7*
High	42.0	43.2	40.3	44.1	40.7	41.8
	40.0–44.1	*39.1–47.3*	*36.0–44.7*	*39.6–48.7*	*36.8–44.6*	*38.1–45.6*
Residential location						
Major city	39.8	41.8	40.7	41.2	37.0	38.1
	38.2–41.3	*38.9–44.6*	*37.9–43.5*	*38.5–44.0*	*34.3–39.8*	*35.2–41.1*
Inner regional	41.6	42.2	39.8	42.0	38.5	45.5
	39.6–43.6	*38.6–45.8*	*36.3–43.4*	*38.2–46.0*	*35.4–41.7*	*41.3–49.7*
Outer regional	39.1	36.7	38.5	40.5	42.5	37.2
	36.3–42.0	*31.2–42.6*	*33.8–43.6*	*36.1–45.0*	*37.6–47.5*	*32.8–41.8*
Remote/Very remote	40.6	49.6	39.2	39.5	43.7	31.1
	34.2–47.4	*33.7–65.6*	*29.0–50.5*	*26.1–54.7*	*32.9–55.0*	*17.2–49.6*
Reason for last dental visit						
Check-up	40.7	41.4	40.3	41.5	39.6	40.9
	39.4–42.0	*38.5–44.2*	*37.8–42.9*	*39.0–44.0*	*37.3–42.0*	*38.3–43.5*
Dental problem	38.7	38.2	42.3	41.2	35.9	34.5
	36.2–41.3	*32.4–44.4*	*37.5–47.4*	*36.6–46.1*	*31.5–40.6*	*28.9–40.6*

Row 1: Proportions were computed using weighted data.
Row 2: 95% CI: Confidence intervals for estimates were computed using weighted data.
Columns are arranged by age at time of Survey.

Table 7-3 shows children who were late with the commencement of toothbrushing. It would be expected that all children would have commenced brushing their teeth with toothpaste by the age of 30 months. However, just over one-quarter of all children in the study had not started brushing their teeth by that age. There was a tendency for a higher percentage of parents of older children to recall late brushing commencement for their children (28.7% and 28.4% of 11–12-year-old and 13–14-year-old children, respectively) than for parents of younger children (22.7% of children aged 5–6 years). Whether this demonstrates changes in late brushing commencement over time or reflects recall error/bias by the parents cannot be determined.

For Indigenous children, 36.5% of parents reported that their child had not commenced brushing by age 30 months. This can be compared to 25.3% of children who identified as non-Indigenous. A consistent pattern was shown for children from socioeconomically disadvantaged backgrounds, with a higher prevalence of delayed toothbrushing compared to children from less disadvantaged backgrounds. Higher prevalence was found for children who had a parent born overseas (33.7%) compared to those with Australian-born parents (21.7%), those whose parents had school-only education (33.4%) compared to those with vocational training (22.3%) or a tertiary education (22.7%), and who were from a low income household (35.0%) compared to children from a medium (21.9%) or high income family (19.7%). There was also an association between reason for last dental visit and late brushing commencement, with children who last visited for a dental problem having a higher percentage reporting late brushing commencement (27.9%) than did children who last visited the dentist for a check-up (23.9%).

Table 7-3: Percentage of children who first brushed teeth with toothpaste at age 30 months or later in the Australian child population

	Population: children aged 5–14 years					
	All ages	5–6	7–8	9–10	11–12	13–14
All	26.1	22.7	25.0	25.8	28.7	28.4
	24.7–27.6	*20.6–25.0*	*22.7–27.5*	*23.5–28.2*	*26.6–31.0*	*25.9–31.0*
Sex						
Male	27.2	24.5	25.7	27.0	29.7	29.4
	25.5–29.0	*21.7–27.5*	*22.6–29.1*	*24.2–30.1*	*26.9–32.7*	*25.9–33.1*
Female	24.9	20.9	24.2	24.5	27.7	27.4
	23.3–26.7	*18.3–23.7*	*21.5–27.2*	*21.8–27.5*	*25.0–30.7*	*24.0–31.2*
Indigenous identity						
Non-Indigenous	25.3	21.8	24.4	24.5	27.8	28.1
	23.9–26.8	*19.7–24.1*	*22.0–26.9*	*22.3–26.9*	*25.7–30.1*	*25.5–30.8*
Indigenous	36.5	33.3	29.7	40.1	42.7	36.9
	31.1–42.2	*24.0–44.0*	*22.8–37.5*	*30.2–50.9*	*32.8–53.3*	*26.7–48.4*
Parents' country of birth						
Australian born	21.7	18.3	20.4	21.6	23.5	24.6
	20.4–23.0	*16.3–20.6*	*18.2–22.8*	*19.3–24.0*	*21.2–25.9*	*21.9–27.5*
Overseas born	33.7	30.3	32.7	32.4	37.5	35.6
	31.2–36.3	*26.3–34.6*	*28.5–37.1*	*28.5–36.6*	*34.0–41.3*	*30.9–40.5*
Parental education						
School	33.4	29.9	33.6	31.0	37.9	34.3
	30.7–36.3	*25.6–34.6*	*28.8–38.7*	*26.4–36.1*	*33.6–42.5*	*29.1–39.8*
Vocational training	22.3	18.8	21.3	22.3	22.3	26.1
	20.3–24.4	*15.2–23.1*	*17.3–26.1*	*18.6–26.4*	*18.7–26.3*	*21.1–31.8*
Tertiary education	22.7	19.7	21.2	23.2	24.4	25.3
	21.3–24.1	*17.4–22.1*	*18.7–24.0*	*20.8–25.9*	*21.9–27.0*	*22.5–28.4*
Household income						
Low	35.0	30.9	35.8	35.3	37.3	35.8
	32.6–37.5	*27.0–35.1*	*31.1–40.6*	*31.0–39.8*	*33.5–41.3*	*31.2–40.6*
Medium	21.9	17.7	20.2	20.7	24.7	26.3
	20.4–23.5	*15.1–20.7*	*17.5–23.3*	*18.1–23.5*	*21.6–28.0*	*22.9–30.0*
High	19.7	17.3	18.9	19.4	20.5	22.9
	18.1–21.5	*14.4–20.7*	*15.7–22.5*	*16.1–23.3*	*17.3–24.0*	*18.9–27.5*
Residential location						
Major city	28.4	24.1	27.6	28.1	31.0	31.8
	26.5–30.5	*21.3–27.1*	*24.4–30.9*	*25.0–31.3*	*28.2–34.1*	*28.4–35.4*
Inner regional	20.4	18.1	19.5	21.1	22.8	20.7
	18.8–22.2	*15.1–21.5*	*16.5–23.0*	*17.8–24.7*	*19.5–26.4*	*17.4–24.4*
Outer regional	21.7	21.7	19.1	19.7	24.2	23.3
	18.7–24.9	*16.8–27.5*	*15.4–23.5*	*15.3–24.9*	*18.8–30.7*	*19.4–27.8*
Remote/Very remote	24.4	23.9	19.7	25.1	33.4	20.2
	16.5–34.4	*14.2–37.5*	*10.9–32.8*	*11.4–46.7*	*25.5–42.3*	*12.0–31.8*
Reason for last dental visit						
Check-up	23.9	19.7	21.6	23.8	25.7	26.9
	22.6–25.2	*17.6–22.1*	*19.4–24.1*	*21.5–26.2*	*23.4–28.2*	*24.1–29.9*
Dental problem	27.9	28.5	25.1	25.8	30.8	30.2
	25.1–30.9	*22.7–35.0*	*20.9–29.9*	*21.4–30.9*	*26.3–35.7*	*24.7–36.3*

Row 1: Proportions were computed using weighted data.
Row 2: 95% CI: Confidence intervals for estimates were computed using weighted data.
Columns are arranged by age at time of Survey.

Australia's fluoride guidelines recommend that teeth should be brushed twice a day from the age of 18 months (Australian Research Centre for Population Oral Health 2012). By age 2–3 years, all children should be brushing their teeth twice a day. However, Table 7-4 shows that only about one-half of all children were brushing the recommended two times per day on average. There was a trend for parents of older children to recall their child brushing twice a day at age 2–3 (55.2% of parents of 13–14 year olds) in comparison to parents of younger children at the time of the study (44.7% of parents with children aged 5–6 years of age).

Children who were identified as Indigenous were considerably less likely to be reported as brushing their teeth twice a day at age 2–3 years (37.5%) than were non-Indigenous children (50.4%). The percentage was also lower for children of parents with school-only education (43.4%) than for children whose parents had either vocational training (50.8%) or a tertiary education (52.9%).

A strong gradient was seen in toothbrushing frequency at age 2–3 years by household income. The percentage of children reported as brushing their teeth twice a day at age 2–3 increased from 42.7% for children from low household incomes, to 50.3% for children from a medium household income family, to 55.4% for children from families with the highest household income.

Children who last visited a dentist because of a dental problem were less likely to have been brushing their teeth at age 2–3 (44.8%) than were children who last visited the dentist for a check-up (53.6%).

Table 7-4: Percentage of children who brushed their teeth at least twice a day with toothpaste at age 2–3 years in the Australian child population

	Population: children aged 5–14 years					
	All ages	5–6	7–8	9–10	11–12	13–14
All	49.7	44.7	46.6	50.0	52.3	55.2
	48.4–51.0	*42.4–47.0*	*44.5–48.7*	*47.6–52.3*	*50.1–54.5*	*52.5–57.7*
Sex						
Male	48.6	42.8	43.7	51.7	51.6	54.0
	47.0–50.2	*39.7–45.9*	*40.8–46.6*	*48.5–54.9*	*48.4–54.9*	*50.3–57.7*
Female	50.8	46.8	49.8	48.3	53.0	56.3
	49.2–52.4	*43.8–49.8*	*46.7–52.9*	*45.2–51.4*	*50.2–55.8*	*52.8–59.7*
Indigenous identity						
Non-Indigenous	50.4	45.7	47.4	50.8	52.9	55.4
	49.2–51.6	*43.4–47.9*	*45.2–49.6*	*48.5–53.1*	*50.7–55.1*	*52.8–58.0*
Indigenous	37.5	30.0	34.2	33.9	44.3	47.3
	32.6–42.6	*21.1–40.8*	*25.8–43.8*	*26.2–42.5*	*34.6–54.5*	*35.3–59.7*
Parents' country of birth						
Australian born	49.3	43.8	45.7	49.2	52.9	55.3
	47.9–50.7	*41.0–46.5*	*43.2–48.2*	*46.4–52.1*	*50.3–55.5*	*52.2–58.4*
Overseas born	50.4	46.6	48.3	51.1	51.4	54.9
	48.4–52.4	*42.9–50.2*	*43.9–52.8*	*47.4–54.8*	*47.6–55.1*	*50.9–58.8*
Parental education						
School	43.4	36.9	38.6	44.2	46.3	50.5
	41.3–45.5	*32.9–41.1*	*34.4–43.0*	*39.5–49.0*	*42.2–50.5*	*45.6–55.5*
Vocational training	50.8	48.9	46.8	48.6	53.0	56.4
	48.5–53.2	*44.1–53.7*	*41.9–51.7*	*43.7–53.5*	*48.4–57.7*	*51.6–61.0*
Tertiary education	52.9	47.5	50.3	53.9	55.8	57.6
	51.3–54.4	*44.6–50.5*	*47.5–53.1*	*50.9–56.9*	*52.8–58.7*	*54.1–61.1*
Household income						
Low	42.7	37.2	38.9	41.7	45.7	49.8
	40.8–44.7	*33.4–41.1*	*35.2–42.8*	*37.6–46.0*	*42.1–49.4*	*45.5–54.1*
Medium	50.3	48.3	48.6	50.3	52.7	51.7
	48.6–52.1	*44.9–51.8*	*45.2–52.1*	*47.0–53.7*	*49.3–56.1*	*47.9–55.6*
High	55.4	49.6	50.4	58.2	57.3	62.6
	53.2–57.5	*45.6–53.7*	*46.1–54.7*	*53.7–62.5*	*53.1–61.5*	*57.5–67.5*
Residential location						
Major city	50.1	45.9	46.4	50.7	52.6	55.3
	48.4–51.7	*43.0–48.7*	*43.6–49.2*	*47.7–53.7*	*49.7–55.4*	*51.7–58.8*
Inner regional	50.4	43.2	49.1	49.0	53.4	57.0
	48.2–52.6	*38.5–48.1*	*45.3–53.0*	*44.2–53.8*	*49.2–57.7*	*53.2–60.8*
Outer regional	46.3	43.4	41.2	48.6	47.3	50.4
	43.6–49.1	*38.1–48.8*	*36.1–46.6*	*43.0–54.2*	*41.9–52.8*	*44.6–56.2*
Remote/Very remote	47.8	28.6	52.9	44.3	56.3	58.1
	41.1–54.6	*20.0–39.2*	*39.3–66.0*	*33.9–55.1*	*41.6–70.0*	*41.4–73.2*
Reason for last dental visit						
Check-up	53.6	51.9	50.5	52.9	54.7	56.8
	52.3–54.9	*49.2–54.6*	*48.0–53.1*	*50.3–55.4*	*52.2–57.1*	*54.0–59.7*
Dental problem	44.8	38.6	43.8	44.5	47.9	48.3
	42.1–47.5	*33.0–44.5*	*39.0–48.7*	*39.6–49.6*	*42.5–53.4*	*41.6–55.1*

Row 1: Proportions were computed using weighted data.
Row 2: 95% CI: Confidence intervals for estimates were computed using weighted data.
Columns are arranged by age at time of Survey.

As noted previously, Australia's fluoride guidelines recommend that teeth should be brushed twice a day from the age of 18 months (Australian Research Centre for Population Oral Health 2012). In addition, teeth should be brushed at least twice a day from the age of 6 years onwards.

Just over two-thirds of children in the study brushed their teeth at least twice a day (Table 7-5). There was a slight increase in the percentage of children reported to be brushing twice daily by child age, with just under two-thirds of children aged 5–6 years brushing twice daily (66.4%) compared to 71.3% of those aged 13–14 years.

There were a number of differences in toothbrushing frequency across demographic and socioeconomic characteristics. Across all age groups, children were more likely to brush their teeth twice a day if they were female (71.1%) than if they were male (66.0%). However, within the two–year age groups, the percentages of male and female children brushing twice daily only differed significantly for the 13–14-year age group, with 13% more female (77.8%) than male children (64.8%) brushing twice a day or more.

Across all age groups except for those aged 13–14 years, non-Indigenous children were more likely to brush their teeth twice a day than their Indigenous counterparts. The difference in percentages was greatest for the 11–12-year age group, with 69.3% of non-Indigenous children and only 44.8% of Indigenous children brushing twice daily or more. Across all age groups combined, 69.5% of non-Indigenous children and 53.5% of Indigenous children brushed at least twice a day.

While approximately two-thirds (66.5%) of Australian born children brushed their teeth at least twice a day, the percentage was higher for children who had overseas-born parents (72.1%). There were also strong socioeconomic gradients in brushing frequency. Brushing twice a day was practiced by 75.0% of children whose parents had a university education, compared to 59.4% of children whose parents had no more than high-school-only education. Similarly, 78.0% of children from high income families brushed their teeth at least twice a day, compared to 69.6% of children from a medium income family and 58.7% of children from a low income family. These social gradients are also observable across all two-year age groups.

Finally, children who had last visited the dentist for a check-up were more likely to brush their teeth at least twice a day (72.6%) compared to children who had last visited the dentist for a dental problem (64.5%).

Table 7-5: Percentage of children who currently brush their teeth at least twice a day with toothpaste in the Australian child population

	Population: children aged 5–14 years					
	All ages	5–6	7–8	9–10	11–12	13–14
All	68.5	66.4	68.4	68.6	67.8	71.3
	67.2–69.8	*64.1–68.6*	*66.0–70.8*	*66.6–70.6*	*65.7–69.8*	*68.7–73.7*
Sex						
Male	66.0	65.4	66.0	67.9	65.8	64.8
	64.4–67.6	*62.4–68.4*	*62.6–69.3*	*65.1–70.7*	*62.9–68.7*	*61.3–68.2*
Female	71.1	67.4	71.1	69.3	69.9	77.8
	69.6–72.6	*64.6–70.2*	*68.2–73.8*	*66.4–72.1*	*67.1–72.6*	*74.5–80.8*
Indigenous identity						
Non-Indigenous	69.5	67.2	69.7	69.8	69.3	71.4
	68.2–70.7	*64.9–69.4*	*67.2–72.1*	*67.7–71.8*	*67.2–71.3*	*68.8–73.9*
Indigenous	53.5	59.2	48.5	52.1	44.8	66.7
	48.2–58.7	*48.7–68.9*	*39.1–58.1*	*43.4–60.7*	*36.1–53.8*	*55.1–76.6*
Parents' country of birth						
Australian born	66.5	65.7	66.0	66.7	65.4	68.8
	65.0–68.0	*62.9–68.4*	*63.2–68.7*	*64.1–69.1*	*62.8–67.9*	*65.6–71.7*
Overseas born	72.1	68.4	72.7	72.2	71.8	75.6
	70.0–74.2	*64.8–71.8*	*68.4–76.6*	*68.5–75.7*	*68.4–74.9*	*71.4–79.4*
Parental education						
School	59.4	55.8	60.5	58.3	58.0	64.2
	57.1–61.6	*51.7–59.9*	*56.2–64.7*	*53.6–62.9*	*54.0–62.0*	*59.2–68.9*
Vocational training	67.0	68.4	65.0	66.4	67.8	67.1
	64.9–68.9	*64.0–72.5*	*60.1–69.6*	*62.3–70.4*	*63.5–71.8*	*62.1–71.7*
Tertiary education	75.0	72.0	74.5	75.8	74.7	78.3
	73.6–76.3	*69.1–74.8*	*71.8–77.0*	*73.2–78.3*	*71.8–77.3*	*75.1–81.1*
Household income						
Low	58.7	58.1	60.2	56.3	56.5	62.6
	56.9–60.6	*54.3–61.8*	*55.9–64.4*	*52.6–60.0*	*53.0–59.9*	*58.3–66.8*
Medium	69.6	69.3	68.1	70.4	71.1	69.0
	67.9–71.3	*66.3–72.1*	*64.4–71.7*	*67.3–73.4*	*68.0–74.1*	*65.1–72.6*
High	78.0	73.7	77.6	79.7	77.4	82.3
	76.1–79.8	*69.1–77.8*	*73.8–80.9*	*76.0–82.9*	*73.8–80.7*	*78.3–85.6*
Residential location						
Major city	69.0	66.2	68.4	69.0	68.7	72.8
	67.3–70.6	*63.2–69.1*	*65.1–71.5*	*66.4–71.4*	*66.0–71.3*	*69.5–75.9*
Inner regional	67.3	67.4	69.7	65.7	65.5	68.1
	64.8–69.6	*63.2–71.3*	*65.4–73.7*	*61.5–69.7*	*61.7–69.1*	*63.3–72.6*
Outer regional	67.9	67.2	66.2	71.3	67.4	67.4
	64.7–70.8	*62.3–71.7*	*60.6–71.4*	*65.6–76.4*	*61.5–72.8*	*62.1–72.2*
Remote/Very remote	67.9	62.1	69.2	71.3	63.7	72.7
	58.1–76.4	*50.3–72.5*	*58.8–78.0*	*53.3–84.4*	*50.7–75.0*	*61.3–81.8*
Reason for last dental visit						
Check-up	72.6	73.8	73.7	71.6	71.3	72.8
	71.2–73.9	*71.1–76.3*	*71.1–76.1*	*69.1–73.9*	*69.1–73.5*	*70.1–75.4*
Dental problem	64.5	62.3	66.1	64.9	62.3	66.8
	62.0–67.0	*56.0–68.3*	*61.2–70.7*	*60.0–69.5*	*57.5–67.0*	*60.7–72.4*

Row 1: Proportions were computed using weighted data.
Row 2: 95% CI: Confidence intervals for estimates were computed using weighted data.
Columns are arranged by age at time of Survey.

Current recommendations for toothpaste use in Australia are for children to use low-fluoride toothpaste up to the age of 6 years, and thereafter standard-strength fluoride toothpaste (Australian Research Centre for Population Oral Health 2012). The rationale for this recommendation comes from studies indicating that early exposure to standard-fluoride toothpaste is a risk factor for dental fluorosis, a mottling of the teeth. Low fluoride children's toothpaste is readily available in Australia and no children should be using standard fluoride toothpaste at age 2–3 years.

Table 7-6 shows the percentages of children reported to be brushing their teeth with standard fluoride toothpaste at age 2–3 years. Overall, the percentages of children brushing with standard fluoride toothpaste at an early age was low. Nonetheless, almost 9% of parents reported that their children were using standard fluoride toothpaste at that age. Parents of older children, who had the longest recall interval, reported higher use of standard fluoride toothpaste (14.2% of children aged 13–14 years at the time of the study) compared to parents of younger children (4.9% of children aged 5–6 years of age at the time of the study).

A higher percentage of Indigenous than non-Indigenous children were reported by their parents to be using a standard fluoride toothpaste at age 2–3. This difference was more than threefold for children aged 7–8 years at the time of the study, with 18.9% of Indigenous children and only 5.7% of non-Indigenous children reported to be using standard fluoride toothpaste at age 2–3 years.

Differences were also seen in early use of standard fluoride toothpaste by other child and parent characteristics. Children of overseas-born parents were more likely to be brushing with a standard fluoride toothpaste at age 2–3 years (10.0%) than were children of Australian-born parents (7.8%). The percentage was also higher for children whose parents had school-level education (11.2%) than for children whose parents had received vocational training (7.4%) or had a tertiary education (7.4%). Children at age 2–3 years were more likely to brush their teeth with a standard fluoride toothpaste if they came from a low income household (11.0%) compared to if they came from a medium (8.1%) or high income household (6.5%).

Finally, a higher percentage of children who had last visited the dentist for a dental problem were brushing with standard fluoride toothpaste at age 2–3 years (11.8%), compared to children who last visited the dentist for a check-up (7.7%).

Table 7-6: Percentage of children who brushed their teeth with standard fluoridated toothpaste at age 2–3 years in the Australian child population

	Population: children aged 5–14 years					
	All ages	5–6	7–8	9–10	11–12	13–14
All	8.6	4.9	6.4	7.3	10.4	14.2
	8.0–9.3	*4.1–5.9*	*5.3–7.8*	*6.4–8.4*	*9.2–11.7*	*12.4–16.1*
Sex						
Male	9.0	4.6	6.2	7.3	10.8	16.3
	8.1–9.9	*3.5–6.0*	*4.6–8.2*	*6.0–8.9*	*9.0–12.8*	*13.8–19.2*
Female	8.3	5.3	6.7	7.3	10.0	12.0
	7.5–9.1	*4.1–6.7*	*5.4–8.4*	*6.0–8.9*	*8.5–11.7*	*9.8–14.6*
Indigenous identity						
Non-Indigenous	8.2	4.6	5.7	6.9	9.8	13.9
	7.6–8.8	*3.8–5.5*	*4.6–6.9*	*6.0–8.0*	*8.6–11.2*	*12.1–15.9*
Indigenous	15.5	7.9	18.9	15.2	17.7	18.7
	11.6–20.4	*3.9–15.2*	*10.2–32.3*	*9.8–22.7*	*12.0–25.4*	*11.6–28.9*
Parents' country of birth						
Australian born	7.8	4.3	6.0	7.0	9.0	12.8
	7.1–8.5	*3.3–5.6*	*4.7–7.7*	*5.8–8.4*	*7.7–10.5*	*11.0–14.9*
Overseas born	10.0	5.9	7.1	7.9	12.7	16.5
	8.9–11.2	*4.6–7.6*	*5.2–9.5*	*6.4–9.6*	*10.2–15.7*	*13.3–20.4*
Parental education						
School	11.2	6.4	8.6	9.0	12.8	18.8
	9.8–12.8	*4.6–8.9*	*5.9–12.2*	*6.8–11.9*	*10.0–16.1*	*15.5–22.7*
Vocational training	7.4	4.6	5.4	6.7	7.4	12.2
	6.3–8.6	*3.0–6.9*	*3.5–8.5*	*5.0–9.0*	*5.5–10.0*	*9.0–16.2*
Tertiary education	7.4	4.1	5.7	6.3	9.7	11.6
	6.6–8.2	*3.2–5.4*	*4.3–7.4*	*5.1–7.7*	*8.1–11.7*	*9.5–14.1*
Household income						
Low	11.0	6.5	8.8	9.6	13.5	16.8
	9.8–12.4	*4.8–8.7*	*6.5–11.7*	*7.7–11.9*	*10.9–16.6*	*13.6–20.5*
Medium	8.1	4.9	4.9	6.8	8.5	15.3
	7.2–9.1	*3.7–6.3*	*3.5–6.9*	*5.5–8.4*	*6.8–10.7*	*12.5–18.6*
High	6.5	2.5	5.6	5.2	8.5	11.1
	5.5–7.6	*1.4–4.3*	*3.7–8.4*	*3.6–7.3*	*6.4–11.4*	*8.3–14.6*
Residential location						
Major city	8.1	4.7	6.2	6.0	10.2	13.9
	7.4–9.0	*3.8–6.0*	*4.8–7.8*	*5.0–7.2*	*8.6–12.0*	*11.6–16.7*
Inner regional	9.1	4.7	6.8	10.1	9.5	14.1
	7.9–10.3	*3.3–6.5*	*4.8–9.6*	*7.7–13.2*	*7.6–11.9*	*11.2–17.5*
Outer regional	10.8	6.7	8.6	10.4	11.9	15.8
	8.8–13.2	*4.0–10.9*	*4.7–15.0*	*7.6–14.0*	*9.5–14.8*	*12.0–20.6*
Remote/Very remote	8.9	4.9	2.5	7.2	16.6	13.8
	5.5–14.0	*1.9–12.4*	*0.8–7.6*	*3.4–14.5*	*7.5–32.8*	*5.8–29.2*
Reason for last dental visit						
Check-up	7.7	3.4	5.1	6.2	8.2	13.5
	7.0–8.4	*2.5–4.6*	*4.0–6.4*	*5.1–7.4*	*7.0–9.6*	*11.6–15.6*
Dental problem	11.8	8.2	7.7	9.6	17.2	16.7
	10.2–13.5	*5.7–11.6*	*5.0–11.7*	*7.3–12.6*	*13.4–21.7*	*12.6–21.9*

Row 1: Proportions were computed using weighted data.
Row 2: 95% CI: Confidence intervals for estimates were computed using weighted data.
Columns are arranged by age at time of Survey.

As noted above, the Australian fluoride guidelines recommend that children should use standard-strength fluoride toothpaste from the age of 6 years onwards (Australian Research Centre for Population Oral Health 2012). However, this study found only a gradual trend away from the use of low-fluoride children's toothpaste and towards standard fluoride toothpaste with increasing child age (Table 7-7). Rather than a large shift at the age group 7–8 years, the percentage of children using standard fluoride toothpaste increased steadily from 24.8% at ages 5–6 to 47.4% at ages 7–8, 74.7% at ages 9–10, 88.0% at ages 11–12 and 94.2% at ages 13–14 years. This indicates that many children are persisting in brushing their teeth with low-fluoride children's toothpaste long past the recommended age of usage cessation.

There were mostly few and small differences in standard fluoride toothpaste use by demographic or socioeconomic characteristics. However, children of overseas-born parents were less likely to be using standard fluoride toothpaste than were children of Australian-born parents, with these differences being significant for the four oldest age groups studied. Also, but only among children aged 7–8 and 9–10 years, the use of standard fluoride toothpaste was more prevalent among female (51.6% and 78.3%, respectively) than among male children (43.7% and 71.1%, respectively).

While there was no effect of Indigenous identity on standard fluoride toothpaste use across all ages, Indigenous children aged 5–6 and 7–8 years were more likely to use standard fluoride toothpaste than were non-Indigenous children. Similarly, and especially around the cut-off age of 5–6 years, a socioeconomic effect could be observed in standard fluoride toothpaste use. The percentage of children using standard fluoride toothpaste at age 5–6 years was highest for those whose parents had school-level education and who were from the lowest household income category.

Also at age 5–6 years, those children who had last visited a dentist for a dental problem were more likely to be using a standard fluoride toothpaste (31.7%) than were those children who last visited the dentist for a check-up (22.6%).

Table 7-7: Percentage of children who currently brush their teeth with standard fluoridated toothpaste in the Australian child population

	Population: children aged 5–14 years					
	All ages	5–6	7–8	9–10	11–12	13–14
All	65.6	24.8	47.4	74.7	88.0	94.2
	64.0–67.1	*22.9–26.8*	*45.4–49.4*	*72.7–76.5*	*86.3–89.4*	*92.9–95.2*
Sex						
Male	63.9	24.6	43.7	71.1	87.9	94.1
	62.1–65.6	*22.2–27.2*	*40.9–46.6*	*68.4–73.7*	*85.6–89.9*	*92.2–95.6*
Female	67.4	25.0	51.6	78.3	88.1	94.2
	65.5–69.2	*22.4–27.7*	*48.8–54.3*	*75.6–80.7*	*86.0–89.9*	*92.2–95.7*
Indigenous identity						
Non-Indigenous	65.5	24.3	46.7	74.5	88.0	94.1
	63.8–67.0	*22.4–26.3*	*44.7–48.7*	*72.5–76.4*	*86.4–89.5*	*92.8–95.2*
Indigenous	68.6	32.2	59.1	77.5	87.9	94.9
	64.2–72.6	*23.7–42.0*	*49.5–68.0*	*70.2–83.4*	*81.5–92.3*	*84.5–98.5*
Parents' country of birth						
Australian born	67.4	25.8	50.1	76.7	90.4	95.6
	65.8–69.0	*23.6–28.1*	*47.6–52.6*	*74.5–78.8*	*88.3–92.1*	*94.3–96.6*
Overseas born	62.4	23.1	42.6	71.2	84.0	91.6
	60.0–64.8	*20.1–26.4*	*39.5–45.8*	*67.8–74.3*	*81.2–86.4*	*88.7–93.8*
Parental education						
School	67.6	31.2	49.6	76.2	86.8	91.9
	65.4–69.7	*27.3–35.4*	*45.4–53.7*	*71.7–80.2*	*83.6–89.4*	*88.8–94.2*
Vocational training	67.4	24.2	43.8	78.3	90.4	95.6
	65.0–69.6	*20.8–28.1*	*38.8–49.0*	*74.4–81.7*	*87.0–93.0*	*93.1–97.3*
Tertiary education	63.9	21.6	47.4	72.3	88.2	95.3
	61.7–66.0	*19.1–24.4*	*45.1–49.8*	*69.4–75.0*	*86.2–90.0*	*93.7–96.5*
Household income						
Low	66.1	28.3	50.1	72.6	85.2	92.6
	63.9–68.2	*24.9–31.9*	*46.5–53.7*	*69.2–75.8*	*82.0–88.0*	*89.7–94.7*
Medium	65.9	23.8	44.3	77.3	88.1	95.5
	64.0–67.7	*21.1–26.7*	*41.0–47.6*	*74.6–79.9*	*85.5–90.4*	*93.6–96.8*
High	65.1	21.7	48.0	75.1	91.4	95.6
	62.4–67.7	*17.9–26.1*	*44.0–51.9*	*70.8–79.0*	*89.1–93.2*	*93.3–97.2*
Residential location						
Major city	64.2	23.8	45.5	73.5	87.0	93.8
	62.1–66.2	*21.5–26.2*	*43.0–48.0*	*70.8–76.0*	*84.8–89.0*	*92.1–95.2*
Inner regional	68.1	26.4	50.6	75.7	91.0	94.9
	65.4–70.6	*22.3–31.0*	*46.8–54.5*	*72.4–78.8*	*88.5–93.0*	*92.4–96.6*
Outer regional	70.5	28.2	55.3	80.9	87.6	94.6
	67.6–73.2	*22.3–34.9*	*50.3–60.2*	*78.0–83.6*	*83.4–90.9*	*92.3–96.2*
Remote/Very remote	65.8	28.0	45.8	74.4	89.5	94.6
	59.0–71.9	*21.6–35.4*	*35.7–56.2*	*66.7–80.8*	*82.5–93.9*	*75.3–99.0*
Reason for last dental visit						
Check-up	68.8	22.6	46.7	74.6	89.2	94.5
	67.0–70.5	*20.2–25.3*	*44.3–49.1*	*72.3–76.7*	*87.5–90.7*	*93.1–95.6*
Dental problem	68.0	31.7	49.3	77.2	84.9	92.9
	65.8–70.1	*27.0–36.9*	*45.3–53.3*	*73.5–80.6*	*80.3–88.6*	*89.1–95.4*

Row 1: Proportions were computed using weighted data.
Row 2: 95% CI: Confidence intervals for estimates were computed using weighted data.
Columns are arranged by age at time of Survey.

Especially in young children, the aim of brushing is to get sufficient exposure to fluoride toothpaste to prevent decay, without excessive exposure which would increase the risk of dental fluorosis in vulnerable populations (Creeth et al. 2013). The amount of toothpaste applied to the brush is an important determinant of fluoride exposure. In Australia, as in most countries, the recommendation is that children should use a pea-sized amount of fluoride toothpaste on their toothbrush when brushing (Australian Research Centre for Population Oral Health 2012), based on the idea that children are brushing their teeth twice daily.

At age 2–3 years, too much fluoride toothpaste increases the risk of dental fluorosis, whereas too little fluoride toothpaste is not as effective for decay prevention. Table 7-8 indicates that just under 40% of children were reported to use a pea-sized amount of toothpaste at age 2–3 years. Non-Indigenous children were more likely to use a pea-sized amount (39.1%) than were Indigenous children (32.6%). Children with a parent born overseas were also more likely to use a pea-sized amount of toothpaste (41.3%) than children whose parents were born in Australia (37.5%), although this difference was only small.

No significant associations were found between toothpaste quantity and parental education, household income, residential location and reason for last dental visit.

Table 7-8: Percentage of children who used a pea-sized amount of toothpaste when brushing their teeth at age 2–3 years in the Australian child population

	Population: children aged 5–14 years					
	All ages	5–6	7–8	9–10	11–12	13–14
All	38.8	35.5	39.0	41.5	37.9	40.1
	37.9–39.7	33.7–37.4	37.1–40.9	39.4–43.6	35.8–40.1	37.7–42.6
Sex						
Male	38.3	34.9	39.1	41.0	37.4	39.5
	37.1–39.6	32.2–37.7	36.5–41.8	38.1–43.9	34.6–40.3	36.5–42.6
Female	39.3	36.2	38.9	42.1	38.4	40.8
	37.8–40.7	33.4–39.0	35.9–42.0	39.1–45.1	35.4–41.5	37.4–44.2
Indigenous identity						
Non-Indigenous	39.1	35.6	39.6	41.9	38.5	40.1
	38.2–40.1	33.7–37.6	37.7–41.6	39.7–44.0	36.3–40.8	37.7–42.5
Indigenous	32.6	31.2	29.6	36.5	28.9	39.1
	28.2–37.4	23.0–40.9	22.0–38.4	27.9–45.9	21.4–37.8	28.4–50.9
Parents' country of birth						
Australian born	37.5	33.6	37.4	40.5	36.0	40.0
	36.2–38.7	31.3–35.9	35.0–40.0	37.9–43.2	33.5–38.6	37.0–43.1
Overseas born	41.3	38.7	42.2	43.6	41.7	40.3
	39.7–42.9	35.3–42.2	38.8–45.7	40.3–47.0	38.1–45.5	36.5–44.2
Parental education						
School	38.6	36.5	38.8	41.2	37.5	39.0
	36.6–40.6	32.4–40.9	34.6–43.2	37.0–45.7	33.7–41.6	33.8–44.4
Vocational training	37.4	35.2	37.4	42.3	34.9	37.1
	35.2–39.7	31.1–39.5	32.8–42.2	37.9–46.9	30.4–39.7	32.0–42.5
Tertiary education	39.4	34.8	39.9	41.3	39.7	42.0
	38.2–40.7	32.4–37.3	37.4–42.4	38.6–44.1	36.7–42.9	39.1–45.0
Household income						
Low	38.1	36.0	38.0	40.1	36.9	39.7
	36.4–39.9	32.5–39.8	34.4–41.7	36.1–44.3	33.4–40.6	35.4–44.2
Medium	37.7	34.4	37.8	39.5	37.4	39.6
	36.2–39.3	31.6–37.3	34.8–40.9	36.4–42.7	34.2–40.6	35.8–43.4
High	40.5	35.4	40.5	46.0	40.7	40.8
	38.7–42.4	31.6–39.4	36.8–44.3	42.0–50.1	36.5–45.1	36.4–45.4
Residential location						
Major city	38.4	35.2	38.0	41.2	38.9	39.1
	37.2–39.6	32.9–37.6	35.6–40.4	38.5–44.0	36.0–41.8	35.9–42.3
Inner regional	39.5	35.7	41.9	42.6	36.1	41.3
	37.6–41.4	32.1–39.5	37.5–46.4	38.8–46.5	32.4–39.9	37.0–45.7
Outer regional	39.2	40.6	39.7	39.5	35.8	40.3
	36.7–41.6	34.6–46.8	35.5–44.0	35.4–43.7	30.4–41.6	36.1–44.7
Remote/Very remote	42.5	24.2	42.0	49.1	37.4	60.6
	34.2–51.2	18.1–31.6	32.5–52.0	30.6–67.8	28.5–47.2	43.3–75.6
Reason for last dental visit						
Check-up	38.8	36.3	38.8	41.3	38.0	39.3
	37.7–40.0	33.9–38.8	36.5–41.1	39.1–43.5	35.5–40.5	36.8–42.0
Dental problem	39.5	34.2	38.7	41.6	37.6	44.9
	37.2–41.8	28.7–40.2	34.6–42.9	36.7–46.7	33.0–42.4	38.3–51.8

Row 1: Proportions were computed using weighted data.
Row 2: 95% CI: Confidence intervals for estimates were computed using weighted data.
Columns are arranged by age at time of Survey.

Across all age groups, only 55.9% of children used a pea-sized amount of toothpaste (Table 7-9). In general, the percentage of children using a pea-sized amount of toothpaste declined across age groups, from 64.1% of 5–6 year olds to 43.8% of 13–14 year olds. Across all age groups, fewer Indigenous children used a pea-sized amount of toothpaste compared to their non-Indigenous counterparts. Although these differences can also be seen in the two-year age groups, because there were relatively few Indigenous children, the wide confidence intervals around the estimates for the two-year age groups make comparisons within age-groups statistically non-significant.

Children from lower income households and whose parents had less schooling were less likely to use a pea-sized amount of toothpaste. Differences in toothpaste quantity across parental education categories are observable from when children are aged 7–8 years. In relation to household income, differences in the use of a pea-sized amount of toothpaste are observable for children aged 9–10, 11–12 and 13–14 years.

Children who last visited the dentist for a problem were also less likely to be using a pea-sized amount of toothpaste, although this difference was relatively small.

Table 7-9: Percentage of children who currently use a pea-sized amount of toothpaste when brushing their teeth in the Australian child population

	Population: children aged 5–14 years					
	All ages	5–6	7–8	9–10	11–12	13–14
All	55.9	64.1	63.0	58.3	50.2	43.8
	54.8–56.9	*62.0–66.1*	*61.1–64.9*	*56.3–60.3*	*48.1–52.3*	*41.5–46.0*
Sex						
Male	55.5	65.0	62.6	57.1	50.0	42.3
	54.0–57.0	*62.0–67.9*	*59.7–65.5*	*54.1–60.0*	*47.2–52.9*	*39.2–45.5*
Female	56.3	63.1	63.5	59.6	50.3	45.2
	54.8–57.7	*60.1–65.9*	*60.9–66.0*	*56.7–62.5*	*47.5–53.2*	*41.5–49.0*
Indigenous identity						
Non-Indigenous	56.5	64.1	63.8	59.3	50.9	44.5
	55.4–57.5	*62.0–66.2*	*61.8–65.7*	*57.2–61.3*	*48.8–53.1*	*42.2–46.8*
Indigenous	45.3	58.6	53.0	43.6	38.8	27.0
	40.9–49.8	*48.2–68.2*	*44.4–61.4*	*35.5–51.9*	*30.4–47.9*	*18.5–37.8*
Parents' country of birth						
Australian born	56.2	63.3	64.8	58.5	50.6	44.0
	55.0–57.4	*60.8–65.8*	*62.4–67.1*	*56.0–60.9*	*48.0–53.1*	*41.2–46.8*
Overseas born	55.3	65.0	60.2	58.1	49.8	43.7
	53.7–57.0	*61.7–68.1*	*56.9–63.5*	*54.6–61.5*	*46.2–53.4*	*39.5–48.0*
Parental education						
School	49.5	62.1	56.0	47.7	45.3	37.1
	47.4–51.5	*57.9–66.1*	*52.0–60.0*	*43.0–52.4*	*41.3–49.4*	*32.8–41.7*
Vocational training	57.0	64.7	66.2	59.6	50.8	45.3
	54.9–59.0	*60.3–68.9*	*61.4–70.7*	*55.1–63.8*	*46.5–55.1*	*40.0–50.7*
Tertiary education	59.1	64.2	65.6	63.6	53.7	47.4
	57.6–60.6	*61.2–67.1*	*63.0–68.2*	*60.7–66.4*	*50.9–56.5*	*44.2–50.7*
Household income						
Low	50.7	62.6	59.9	50.1	45.0	37.2
	48.9–52.5	*58.9–66.1*	*56.4–63.4*	*46.5–53.6*	*41.3–48.7*	*33.3–41.2*
Medium	57.9	66.9	65.4	58.7	52.7	46.0
	56.4–59.3	*63.9–69.7*	*62.3–68.3*	*55.6–61.8*	*49.4–56.0*	*42.5–49.6*
High	59.3	61.9	64.7	66.3	54.8	48.6
	57.2–61.4	*57.8–65.8*	*60.5–68.7*	*62.2–70.1*	*50.4–59.0*	*44.3–52.9*
Residential location						
Major city	55.8	63.7	62.0	58.2	49.9	44.6
	54.5–57.1	*61.1–66.2*	*59.4–64.6*	*55.7–60.8*	*47.1–52.6*	*41.5–47.7*
Inner regional	56.3	65.5	65.7	58.2	49.5	43.6
	54.4–58.3	*61.3–69.5*	*62.7–68.6*	*53.9–62.4*	*45.8–53.2*	*39.6–47.7*
Outer regional	55.0	63.9	64.8	55.6	53.3	39.8
	52.1–57.8	*59.5–68.1*	*60.4–68.9*	*51.4–59.7*	*48.1–58.4*	*35.1–44.6*
Remote/Very remote	58.3	63.8	62.5	71.2	51.3	40.1
	50.6–65.7	*53.5–72.9*	*49.7–73.7*	*53.8–84.0*	*37.9–64.6*	*28.7–52.7*
Reason for last dental visit						
Check-up	56.6	65.1	65.1	60.3	52.2	45.1
	55.4–57.8	*62.0–68.1*	*62.6–67.6*	*58.0–62.6*	*49.8–54.6*	*42.5–47.7*
Dental problem	52.8	65.4	59.9	55.1	45.6	37.5
	50.3–55.2	*59.8–70.7*	*55.5–64.2*	*50.5–59.6*	*40.6–50.7*	*31.9–43.5*

Row 1: Proportions were computed using weighted data.
Row 2: 95% CI: Confidence intervals for estimates were computed using weighted data.
Columns are arranged by age at time of Survey.

One risk factor for dental fluorosis is the eating or licking of toothpaste (Do & Spencer 2007). Children who eat fluoride toothpaste may be exposing themselves to more than the recommended intake of fluoride, increasing the likelihood of developing dental fluorosis. Australia's fluoride guidelines specifically state that, 'Young children should not be permitted to lick or eat toothpaste' (Australian Research Centre for Population Oral Health 2012).

Some toothpastes are more flavoursome and have increased appeal with younger children, and this might be encouraging children to consume toothpaste other than what is required for toothbrushing.

Among all children, 50.9% were reported by their parents to have never eaten or licked toothpaste at age 2–3 years. Parents of older children were more likely to report their child not eating or licking toothpaste at age 2–3 (61.3% of children aged 13–14 at the time of the study) than were parents of younger children (35.7% of children aged 5–6 at the time of the study).

Overall, a higher percentage of non-Indigenous children did not consume toothpaste at age 2–3 years (51.3%) than did Indigenous children (43.3%). This difference, however, was only evident in the recall of parents of older children and there were no significant differences in the recalled toothpaste consumption at age 2–3 years for the youngest three age groups.

There was also a trend for a greater percentage of children from higher income households to not be eating or licking toothpaste at age 2–3 years, compared to children from lower income households at that age. Significant differences could be seen for children who were aged 9–10, 11–12 and 12–13 years at the time of the study.

Table 7-10: Percentage of children who never ate or licked toothpaste at age 2–3 years in the Australian child population

	Population: children aged 5–14 years					
	All ages	5–6	7–8	9–10	11–12	13–14
All	50.9	35.7	47.1	53.5	57.8	61.3
	49.8–52.0	*33.9–37.6*	*45.0–49.1*	*51.2–55.8*	*55.7–59.9*	*59.0–63.6*
Sex						
Male	50.7	36.7	46.6	53.5	57.9	60.2
	49.3–52.2	*34.0–39.4*	*43.8–49.4*	*50.4–56.5*	*54.8–60.9*	*56.7–63.6*
Female	51.2	34.7	47.6	53.5	57.7	62.5
	49.8–52.6	*32.2–37.3*	*44.8–50.5*	*50.1–56.8*	*55.0–60.4*	*59.6–65.3*
Indigenous identity						
Non-Indigenous	51.3	35.8	47.3	53.3	58.8	62.0
	50.2–52.4	*33.9–37.7*	*45.3–49.4*	*50.9–55.7*	*56.6–60.9*	*59.5–64.3*
Indigenous	43.3	32.8	44.7	54.9	41.5	44.2
	38.9–47.8	*24.5–42.3*	*35.9–53.9*	*46.0–63.5*	*33.1–50.5*	*32.3–56.8*
Parents' country of birth						
Australian born	51.5	35.4	47.2	54.2	58.6	63.1
	50.2–52.8	*32.9–38.0*	*44.9–49.5*	*51.6–56.8*	*56.0–61.1*	*60.1–66.0*
Overseas born	49.7	36.0	46.8	52.4	56.3	57.4
	47.9–51.5	*32.9–39.2*	*43.3–50.3*	*48.7–56.1*	*52.6–59.9*	*53.5–61.3*
Parental education						
School	52.1	38.8	52.3	52.1	55.5	61.6
	50.0–54.1	*34.9–42.7*	*48.3–56.3*	*47.0–57.2*	*51.3–59.6*	*57.0–66.0*
Vocational training	49.1	30.2	44.2	54.1	60.0	56.0
	46.9–51.3	*26.0–34.8*	*39.3–49.2*	*49.7–58.3*	*55.3–64.6*	*50.7–61.2*
Tertiary education	51.2	36.0	46.3	54.1	58.1	63.7
	49.6–52.7	*33.4–38.6*	*43.6–49.1*	*50.9–57.3*	*55.3–60.8*	*60.5–66.8*
Household income						
Low	47.9	33.7	45.3	49.0	52.7	58.7
	45.9–49.8	*30.2–37.3*	*41.1–49.6*	*45.1–53.0*	*48.7–56.6*	*54.7–62.6*
Medium	50.5	35.1	47.8	53.0	56.6	60.4
	49.0–52.1	*32.1–38.2*	*44.7–50.9*	*49.2–56.7*	*53.3–59.8*	*56.9–63.8*
High	54.3	36.4	49.1	58.7	64.7	65.4
	52.1–56.5	*32.6–40.4*	*45.1–53.0*	*54.1–63.2*	*60.6–68.6*	*61.1–69.5*
Residential location						
Major city	51.2	37.2	47.7	53.3	57.8	61.1
	49.7–52.6	*34.9–39.6*	*45.1–50.4*	*50.3–56.3*	*55.0–60.6*	*58.0–64.2*
Inner regional	50.7	31.5	45.9	52.8	59.3	63.8
	48.5–52.9	*27.6–35.7*	*41.8–50.1*	*48.3–57.3*	*55.2–63.2*	*59.6–67.7*
Outer regional	50.9	34.8	49.0	52.6	56.8	59.3
	48.5–53.4	*31.1–38.8*	*44.9–53.1*	*47.8–57.4*	*51.5–61.9*	*54.1–64.3*
Remote/Very remote	46.1	29.7	30.7	66.2	49.2	55.1
	40.9–51.4	*22.4–38.1*	*20.9–42.7*	*52.7–77.5*	*39.0–59.4*	*43.1–66.5*
Reason for last dental visit						
Check-up	52.9	37.2	47.6	54.3	58.5	61.9
	51.6–54.1	*34.6–40.0*	*45.2–50.1*	*51.7–56.8*	*56.1–60.9*	*59.2–64.5*
Dental problem	49.5	34.6	44.2	51.0	55.5	61.0
	47.0–52.0	*29.4–40.1*	*39.6–48.9*	*46.4–55.6*	*50.4–60.6*	*54.8–66.8*

Row 1: Proportions were computed using weighted data.
Row 2: 95% CI: Confidence intervals for estimates were computed using weighted data.
Columns are arranged by age at time of Survey.

There is evidence that eating or licking toothpaste is relatively common, especially among the youngest children surveyed, with only 60.6% of children aged 5–6 years never eating or licking toothpaste (Table 7-11). Few older children, however, were believed to be still eating or licking toothpaste even a little bit.

Especially among younger age groups, children identified as Indigenous were more likely to be eating or licking toothpaste. However, there were few differences in the eating or licking of toothpaste by parent country of birth or parental education, household income, residential location or reason for child's last dental visit.

Table 7-11: Percentage of children who currently never eat or lick toothpaste in the Australian child population

	Population: children aged 5–14 years					
	All ages	5–6	7–8	9–10	11–12	13–14
All	81.3	60.7	75.3	85.4	91.4	94.2
	80.4–82.2	*58.8–62.5*	*73.5–77.0*	*84.0–86.7*	*90.3–92.4*	*93.0–95.2*
Sex						
Male	80.3	60.2	74.2	84.4	89.9	93.6
	79.2–81.4	*57.6–62.8*	*71.6–76.6*	*82.2–86.3*	*88.1–91.5*	*91.7–95.1*
Female	82.4	61.2	76.4	86.5	92.9	94.7
	81.1–83.5	*58.5–63.8*	*73.7–79.0*	*84.2–88.4*	*91.4–94.2*	*93.0–96.0*
Indigenous identity						
Non-Indigenous	81.8	61.0	75.9	85.9	91.9	94.5
	80.9–82.7	*59.0–62.9*	*74.1–77.6*	*84.4–87.3*	*90.8–92.8*	*93.3–95.5*
Indigenous	73.0	51.6	65.8	79.8	85.4	87.7
	68.7–76.9	*41.3–61.8*	*56.6–73.9*	*72.0–85.8*	*77.9–90.7*	*75.6–94.3*
Parents' country of birth						
Australian born	80.7	60.0	74.2	84.8	91.2	93.9
	79.6–81.7	*57.6–62.4*	*72.0–76.2*	*83.0–86.4*	*89.8–92.5*	*92.4–95.1*
Overseas born	82.4	61.5	77.2	86.8	91.8	94.6
	81.0–83.7	*57.9–65.0*	*74.1–80.0*	*84.5–88.8*	*90.0–93.3*	*92.4–96.2*
Parental education						
School	81.1	61.1	78.4	82.1	90.6	92.1
	79.4–82.6	*56.9–65.0*	*74.7–81.6*	*78.7–85.0*	*88.2–92.5*	*89.2–94.3*
Vocational training	80.2	56.1	73.0	85.2	91.1	93.4
	78.4–81.9	*51.3–60.8*	*68.5–77.1*	*82.0–87.9*	*88.5–93.2*	*90.3–95.6*
Tertiary education	82.2	61.6	76.0	87.5	92.2	95.9
	80.9–83.5	*59.0–64.2*	*73.6–78.3*	*85.7–89.1*	*90.7–93.5*	*94.5–97.0*
Household income						
Low	79.2	56.8	75.4	81.8	89.2	91.9
	77.5–80.7	*53.2–60.4*	*71.8–78.6*	*78.7–84.5*	*86.9–91.1*	*88.9–94.1*
Medium	81.8	60.5	75.0	86.7	91.6	94.8
	80.5–82.9	*57.5–63.4*	*72.4–77.4*	*84.5–88.6*	*89.6–93.1*	*92.8–96.3*
High	83.3	62.8	78.3	88.1	94.3	95.8
	81.5–84.9	*59.0–66.4*	*74.6–81.6*	*85.3–90.4*	*92.3–95.7*	*93.1–97.4*
Residential location						
Major city	82.1	62.1	76.8	86.5	91.5	94.8
	81.0–83.2	*59.7–64.4*	*74.6–78.8*	*84.8–88.1*	*90.1–92.7*	*93.2–96.0*
Inner regional	80.0	57.9	73.5	82.6	91.7	93.7
	78.1–81.8	*54.0–61.7*	*69.7–77.0*	*79.7–85.2*	*89.6–93.3*	*91.3–95.4*
Outer regional	79.7	54.5	74.3	83.2	91.0	92.0
	77.6–81.7	*50.7–58.2*	*69.7–78.3*	*80.0–86.0*	*87.8–93.4*	*87.7–94.8*
Remote/Very remote	75.8	65.1	52.1	86.2	86.9	91.5
	69.0–81.5	*57.2–72.3*	*36.1–67.8*	*70.7–94.1*	*69.3–95.1*	*77.4–97.1*
Reason for last dental visit						
Check-up	83.1	61.2	75.5	85.2	91.8	94.5
	82.1–84.1	*58.7–63.7*	*73.3–77.5*	*83.5–86.8*	*90.5–92.9*	*93.1–95.6*
Dental problem	81.9	62.9	76.6	84.1	90.2	93.1
	80.2–83.5	*57.3–68.2*	*72.5–80.3*	*80.7–87.0*	*87.0–92.6*	*89.1–95.7*

Row 1: Proportions were computed using weighted data.
Row 2: 95% CI: Confidence intervals for estimates were computed using weighted data.
Columns are arranged by age at time of Survey.

It is recommended that parents assist children aged up to 6 years of age with their toothbrushing (Australian Research Centre for Population Oral Health 2012). It is likely that the form of toothbrushing assistance changes for children of different ages, moving from manual assistance for younger children to verbal reminders for older children. However, information was not collected on the type of parental assistance.

Overall, 87.0% of parents helped their children aged 5–6 years in some way with their toothbrushing, and about half (50.6%) still assisted in some way when their children were aged 9–10 years (Table 7-12).

Especially for the older age groups, male children were more likely to be helped in some way with toothbrushing than were female children and children from families with lower household incomes were more likely to be helped than were children from high household incomes.

There were few and small differences in parental assistance by parental education, residential location and reason for child's last dental visit.

Table 7-12: Percentage of children whose parents currently help in some way with toothbrushing in the Australian child population

| | Population: children aged 5–14 years | | | | | |
	All ages	5–6	7–8	9–10	11–12	13–14
All	48.7	87.0	68.9	46.3	26.7	14.3
	47.1–50.3	*85.3–88.5*	*67.0–70.8*	*44.3–48.3*	*24.9–28.5*	*12.8–16.0*
Sex						
Male	51.8	88.2	71.1	50.6	30.7	16.9
	49.9–53.6	*85.7–90.3*	*68.3–73.8*	*47.9–53.2*	*28.1–33.5*	*14.7–19.4*
Female	45.5	85.7	66.5	42.0	22.3	11.7
	43.5–47.5	*83.5–87.7*	*64.0–68.9*	*39.3–44.7*	*20.1–24.7*	*9.8–14.0*
Indigenous identity						
Non-Indigenous	48.4	86.9	68.7	46.2	26.3	14.2
	46.7–50.0	*85.1–88.4*	*66.7–70.6*	*44.2–48.3*	*24.5–28.1*	*12.7–15.9*
Indigenous	54.2	87.9	73.1	49.2	33.5	15.7
	49.5–58.9	*81.2–92.4*	*63.9–80.6*	*40.3–58.1*	*24.5–43.9*	*9.2–25.5*
Parents' country of birth						
Australian born	48.7	87.5	70.3	45.9	25.7	13.5
	47.0–50.5	*85.5–89.2*	*67.9–72.6*	*43.4–48.4*	*23.6–28.0*	*11.7–15.5*
Overseas born	48.5	86.0	66.3	47.0	28.1	15.7
	46.2–50.8	*82.8–88.6*	*63.1–69.4*	*43.7–50.4*	*25.2–31.3*	*12.9–18.9*
Parental education						
School	49.5	88.7	67.7	50.5	28.8	15.5
	47.0–51.9	*85.7–91.2*	*63.3–71.8*	*45.9–55.1*	*25.5–32.5*	*12.5–19.0*
Vocational training	48.2	86.4	68.6	47.2	26.2	17.0
	45.7–50.6	*82.7–89.4*	*64.0–72.9*	*42.8–51.7*	*22.6–30.3*	*13.5–21.1*
Tertiary education	48.1	86.3	69.3	43.6	24.8	11.5
	46.1–50.1	*83.7–88.5*	*66.7–71.8*	*40.8–46.5*	*22.5–27.3*	*9.8–13.4*
Household income						
Low	51.1	87.7	70.9	51.0	32.3	16.8
	48.8–53.4	*84.9–90.0*	*67.3–74.2*	*47.1–54.9*	*29.1–35.7*	*13.9–20.2*
Medium	47.9	87.5	69.1	45.1	25.0	13.7
	45.9–50.0	*85.1–89.6*	*66.1–72.0*	*41.5–48.8*	*22.5–27.6*	*11.4–16.3*
High	46.9	85.7	68.1	42.9	21.2	11.1
	44.4–49.5	*81.8–88.9*	*64.4–71.5*	*38.6–47.3*	*18.2–24.5*	*8.4–14.5*
Residential location						
Major city	48.5	86.4	68.7	45.8	26.0	13.8
	46.4–50.6	*84.1–88.4*	*66.2–71.1*	*43.3–48.4*	*23.9–28.4*	*11.8–16.0*
Inner regional	49.7	89.1	70.0	47.4	27.5	16.4
	46.7–52.6	*86.6–91.1*	*65.9–73.8*	*43.4–51.4*	*23.9–31.5*	*13.5–19.7*
Outer regional	48.1	87.9	69.2	49.2	27.9	13.7
	44.8–51.5	*84.5–90.7*	*65.0–73.2*	*43.4–54.9*	*23.4–32.8*	*11.1–16.8*
Remote/Very remote	47.8	84.8	65.3	38.8	32.4	15.1
	39.5–56.3	*72.6–92.2*	*57.8–72.2*	*28.5–50.1*	*22.9–43.6*	*7.7–27.7*
Reason for last dental visit						
Check-up	45.0	87.2	70.0	45.7	25.5	13.7
	43.2–46.8	*85.0–89.2*	*67.5–72.3*	*43.3–48.1*	*23.6–27.5*	*12.2–15.4*
Dental problem	48.9	87.6	68.8	48.2	28.5	13.7
	46.5–51.4	*82.7–91.2*	*64.5–72.7*	*43.9–52.4*	*24.0–33.5*	*10.3–18.0*

Row 1: Proportions were computed using weighted data.
Row 2: 95% CI: Confidence intervals for estimates were computed using weighted data.
Columns are arranged by age at time of Survey.

7.2 Patterns of other discretionary preventive behaviours

A high percentage of Australian children live in areas where the tap water contains an amount of fluoride that is beneficial for oral health. The process of adding fluoride compounds to public water supplies, termed water fluoridation, has long been hailed as an extremely important and effective public health measure for improving the oral health of both children and adults. Every Australian capital city had introduced fluoridated tap water by the 1970s with the exception of Brisbane, which commenced water fluoridation in late 2008. However, large areas of rural and remote Australia have not historically had fluoridated water. Throughout Queensland and elsewhere in rural Australia, children who could not obtain the benefits of consuming fluoridated water have frequently been recommended to use fluoride tablets or drops as a substitute for fluoridated water. However, the evidence for the effectiveness of fluoride supplements in the form of tablets or drops is quite limited, and there are studies showing that their consumption is associated with an increased risk of dental fluorosis (Australian Research Centre for Population Oral Health 2006). The Australian guidelines on the use of fluorides therefore recommended that tablets or drops that are chewed or swallowed, rather than mixed into drinking water at an optimum concentration, should not be consumed (Australian Research Centre for Population Oral Health 2012).

Given the high percentage of the Australian population with access to fluoridated public water, it is not surprising that only a low percentage of children had ever consumed fluoride tablets or drops (Table 7-13). Children from low income families and whose parents had the least schooling were less likely to have consumed fluoride tablets or drops. Children from Outer regional locations were almost twice as likely to have used fluoride tablets or drops compared to children from a Major city.

Table 7-13: Percentage of children who have used fluoride tablets or drops at any time in their life in the Australian child population

	Population: children aged 5–14 years					
	All ages	5–6	7–8	9–10	11–12	13–14
All	6.4	3.4	5.9	5.7	8.3	8.6
	5.8–7.0	2.7–4.3	5.0–7.0	4.9–6.7	7.2–9.5	7.4–9.9
Sex						
Male	6.2	3.2	6.3	6.1	7.6	8.1
	5.5–7.0	2.4–4.3	5.0–7.9	4.9–7.5	6.3–9.1	6.5–9.9
Female	6.5	3.6	5.4	5.4	9.0	9.1
	5.8–7.3	2.7–4.8	4.2–7.0	4.3–6.7	7.5–10.7	7.4–11.1
Indigenous identity						
Non-Indigenous	6.4	3.4	5.9	5.9	8.5	8.4
	5.8–7.1	2.7–4.3	4.9–7.0	5.0–7.0	7.4–9.8	7.2–9.8
Indigenous	4.7	3.7	5.0	2.4	4.7	8.7
	3.2–6.8	1.5–9.0	1.9–12.5	1.1–5.3	2.3–9.2	4.1–17.3
Parents' country of birth						
Australian born	6.9	3.3	6.8	5.9	9.8	9.0
	6.3–7.7	2.5–4.3	5.5–8.3	4.9–7.2	8.3–11.4	7.5–10.7
Overseas born	5.3	3.6	4.1	5.5	5.9	7.4
	4.6–6.1	2.5–5.1	3.0–5.6	4.2–7.1	4.7–7.4	5.8–9.5
Parental education						
School	4.6	2.1	3.2	3.7	7.1	6.7
	3.9–5.5	1.2–3.5	2.1–4.9	2.5–5.3	5.5–9.1	4.9–9.1
Vocational training	6.9	2.3	7.9	6.6	7.2	9.9
	5.9–8.0	1.4–3.9	5.7–10.9	4.9–8.9	5.5–9.4	7.5–12.9
Tertiary education	7.1	4.6	6.4	6.4	9.5	9.1
	6.3–8.1	3.5–5.9	5.2–7.9	5.2–7.9	7.9–11.3	7.5–11.1
Household income						
Low	4.9	2.1	4.5	4.8	6.3	6.9
	4.2–5.7	1.3–3.4	3.2–6.4	3.5–6.6	4.9–7.9	5.2–9.1
Medium	7.0	3.8	6.2	6.4	9.4	9.4
	6.2–7.9	2.8–5.0	4.8–8.0	5.0–8.0	7.7–11.4	7.5–11.6
High	7.1	4.5	6.5	6.2	9.1	9.5
	6.0–8.4	3.0–6.7	4.7–8.8	4.8–8.1	7.1–11.6	7.3–12.4
Residential location						
Major city	5.5	3.1	5.7	5.1	6.7	7.1
	4.9–6.3	2.3–4.1	4.6–7.1	4.1–6.3	5.5–8.2	5.7–8.8
Inner regional	8.1	4.4	6.5	6.8	11.6	10.7
	6.8–9.6	2.9–6.7	4.6–9.1	5.1–8.9	9.1–14.5	8.4–13.6
Outer regional	9.0	4.3	6.0	8.8	10.8	14.1
	7.5–10.8	2.9–6.3	3.7–9.4	5.8–13.2	8.3–14.0	10.8–18.3
Remote/Very remote	5.7	2.0	6.1	3.1	12.7	5.0
	3.2–9.9	0.6–6.5	1.5–22.4	1.1–8.8	5.5–26.6	2.2–11.0
Reason for last dental visit						
Check-up	7.4	4.7	6.8	6.3	9.2	8.9
	6.7–8.2	3.6–6.0	5.6–8.3	5.3–7.5	7.9–10.7	7.6–10.5
Dental problem	5.9	2.2	6.5	5.6	6.8	7.8
	4.9–7.0	1.2–4.1	4.5–9.3	4.0–7.9	4.8–9.5	5.3–11.3

Row 1: Proportions were computed using weighted data.
Row 2: 95% CI: Confidence intervals for estimates were computed using weighted data.
Columns are arranged by age at time of Survey.

Mouth rinses are liquid solutions, sometimes containing fluoride, which are promoted as contributing to better oral health. There is evidence that mouth rinses can be effective at killing oral bacteria involved in diseases of the gums and teeth. In particular, mouth rinses with added fluoride are beneficial in reducing dental decay (Marinho et al. 2003b). In this Study, parents were specifically asked whether or not their child used a fluoride mouth rinse.

The proportion of children who had ever used a fluoride mouth rinse was reasonably low, but increased relatively consistently across increasing age groups, from 10.9% of children aged 5–6 years to 45.6% of those aged 13–14 years (Table 7-14).

Children from high income households and whose parents had a tertiary education were less likely to have used a fluoride mouth rinse at any time in their life. Across all children, 25.9% of children from a high income household had ever used mouth rinse, compared to 33.0% of children from a low income household. Again, across all children, 27.6% of children whose parents had a tertiary education had ever used mouth rinse, compared to 33.7% of children whose parents had vocational training and 32.5% whose parents had school-level education.

Children who last visited the dentist for a dental problem were more likely to have ever used mouth rinse, although this difference was relatively small.

Table 7-14: Percentage of children who have used fluoride mouth rinse at any time in their life in the Australian child population

	Population: children aged 5–14 years					
	All ages	5–6	7–8	9–10	11–12	13–14
All	30.5	10.9	20.9	34.9	40.5	45.6
	29.3–31.7	*9.6–12.3*	*19.3–22.6*	*32.7–37.2*	*38.5–42.5*	*43.0–48.2*
Sex						
Male	29.9	10.1	20.4	33.5	41.2	45.2
	28.4–31.4	*8.3–12.2*	*18.2–22.9*	*30.8–36.4*	*38.3–44.1*	*41.6–48.8*
Female	31.1	11.7	21.4	36.4	39.7	46.0
	29.7–32.6	*10.1–13.6*	*19.0–23.9*	*33.4–39.4*	*37.1–42.4*	*42.3–49.7*
Indigenous identity						
Non-Indigenous	30.5	10.8	20.7	34.7	40.2	45.8
	29.3–31.7	*9.5–12.3*	*19.0–22.5*	*32.6–37.0*	*38.2–42.3*	*43.2–48.5*
Indigenous	30.2	13.0	21.1	37.1	45.5	36.8
	25.7–35.0	*8.2–19.9*	*15.3–28.3*	*28.4–46.7*	*36.6–54.7*	*26.4–48.7*
Parents' country of birth						
Australian born	29.7	10.5	20.0	34.2	40.2	44.1
	28.4–31.1	*9.0–12.2*	*18.1–22.1*	*31.5–37.1*	*37.8–42.6*	*41.0–47.1*
Overseas born	31.7	11.5	21.9	36.0	40.9	48.0
	29.8–33.5	*9.4–14.0*	*19.0–25.0*	*32.5–39.7*	*37.6–44.3*	*43.5–52.5*
Parental education						
School	32.5	13.1	23.1	38.0	42.5	45.0
	30.5–34.5	*10.5–16.1*	*19.6–26.9*	*33.8–42.3*	*38.5–46.5*	*40.3–49.7*
Vocational training	33.7	11.5	20.3	40.1	42.7	50.7
	31.5–36.0	*8.8–14.9*	*16.8–24.3*	*35.5–44.8*	*38.3–47.3*	*45.7–55.8*
Tertiary education	27.6	9.3	19.8	30.7	37.9	42.7
	26.2–29.1	*7.6–11.2*	*17.7–22.0*	*27.9–33.6*	*35.3–40.5*	*39.3–46.2*
Household income						
Low	33.0	14.1	22.1	37.4	44.9	45.5
	31.3–34.9	*11.5–17.2*	*19.2–25.2*	*33.9–41.0*	*41.2–48.7*	*41.3–49.8*
Medium	31.8	11.6	21.5	37.3	40.8	47.0
	30.1–33.5	*9.3–14.3*	*19.2–24.1*	*33.7–41.1*	*37.5–44.2*	*43.3–50.7*
High	25.9	7.4	18.5	28.5	35.1	42.2
	24.0–27.9	*5.6–9.7*	*15.7–21.8*	*25.0–32.3*	*31.3–39.0*	*37.1–47.4*
Residential location						
Major city	30.6	10.7	20.7	34.8	41.1	46.9
	29.1–32.2	*9.1–12.6*	*18.7–22.9*	*32.0–37.8*	*38.5–43.8*	*43.4–50.3*
Inner regional	31.2	11.8	20.6	35.5	40.6	46.2
	29.3–33.1	*9.2–15.1*	*17.3–24.3*	*31.3–39.9*	*37.0–44.2*	*42.6–49.9*
Outer regional	29.7	11.5	24.1	35.6	37.1	38.0
	27.5–32.1	*9.0–14.5*	*20.6–27.9*	*30.6–41.0*	*32.6–41.9*	*33.2–43.1*
Remote/Very remote	24.4	5.7	15.3	30.8	34.0	37.6
	18.5–31.4	*2.1–14.6*	*8.5–26.1*	*18.9–46.1*	*25.3–43.9*	*23.4–54.3*
Reason for last dental visit						
Check-up	31.4	10.4	20.4	33.6	39.3	45.2
	30.1–32.8	*8.8–12.2*	*18.5–22.4*	*31.0–36.2*	*37.0–41.6*	*42.4–48.1*
Dental problem	35.4	14.1	25.8	41.3	46.4	45.4
	33.0–37.8	*10.5–18.6*	*21.9–30.1*	*36.7–46.1*	*41.8–51.0*	*39.4–51.4*

Row 1: Proportions were computed using weighted data.
Row 2: 95% CI: Confidence intervals for estimates were computed using weighted data.
Columns are arranged by age at time of Survey.

Topical fluorides, in the form of varnishes or gels, can be applied to the teeth and provide protection against the development of caries. Australia's fluoride guidelines state that 'High concentration fluoride gels and foams (those containing more than 1.5mg/g fluoride ion) may be used for people aged 10 years or more who are at an elevated risk of developing caries in situations where other fluoride vehicles may be unavailable or impractical' (Australian Research Centre for Population Oral Health 2012).

Reported receipt of topical fluoride applications increased across successive child age groups, reaching 37.4% for those aged 13–14 years (Table 7-15). Despite recommendations to the contrary, one-quarter of children aged 7–8 years had received a topical fluoride application and 13.8% of those aged 5–6 years were also reported to have received a fluoride application from a dentist or oral health therapist.

There were obvious socioeconomic gradients in the receipt of topical fluoride applications. Non-Indigenous children were considerably more likely to have had a topical fluoride application (28.8%) than were Indigenous children (19.2%). Children from higher income families were twice as likely to have received a topical fluoride application (39.8%) than were children from a low-income family (19.0%) and more children whose parents had a tertiary education (34.7%) had received a fluoride application than children whose parents had school-only education (18.7%). Higher prevalence of fluoride applications was also shown for children from a Major city residence and who had last visited a dentist for a check-up.

Differences in the receipt of a topical fluoride application can be observed across most of the two-year child age groups.

Table 7-15: Percentage of children who have had fluoride applied to their teeth by a dentist or oral health therapist in the Australian child population

	Population: children aged 5–14 years					
	All ages	5–6	7–8	9–10	11–12	13–14
All	28.2	14.8	24.2	29.0	35.2	37.8
	26.6–29.7	*13.1–16.7*	*21.8–26.7*	*26.8–31.3*	*32.7–37.7*	*34.8–40.9*
Sex						
Male	27.4	13.7	24.3	27.2	34.8	37.2
	25.6–29.2	*11.7–16.0*	*21.6–27.2*	*24.4–30.2*	*31.8–37.9*	*33.5–41.0*
Female	29.0	15.9	24.0	30.8	35.6	38.5
	27.1–31.0	*13.5–18.6*	*21.1–27.3*	*27.9–33.9*	*32.3–39.0*	*34.2–43.0*
Indigenous identity						
Non-Indigenous	28.8	15.3	24.4	29.8	35.9	38.7
	27.2–30.4	*13.5–17.2*	*21.9–27.0*	*27.4–32.3*	*33.3–38.5*	*35.5–41.9*
Indigenous	19.2	9.3	21.9	17.4	28.0	19.1
	15.8–23.1	*5.1–16.2*	*14.9–31.0*	*12.2–24.2*	*21.1–36.0*	*11.7–29.8*
Parents' country of birth						
Australian born	28.2	14.9	23.6	28.4	35.8	38.6
	26.6–30.0	*12.8–17.4*	*21.1–26.3*	*25.8–31.2*	*32.9–38.8*	*34.9–42.4*
Overseas born	28.3	14.8	25.2	30.4	34.7	36.3
	26.2–30.4	*12.5–17.4*	*21.4–29.5*	*27.1–33.8*	*31.1–38.5*	*32.2–40.6*
Parental education						
School	18.7	8.8	13.9	20.8	25.0	24.1
	16.8–20.6	*6.7–11.4*	*11.3–17.1*	*17.2–25.0*	*21.5–28.9*	*20.1–28.6*
Vocational training	27.5	13.6	21.8	25.4	34.7	40.0
	25.3–29.8	*10.7–17.2*	*17.9–26.3*	*21.7–29.5*	*29.9–39.8*	*34.9–45.4*
Tertiary education	34.7	19.2	30.7	36.5	42.9	46.0
	32.7–36.8	*16.5–22.1*	*27.4–34.3*	*33.5–39.6*	*39.6–46.2*	*42.0–50.1*
Household income						
Low	19.0	7.7	15.2	19.2	24.1	28.1
	17.4–20.7	*6.1–9.7*	*12.6–18.1*	*16.6–22.1*	*21.2–27.4*	*24.4–32.2*
Medium	28.9	17.5	23.5	29.1	35.8	38.2
	27.1–30.7	*14.9–20.5*	*20.5–26.8*	*26.2–32.3*	*32.1–39.7*	*34.2–42.3*
High	39.8	21.5	35.3	42.1	50.6	51.7
	37.1–42.5	*18.0–25.4*	*30.4–40.4*	*37.7–46.7*	*46.2–55.0*	*46.1–57.2*
Residential location						
Major city	31.0	16.6	26.9	31.9	39.2	41.1
	28.9–33.1	*14.4–19.0*	*23.8–30.3*	*28.9–35.1*	*35.8–42.6*	*37.1–45.2*
Inner regional	21.6	10.7	19.7	20.9	25.8	30.3
	19.5–23.8	*8.3–13.8*	*16.4–23.5*	*17.8–24.3*	*22.2–29.9*	*25.7–35.3*
Outer regional	23.7	9.8	15.9	27.4	29.1	34.0
	20.9–26.7	*6.8–14.1*	*12.7–19.8*	*22.9–32.5*	*24.3–34.3*	*28.8–39.5*
Remote/Very remote	21.2	14.0	16.6	21.3	28.4	26.6
	16.1–27.4	*5.1–33.2*	*8.0–31.2*	*16.0–27.9*	*17.0–43.4*	*17.0–39.2*
Reason for last dental visit						
Check-up	33.8	22.2	29.3	33.1	39.5	40.6
	32.1–35.6	*19.6–25.1*	*26.2–32.5*	*30.4–35.8*	*36.7–42.4*	*37.4–43.9*
Dental problem	24.6	15.7	24.6	24.9	27.4	28.8
	22.4–26.9	*11.9–20.3*	*20.6–29.1*	*21.4–28.8*	*23.1–32.2*	*23.5–34.7*

Row 1: Proportions were computed using weighted data.
Row 2: 95% CI: Confidence intervals for estimates were computed using weighted data.
Columns are arranged by age at time of Survey.

Table 7-16: Oral health behaviours by state/territory in the Australian child population

				Population: children aged 5–14 years					
	Aus	ACT	NSW	NT	Qld	SA	Tas	Vic	WA
Starting toothbrushing with toothpaste before 18 months	33.8	31.5	28.9	30.7	48.2	30.3	36.1	28.1	34.9
	32.6–35.0	28.8–34.3	26.7–31.3	24.2–38.0	46.0–50.5	27.8–33.0	33.3–38.9	26.1–30.3	32.3–37.5
Started toothbrushing between 18 and 30 months	40.1	45.1	40.1	35.1	34.0	45.4	45.8	43.1	40.6
	38.9–41.2	42.0–48.3	37.5–42.7	29.9–40.6	32.0–36.0	42.3–48.6	42.2–49.5	41.0–45.2	37.9–43.4
Started toothbrushing after 30 months	26.1	23.4	31.0	34.2	17.8	24.3	18.1	28.8	24.6
	24.7–27.6	21.0–25.9	27.6–34.6	25.4–44.2	15.8–20.0	21.1–27.8	15.2–21.6	26.2–31.6	21.6–27.8
Toothbrushing at least twice a day	49.7	48.8	48.1	45.2	53.4	47.3	52.2	49.4	48.7
	48.4–51.0	45.5–52.2	45.4–50.9	39.0–51.6	51.0–55.8	44.9–49.6	47.7–56.6	46.8–52.1	45.5–52.0
Toothbrushing with standard fluoridated toothpaste at age 2–3 years	8.6	6.5	8.4	8.6	11.6	7.6	6.5	7.4	7.0
	8.0–9.3	5.1–8.3	7.3–9.6	6.0–12.2	10.1–13.3	6.1–9.5	4.9–8.6	6.1–9.0	5.8–8.4
Using pea-sized amount of toothpaste at age 2–3 years	38.8	39.1	40.4	33.9	38.9	37.1	37.4	37.3	39.1
	37.9–39.7	35.8–42.4	38.6–42.2	28.9–39.4	36.9–40.9	34.3–40.0	34.0–40.8	35.3–39.3	36.4–41.9
Eating or licking toothpaste at age 2–3 years	50.9	52.1	52.2	47.4	49.3	54.3	47.3	50.7	50.0
	49.8–52.0	49.0–55.1	49.8–54.6	40.5–54.4	47.2–51.3	51.3–57.2	43.7–50.9	48.4–53.1	47.2–52.9
Parents helping with toothbrushing at age 2–3 years	99.3	99.6	99.4	96.2	98.9	99.6	99.3	99.5	99.8
	99.1–99.5	99.2–99.8	98.9–99.7	81.0–99.4	98.2–99.3	99.3–99.8	98.1–99.8	99.2–99.7	99.4–99.9
Use of fluoride tablets or drops	6.4	3.6	3.8	3.5	15.5	3.9	3.0	4.2	3.9
	5.8–7.0	2.8–4.6	3.0–4.7	2.1–5.8	13.8–17.4	2.9–5.4	2.0–4.7	3.4–5.1	3.0–5.1
Use of fluoridated mouth rinse	30.5	35.7	33.2	23.9	23.4	32.5	22.6	29.7	38.3
	29.3–31.7	31.5–40.2	30.6–35.9	17.8–31.2	22.1–24.8	29.6–35.6	19.2–26.5	27.2–32.4	35.0–41.7
Professional application of fluoride	28.2	26.9	38.1	22.5	27.1	39.7	17.2	18.2	18.1
	26.6–29.7	23.4–30.8	34.5–41.7	17.2–28.9	24.4–29.9	36.6–42.9	14.6–20.2	16.4–20.2	15.9–20.6

Row 1: Proportions were computed using weighted data.
Row 2: 95% CI: Confidence intervals for estimates were computed using weighted data.
Columns are arranged by age at time of Survey.

Summary

Much of this chapter has concerned itself with whether the oral health behaviours of Australian children are in accord with the recommendations published by ARCPOH in consultation with a panel of relevant experts (Australian Research Centre for Population Oral Health 2012). These guidelines are concerned with fluoride use, but as oral health behaviours such as toothbrushing are fundamentally related to the application of fluoride to the teeth as a primary decay preventive measure, the fluoride exposure guidelines necessarily also relate to behaviours surrounding these behaviours, for example, parental supervision of child toothbrushing.

The summary Table 7-16 shows descriptive findings for Australia as a whole and for individual Australian states and territories. Presented results are for combined ages 5–14 years and oral health behaviours which do not change dramatically on the basis of child age. Overall, there was generally poor compliance with recommendations regarding oral health behaviours.

In relation to toothbrushing, the Australian fluoride exposure guidelines recommend twice daily brushing with a pea-sized amount of fluoride toothpaste (low fluoride toothpaste from 18 months to 5 years inclusive), that children should spit out, not swallow and not rinse, and that there should be adult supervision to the age of 6 years. However, findings of the study indicate that about one-third of children (33.8%) commence toothbrushing before the age 18 months and that one-quarter of children (26.1%) do not start toothbrushing until age 30 months or later (Table 7-16). Only 40.1% of children start brushing at the recommended time (+/- 6 months). Persistent associations between time starting toothbrushing and socioeconomic disadvantage and demographic characteristics were also found (Table 7-1 to Table 7-3).

Also inconsistent with Australia's fluoride guidelines, some children (8.6%) were found to have been brushing their teeth with standard fluoride toothpaste at age 2–3 years (Table 7-16) while many older children were still using low fluoride toothpaste well past the recommended cut-off age of 6 years, over 50% at age 7–8 years and almost one-quarter of children at age 9–10 years (Table 7-7).

Only about 40% of children brush their teeth at least twice a day, despite long-standing recommendations in Australia from oral health professionals and on toothpaste packets (Table 7-16). Similarly, just under 40% of children use the recommended pea-sized amount of toothpaste, and over 50% of children were recalled to be eating or licking toothpaste at age 2–3 years, which are recognised risk factors for developing dental fluorosis.

In Australia, only 6.4% of children had ever consumed fluoride tablets or drops (Table 7-16), and this was predominantly in jurisdictions where water fluoridation coverage has traditionally been low, such as Queensland where 15.5% of children had used fluoride tablets or drops.

Use of fluoridated mouth rinse was relatively low across Australia with only 1 in 3 children having ever used mouth rinse (Table 7-16). Some variation in mouth rinse use across states and territories was observable, with percentages ranging from a low of 22.6% in Tasmania to 38.3% in Western Australia.

Over one-quarter (28.2%) of Australian children had received at least one topical fluoride application from a dentist or oral health therapist (Table 7-16). Variations by state and territory most likely reflect differences in policies regarding the application of topical fluorides within School Dental Services, as well as differences in dental disease and risk management across jurisdictions.

References

Australian Research Centre for Population Oral Health 2012. Outcome of fluoride consensus workshop 2012 to review Fluoride Guidelines from 2005. Available at: https://www.adelaide.edu.au/arcpoh/dperu/fluoride/Outcome_of_fluoride_consensus_workshop_2012.pdf.

Australian Research Centre for Population Oral Health 2006. The use of fluorides in Australia: guidelines. Australian Dental Journal 51:195–9.

Armfield JM & Spencer AJ 2012. Dental health behaviours among children 2002-2004: the use of fluoride toothpaste, fluoride tablets and drops, and fluoride mouth rinse. Dental statistics and research series no. 56. Cat. no. DEN 215. Canberra: Australian Institute of Health and Welfare.

Creeth J, Bosma ML & Govier K 2013. How much is a 'pea-sized amount'? A study of dentifrice dosing by parents in three countries. International Dental Journal 63 Suppl 2:25–30.

Do LG & Spencer AJ 2007. Risk-benefit balance in the use of fluoride among young children. Journal of Dental Research 86:723–8.

Marinho VC, Higgins JP, Sheiham A & Logan S 2003a. Fluoride toothpastes for preventing dental caries in children and adolescents. Cochrane Database of Systematic Reviews Issue 1: Art. No. CD002278.

Marinho VC, Higgins JP, Logan S & Sheiham AF 2003b. Fluoride mouth rinses for preventing dental caries in children and adolescents. Cochrane Database of Systematic Reviews Issue 3: Art. No. CD002284.

McLellan L, Rissel C, Donnelly N & Bauman A 1999. Health behaviour and the school environment in New South Wales, Australia. Social Science & Medicine 49:611–9.

Slade GD, Davies JM, Spencer AJ & Stewart JF 1995. Associations between exposure to fluoridated drinking water and dental caries experience among children in two Australian states. Journal of Public Health Dentistry 55:218–28.

Slade GD, Sanders AE, Bill CJ & Do LG 2006. Risk factors for dental caries in the five-year-old South Australian population. Australian Dental Journal 51:130–9.

Walsh T, Sorthington HV, Glenny AM, Appelbe P, Marinho VC & Shi X 2010. Fluoride toothpastes of different concentrations for preventing dental caries in children and adolescents. Cochrane Database of Systematic Reviews Issue 1: Art. No. CD007868.

8 Australian children's general health behaviours

LG Do, JE Harford, DH Ha and AJ Spencer

Oral health is an integral part of general health and shares a number of common determinants with general health. Those common determinants are mostly related to diet. General health behaviours that affect child oral health centre largely on consumption of water and of drinks and foods containing sugar.

Water consumption can affect oral health in two ways. First, water is a 'tooth friendly' drink. Water contains no decay-causing sugar and is generally in the range of acidity that is safe for teeth. Second, water is the main way in which fluoride is accessible to the whole community, irrespective of their individual oral hygiene behaviours. Multiple studies from more than 20 countries have shown that fluoridation reduces dental caries (National Health and Medical Research Council 2007; Rugg-Gunn and Do 2012; Iheozor-Ejiofor et al. 2015), which explains the high priority given to water fluoridation by public health authorities. Water fluoridation provides the greatest benefit to those who can least afford professional dental care (Slade et al. 1995b; Burt 2002). This chapter examines children's consumption of mains and tap water as well as bottled water to assess the extent to which children are likely to receive the benefits to their oral health than can be gained from the fluoridation of reticulated water.

Consumption of sugar is a key risk factor for dental caries (Moynihan and Kelly 2014; Sheiham and James 2014). The impact of sugar on oral health depends in large part on the type, quantity and pattern of consumption. For oral health purposes, sugar that does not occur naturally in milk or in whole fruit or vegetables can contribute to a child's risk of experiencing tooth decay. These sugars are known as 'free sugars' and are defined as 'monosaccharides and disaccharides added to foods and beverages by the manufacturer, cook or consumer, and sugars naturally present in honey, syrups, fruit juices and fruit juice concentrates' (Rosenberg et al. 2005). Dietary guidelines for Australia recommend that Australians 'Limit intake of foods and drinks containing added sugars such as confectionary, sugar-sweetened soft drinks and cordials, fruit drinks, vitamin waters, energy and sports drinks' (National Health and Medical Research Council 2013). More recently, the World Health Organization has issued a strong recommendation that free sugar intake be limited to 10% of total energy intake and that a limit of 5% of total energy be considered on the basis of the potential impact on oral health of lowering sugar consumption (Rosenberg et al. 2005).

This chapter examines children's patterns of intake of water and free sugars intake. Free sugar intake was evaluated from a number of sugar-sweetened beverages (SSBs), drinks that contain any free sugars, sugary snacks and added table sugar.

8.1 Patterns of water consumption

Patterns of water consumption are important for oral health because reticulated water is a key source of fluoride for Australian children (Spencer et al. 1996). There was evidence that dental caries experience in the primary teeth increased with decreasing use of non-fluoridated water (Armfield and Spencer 2004). There has been concern in recent years that the growing popularity of un-fluoridated bottled water may displace consumption of fluoridated water and contribute to a stalling or reversal in gains in child oral health.

The majority of children (91.6%) usually drank at least one glass of tap/public water each day (Table 8-1). However, over one in four children (28.7%) drank at least one glass of bottled water a day.

Small differences in tap water consumption were evident across levels of parental education and household income. Children of parents with higher levels of education or income were more likely to consume tap water daily. Larger variation was evident for residential location with children in Inner Regional and Outer Regional areas less likely than children in Major city areas to usually consume tap water daily.

There was considerable variation in bottled water consumption by Indigenous children with around 30% more likely to consume bottled water than non-Indigenous children. Significant variations were observed by parental education, household income and residential location. Approximately two-fold or more differences were evident across groups by parental education, household income and residential location. Children whose parents had the least education (38.2%), or the lowest income (37.3%) were the most likely to consume bottled water while children who lived Major city areas were least likely (19.8%).

In summary, while the consumption of tap/public water was high, a sizeable proportion of Australian children consumed bottled water every day. More significantly, Australian children from lower socioeconomic backgrounds were more likely to consume bottled water than their counterparts in higher socioeconomic groups.

Table 8-1: Percentage of children drank at least one glass of tap/public water or bottled water in a usual day in the Australian child population

	Population: children aged 5–14 years	
	Tap/public water	**Bottled water**
All	91.6	28.7
	90.6–92.4	*26.8–30.7*
Sex		
Male	91.4	28.7
	90.3–92.4	*26.6–31.0*
Female	91.7	28.8
	90.7–92.7	*26.6–31.0*
Indigenous identity		
Non-Indigenous	91.6	28.2
	90.6–92.5	*26.3–30.2*
Indigenous	90.4	37.9
	87.5–92.8	*32.2–43.9*
Parents' country of birth		
Australian born	90.5	29.6
	89.3–91.6	*27.4–32.0*
Overseas born	93.4	26.9
	92.4–94.3	*24.6–29.3*
Parental education		
School	89.8	38.2
	88.3–91.2	*35.5–40.9*
Vocational training	89.8	33.1
	88.2–91.1	*30.0–36.2*
Tertiary education	93.3	20.8
	92.3–94.3	*18.9–23.0*
Household income		
Low	90.1	37.3
	88.7–91.4	*34.7–40.0*
Medium	90.2	28.9
	89.0–91.4	*26.4–31.4*
High	94.5	18.7
	93.3–95.5	*16.3–21.3*
Residential location		
Major city	95.4	19.8
	94.6–96.0	*18.0–21.7*
Inner regional	83.0	45.7
	79.8–85.7	*41.4–50.1*
Outer regional	81.0	48.1
	78.2–83.6	*44.3–52.0*
Remote/Very remote	90.3	47.0
	82.6–94.8	*30.3–64.4*
Reason for last dental visit		
Check-up	92.0	27.4
	91.1–92.9	*25.4–29.6*
Dental problem	90.1	32.1
	88.3–91.7	*29.1–35.4*

Row 1: Proportions were computed using weighted data.
Row 2: 95% CI: Confidence intervals for estimates were computed using weighted data.
Columns are arranged by age at time of Survey.

Consumption of tap/public water during different life periods may reflect behaviours toward or availability of tap/public water. Parents were asked to indicate approximate proportion of tap/public water consumption for three different life periods of their children. The majority of children consumed almost all of their drinking water from a tap or public supply at all ages (Table 8-2). Children were most likely to consume almost none (0–19%) of their drinking water from tap or public supples in the first year of life. This proportion declined and remained just under 10% during the later life periods. Conversely, a large and increasing proportion of children reportedly consumed almost only tap/public water during the three periods of life.

Table 8-2: Percentage of children with different levels of tap/public water consumption during different life periods in the Australian child population

Age period	Population: children aged 5–14 years				
	Proportion of tap/public water consumption				
	0–19%	20–39%	40–59%	60–79%	80–100%
Birth–12 months	24.6	7.0	5.1	4.3	59.0
	23.5-25.8	6.5-7.6	4.6-5.7	3.8-4.8	57.5-60.5
1–4 years	9.1	6.3	9.8	8.9	65.9
	8.2-10.0	5.7-6.9	9.2-10.6	8.3-9.6	64.3-67.4
5 years–now	8.0	4.9	6.5	10.0	70.7
	7.2-9.0	4.4-5.4	6.0-7.1	9.2-10.6	69.2-72.2

Row 1: Proportions were computed using weighted data.
Row 2: 95% CI: Confidence intervals for estimates were computed using weighted data.

Consuming tap/public water is an important health behaviour. Those who reportedly mostly drank tap/public water as their drinking water in a usual day were further investigated (Table 8-3). Variations in mainly consuming tap/public water across all indicators, except for sex, established early in life and mostly remained across time. Indigenous children and children with a parent born overseas were less likely to have almost all tap/public water for drinking water than their counterparts during the two early life periods, although the difference was smaller after the age of 5 years. The variations by parental education, household income and residential location established early in life and remained so across all life periods. Those children whose parents had a tertiary education were 1.2 to 1.3 times more likely to have almost all tap/public water for drinking than those with a parent who had school-only education. Likewise, the relative differences between those from high income households and low income households were 1.2 to 1.4 times. Children outside of Major city areas were less likely to mostly use public water for drinking than their counterparts. Furthermore, children who had dental problems were less likely to consume tap/public water than those who visited for check-up since an early age and this remained over time.

Table 8-3: Percentage of children who had almost all tap/public water as their daily drinking water during different life periods in the Australian child population

	Population: children aged 5–14 years		
	Birth–12 months	1–4 years	5 years–now
All	59.0	65.9	70.7
	57.5–60.5	*64.3–67.4*	*69.2–72.2*
Sex			
Male	58.9	66.0	70.8
	57.0–60.7	*64.0–67.8*	*69.0–72.6*
Female	59.1	65.8	70.6
	57.4–60.8	*64.0–67.5*	*68.9–72.2*
Indigenous identity			
Non-Indigenous	59.7	66.5	71.0
	58.2–61.1	*65.0–68.0*	*69.5–72.5*
Indigenous	48.0	56.1	66.1
	41.5–54.6	*49.4–62.6*	*60.1–71.7*
Parents' country of birth			
Australian born	61.0	67.3	70.6
	59.3–62.6	*65.5–69.0*	*68.7–72.4*
Overseas born	55.6	63.5	70.9
	53.3–57.9	*61.2–65.7*	*69.0–72.8*
Parental education			
School	50.4	56.4	64.4
	48.1–52.8	*53.9–58.8*	*62.1–66.6*
Vocational training	58.7	64.1	66.5
	56.2–61.2	*61.8–66.4*	*64.0–68.8*
Tertiary education	64.4	72.5	76.6
	62.7–66.1	*70.8–74.2*	*74.9–78.3*
Household income			
Low	48.7	56.2	64.8
	46.5–50.8	*54.1–58.3*	*62.7–66.8*
Medium	60.5	67.1	70.2
	58.6–62.4	*65.2–69.0*	*68.2–72.1*
High	69.1	76.1	78.7
	66.9–71.2	*74.0–78.1*	*76.6–80.7*
Residential location			
Major city	62.8	71.0	76.8
	61.0–64.6	*69.2–72.7*	*75.2–78.3*
Inner regional	52.0	55.3	57.6
	49.3–54.7	*52.4–58.1*	*54.2–61.0*
Outer regional	48.2	53.4	56.0
	44.7–51.8	*49.8–57.0*	*52.6–59.4*
Remote/Very remote	42.5	48.4	54.6
	36.3–49.0	*41.7–55.1*	*47.0–62.0*
Reason for last dental visit			
Check-up	61.0	68.1	72.0
	59.5–62.5	*66.6–69.6*	*70.4–73.6*
Dental problem	53.7	60.2	66.0
	51.1–56.4	*57.6–62.7*	*63.4–68.4*

Row 1: Proportions were computed using weighted data.
Row 2: 95% CI: Confidence intervals for estimates were computed using weighted data.
Columns are arranged by age at time of Survey.

8.2 Patterns of sugary drink consumption

Beverages are an important source of sugar in the diets of Australian children (Australian Bureau of Statistics 2015). Sugar-sweetened beverages (SSBs) include sweetened soft drinks, sweetened energy drinks, sweetened cordials and sweetened fruit juices. They are a significant source of refined sugar and consumption has been implicated in the increase in childhood overweight, obesity and lifestyle-related disease in SSBs, which are of considerable interest for dental health. Parents of children in the Survey were asked to provide the number of serves of different beverages their child consumed on a usual day. Percentages of children consuming different levels of SSBs as well as average number of SSBs consumed per day are reported below.

Half of all children (50.9%) usually drank one or more glass of SSBs on a usual day and this increased from 41.5% in children aged 5–6 years to 58.7% in those aged 13–14 years (Table 8-4). For all ages, the proportion was higher for Indigenous children (73.1%) and lowest among children from high income households (36.5%). Largest variations were found associated with Indigenous identity, parental education, household income and reason for last dental visit. Indigenous children were 1.5 times more likely to usually consume SSBs than their non-Indigenous counterparts. Children of parents with a school-only education or lowest income households were 1.7 times more likely than those with the highest levels to usually consume SSBs. That percentage was 1.3 times higher among children who last visited for a dental problem compared with those who last visited for a check-up.

The variations for Indigenous identity, parental education, household income and reason for last dental visit were evident in every age group. Largest variations were observed among the 5–6-year age group. In this age group, children whose parents had school-only education or who were from low income households were more than twice as likely to usually consume SSBs. Children aged 5–6 years who last visited for a dental problem were almost twice as likely to drink SSBs in a usual day.

In summary, a large proportion of Australian children consumed sugar-sweetened beverages in a usual day. This proportion was driven by children from lower socioeconomic backgrounds. It was also associated with problem-based dental visiting.

Table 8-4: Percentage of children who drink one or more glass of sugar-sweetened beverages (SSB) in a usual day in the Australian child population

| | Population: children aged 5–14 years | | | | | |
	All ages	5–6	7–8	9–10	11–12	13–14
All	50.9	41.5	45.9	50.6	57.7	58.7
	49.0–52.7	*38.5–44.6*	*42.9–48.9*	*47.9–53.4*	*55.1–60.1*	*55.7–61.7*
Sex						
Male	52.8	42.1	46.8	52.6	58.7	63.7
	50.6–54.9	*38.3–46.1*	*43.1–50.6*	*49.5–55.7*	*55.5–61.8*	*59.8–67.5*
Female	48.9	40.8	44.8	48.7	56.5	53.5
	46.7–51.1	*37.2–44.5*	*41.0–48.6*	*44.8–52.6*	*53.3–59.7*	*49.4–57.6*
Indigenous identity						
Non-Indigenous	49.5	39.5	44.1	49.3	56.4	58.2
	47.7–51.4	*36.5–42.6*	*41.1–47.1*	*46.5–52.1*	*53.8–58.9*	*55.2–61.2*
Indigenous	73.1	70.9	71.7	71.7	77.8	73.0
	67.6–77.9	*61.8–78.6*	*60.8–80.5*	*61.9–79.8*	*68.4–85.1*	*60.3–82.8*
Parents' country of birth						
Australian born	49.4	39.7	44.0	49.2	56.8	57.3
	47.6–51.2	*36.7–42.8*	*40.8–47.3*	*45.9–52.5*	*54.0–59.6*	*53.8–60.7*
Overseas born	53.3	44.8	48.6	53.1	58.8	61.2
	50.5–56.1	*39.9–49.8*	*44.1–53.2*	*48.8–57.4*	*54.9–62.6*	*56.5–65.7*
Parental education						
School	67.8	61.2	66.2	67.4	71.3	72.7
	65.4–70.1	*56.7–65.6*	*61.5–70.5*	*62.7–71.7*	*67.1–75.2*	*68.0–76.9*
Vocational training	52.4	42.7	44.4	54.4	58.0	60.7
	49.9–54.8	*38.2–47.4*	*39.5–49.4*	*49.7–59.0*	*52.9–62.9*	*55.8–65.3*
Tertiary education	38.8	28.2	34.2	38.2	46.8	47.6
	36.6–41.0	*24.9–31.7*	*30.8–37.8*	*34.8–41.8*	*43.7–49.9*	*43.4–51.7*
Household income						
Low	64.8	57.9	63.0	64.6	71.6	66.8
	62.7–67.0	*53.5–62.2*	*58.4–67.4*	*60.9–68.1*	*68.1–74.8*	*62.0–71.3*
Medium	48.5	38.7	40.1	48.8	56.1	58.8
	46.6–50.4	*35.0–42.5*	*36.5–43.7*	*45.0–52.6*	*52.5–59.6*	*54.9–62.6*
High	36.5	24.0	32.9	35.7	42.1	48.3
	33.6–39.4	*20.3–28.0*	*28.0–38.3*	*30.6–41.1*	*37.9–46.3*	*42.6–54.1*
Residential location						
Major city	50.2	40.3	44.9	49.3	57.3	59.4
	47.7–52.7	*36.3–44.4*	*41.0–48.9*	*45.7–52.9*	*54.0–60.6*	*55.4–63.3*
Inner regional	49.7	39.5	44.7	53.9	56.4	53.7
	46.9–52.5	*34.8–44.3*	*39.1–50.4*	*49.5–58.2*	*52.3–60.3*	*48.1–59.2*
Outer regional	54.9	49.1	51.4	51.5	59.4	61.8
	50.5–59.3	*42.9–55.3*	*44.6–58.2*	*45.4–57.6*	*52.7–65.8*	*56.4–67.0*
Remote/Very remote	63.1	63.6	57.8	57.4	70.7	67.1
	53.5–71.8	*51.8–74.0*	*40.9–73.0*	*40.4–72.9*	*60.9–78.9*	*50.9–80.0*
Reason for last dental visit						
Check-up	46.8	32.4	39.7	46.9	53.2	56.3
	44.9–48.8	*29.3–35.5*	*36.5–43.0*	*43.6–50.2*	*50.5–55.9*	*53.0–59.5*
Dental problem	60.8	59.2	54.5	56.8	67.1	68.7
	58.1–63.6	*52.2–65.9*	*49.3–59.5*	*51.6–61.8*	*62.4–71.4*	*62.5–74.4*

Row 1: Proportions were computed using weighted data.
Row 2: 95% CI: Confidence intervals for estimates were computed using weighted data.
Columns are arranged by age at time of Survey.

There is a dose-response relationship between sugar consumption and caries experience (Moynihan & Kelly 2014). Table 8-4 to Table 8-7 examine variations in the quantity of SSBs consumed.

One in four children (24.7%) consumed at least two SSBs on a usual day with around half of these (11.6% of all children) consuming at least three SSBs (Table 8-5). More males, children with a parent born overseas and children who last visited for a dental problem than females, children with Australian-born parents and children who last visited for a dental check-up consumed SSBs. Indigenous children were twice as likely as non-Indigenous children to do so. There were strong gradients in consumption of SSBs related to parental education and household income. Children with a parent whose highest level of education was vocational training or school were 1.5 and 2.6 times more likely to consume two or more SSBs daily, and 1.7 and 2.3 times more likely to usually consume three or more glasses of SSBs. Similar differences in consumption of three or more SSBs were evident across levels of household income with the exception of three or more SSBs, for which children from the lowest income households were almost four times more likely to consume this level of SSBs.

Table 8-5: Percentage of children who drink two or more glasses of sugar-sweetened beverages (SSB) in a usual day in the Australian child population

	Population: children aged 5–14 years	
	2+ SSB	3+ SSB
All	24.7	11.6
	23.3–26.2	*10.5–12.7*
Sex		
Male	27.1	13.0
	25.3–28.9	*11.7–14.4*
Female	22.3	10.0
	20.6–24.0	*8.9–11.3*
Indigenous identity		
Non-Indigenous	23.5	10.8
	22.1–25.0	*9.8–11.8*
Indigenous	46.2	25.5
	40.3–52.2	*20.3–31.5*
Parents' country of birth		
Australian born	22.5	9.6
	21.0–24.0	*8.6–10.6*
Overseas born	28.5	15.0
	26.2–30.9	*13.2–16.9*
Parental education		
School	39.8	19.9
	37.5–42.2	*17.9–22.1*
Vocational training	23.2	10.4
	21.3–25.3	*9.1–12.0*
Tertiary education	15.4	6.3
	14.1–16.9	*5.5–7.3*
Household income		
Low	37.3	18.8
	35.2–39.4	*17.0–20.8*
Medium	20.5	8.6
	19.1–21.9	*7.6–9.8*
High	13.5	4.9
	11.8–15.5	*4.0–6.0*
Residential location		
Major city	24.5	11.7
	22.7–26.5	*10.4–13.2*
Inner regional	23.1	9.8
	20.7–25.7	*8.4–11.3*
Outer regional	27.3	12.6
	23.3–31.7	*9.6–16.5*
Remote/Very remote	32.7	17.8
	23.7–43.1	*12.1–25.5*
Reason for last dental visit		
Check-up	21.2	9.3
	19.8–22.7	*8.4–10.3*
Dental problem	32.5	16.0
	29.9–35.2	*13.9–18.2*

Row 1: Proportions were computed using weighted data.
Row 2: 95% CI: Confidence intervals for estimates were computed using weighted data.
Columns are arranged by age at time of Survey.

Average number of sugar-sweetened beverages per day can be an indicator of sugar consumption. On average, Australian children drank 1.1 glasses of SSBs on a usual day (Table 8-6). This varied from 0.8 glasses in children aged 5–6 years to 1.3 glasses in children aged 13-14 years.

For all ages, Indigenous children had the highest average number of SSBs a day (1.9) while children from the high income households had the lowest (0.6). Gradients were observed across groups by Indigenous identity, parental country of birth, parental education, household income and reason for last dental visit. Children of low income households had, on average, 2.5 times higher number of SSBs a day than children from high income households. The difference between children of a parent with school-only education and children whose parents had a tertiary education was 2.3 times. The differences were around 1.5 times for children with a parent who had a vocational education compared to tertiary education and for children in the medium income group compared to the highest income group. Children who had dental problems had 1.5 times higher number of SSBs a day than those who visited for a check-up.

The gradients were also consistent within age groups. The differences in average number of SSBs were mostly largest in the youngest age groups. The average number of SSBs consumed a day by children aged 5–6 years from the lowest income group were more than 3 times higher than that of children of the same age from the highest income group. Such relative difference was more than 2 times between Indigenous and non-Indigenous children in the 5–6-year age group. The gradient by parental education was consistent within all age groups.

In summary, the amount of sugar-sweetened beverages varied greatly across socioeconomic and dental visiting indicators. Such gradients were established from an early age and remained consistent with age.

Table 8-6: Average number of sugar-sweetened beverages (SSB) per day in a usual day among the Australian child population

	Population: children aged 5–14 years					
	All ages	5–6	7–8	9–10	11–12	13–14
All	1.1	0.8	0.9	1.0	1.2	1.3
	1.0–1.1	*0.7–0.9*	*0.8–1.0*	*0.9–1.1*	*1.2–1.3*	*1.2–1.4*
Sex						
Male	1.1	0.9	1.0	1.1	1.3	1.5
	1.1–1.2	*0.8–1.0*	*0.9–1.1*	*1.0–1.2*	*1.2–1.4*	*1.3–1.7*
Female	1.0	0.8	0.9	0.9	1.2	1.1
	0.9–1.0	*0.7–0.9*	*0.8–1.0*	*0.8–1.0*	*1.1–1.3*	*1.0–1.2*
Indigenous identity						
Non-Indigenous	1.0	0.8	0.9	1.0	1.2	1.3
	1.0–1.1	*0.7–0.8*	*0.8–1.0*	*0.9–1.0*	*1.1–1.3*	*1.2–1.4*
Indigenous	1.9	1.7	1.7	1.7	2.2	1.9
	1.6–2.1	*1.3–2.2*	*1.3–2.1*	*1.4–2.1*	*1.8–2.7*	*1.5–2.3*
Parents' country of birth						
Australian born	1.0	0.7	0.8	0.9	1.1	1.2
	0.9–1.0	*0.6–0.8*	*0.7–0.9*	*0.8–1.0*	*1.0–1.2*	*1.1–1.3*
Overseas born	1.3	1.0	1.1	1.2	1.4	1.5
	1.1–1.4	*0.8–1.2*	*1.0–1.3*	*1.0–1.3*	*1.3–1.6*	*1.3–1.7*
Parental education						
School	1.6	1.3	1.6	1.6	1.8	1.8
	1.5–1.7	*1.2–1.5*	*1.4–1.7*	*1.4–1.7*	*1.6–1.9*	*1.6–2.0*
Vocational training	1.0	0.8	0.8	1.0	1.1	1.3
	0.9–1.1	*0.7–0.9*	*0.7–0.9*	*0.8–1.1*	*1.0–1.3*	*1.1–1.6*
Tertiary education	0.7	0.5	0.6	0.7	0.9	0.9
	0.7–0.8	*0.4–0.6*	*0.5–0.7*	*0.6–0.8*	*0.8–1.0*	*0.8–1.0*
Household income						
Low	1.5	1.3	1.4	1.5	1.8	1.6
	1.4–1.6	*1.1–1.4*	*1.2–1.6*	*1.4–1.7*	*1.6–1.9*	*1.4–1.8*
Medium	0.9	0.7	0.8	0.8	1.1	1.1
	0.8–0.9	*0.6–0.7*	*0.7–0.8*	*0.7–0.9*	*1.0–1.2*	*1.0–1.2*
High	0.6	0.4	0.5	0.6	0.7	1.0
	0.6–0.7	*0.3–0.5*	*0.4–0.6*	*0.5–0.6*	*0.6–0.8*	*0.8–1.1*
Residential location						
Major city	1.1	0.8	0.9	1.0	1.3	1.3
	1.0–1.1	*0.7–0.9*	*0.8–1.1*	*0.9–1.1*	*1.1–1.4*	*1.2–1.5*
Inner regional	1.0	0.7	0.9	1.0	1.1	1.1
	0.9–1.0	*0.6–0.8*	*0.7–1.0*	*0.9–1.1*	*1.0–1.3*	*0.9–1.2*
Outer regional	1.1	1.0	1.0	1.0	1.3	1.4
	1.0–1.3	*0.7–1.3*	*0.7–1.2*	*0.8–1.2*	*1.0–1.5*	*1.2–1.5*
Remote/Very remote	1.4	1.3	1.4	1.2	1.5	1.5
	1.1–1.6	*0.8–1.8*	*0.8–2.0*	*0.7–1.6*	*1.2–1.8*	*1.1–1.9*
Reason for last dental visit						
Check-up	0.9	0.6	0.7	0.9	1.1	1.2
	0.9–1.0	*0.5–0.6*	*0.7–0.8*	*0.8–0.9*	*1.0–1.2*	*1.1–1.3*
Dental problem	1.4	1.3	1.2	1.2	1.4	1.7
	1.2–1.5	*1.1–1.5*	*1.0–1.3*	*1.1–1.4*	*1.3–1.6*	*1.4–2.1*

Row 1: Means were computed using weighted data.
Row 2: 95% CI: Confidence intervals for estimates were computed using weighted data.
Columns are arranged by age at time of Survey.

Children's consumption of sugar can be increased by consuming fruit juices and sweetened, flavoured milk drinks. While fruit juices and flavoured milks are often consumed as a healthy alternative to SSBs, the sugar in them is the same in terms of its effect on oral health. Four glasses of either SSBs, fruit juice or flavoured milk drinks exceed the maximum amount of sugar that any child of any activity level can consume to comply with WHO guidelines for 10% of energy to be from free sugars.

Around one in five children usually drank four or more glasses of any drink that contained free sugar (Table 8-7). The proportion with this level of consumption increased across age groups and was lowest in children aged 5–6 years (15.3%) and highest in children aged 13–14 years (23.7%).

Across all ages, the proportion with this level of consumption was highest among Indigenous children (37.3%) and lowest among children from high income households (10%). There were also variations in consumption by Indigenous identity, parental country of birth, parental education, household income and reason for last dental visit. Indigenous children were more than twice as likely to consume four or more glasses of sugar-containing drinks than non-Indigenous children. The gradient was strong between groups by household income, with the lowest income group being more than 3 times and 2 times likely to have this level of sugar consumption than the high and medium income groups. The medium income group also had a 1.5 times higher rate of consumption at this level than the high income group. Children whose last dental visit was for a dental problem were 1.6 times more likely to consume four or more glasses of sugar-containing drinks than those who visited for a check-up.

For all of these comparisons, the differences were evident in all age groups both in relative and absolute terms. The relative differences were mostly largest in the youngest age groups across the indicators. The relative difference between the low and high income group was almost 5 times in the 5–6-year age group and 1.8 times in the 13–14-year age group. However, the absolute difference remained consistent. Likewise, children aged 5–6 years who last visited for a dental problem were 2.5 times more likely to consume four or more glasses of sugary drinks than children of the same age whose last dental visit was for a check-up. Children aged 5–10 years whose parents had a school-only education were more than 3 times more likely to consume this level of sugary drinks than those whose parents were tertiary educated.

In summary, almost one-fifth of Australian children were likely to consume an amount of free sugar exceeding 10% of energy intake from drinks alone. This proportion was strongly associated with socioeconomic indicators and dental visiting pattern. This pattern of sugar consumption was also established early in age and remained consistent with age.

Table 8-7: Percentage of children who drink four or more glasses of any drinks that contain sugar in a usual day in the Australian child population (includes SSB, fruit juice, flavoured milk)

	Population: children aged 5–14 years					
	All ages	5–6	7–8	9–10	11–12	13–14
All	19.6	15.3	17.5	18.4	22.8	23.7
	18.3–20.9	*13.5–17.3*	*15.5–19.8*	*16.5–20.5*	*20.8–24.9*	*21.6–25.8*
Sex						
Male	21.0	16.5	18.0	19.3	23.8	27.3
	19.4–22.6	*14.1–19.2*	*15.4–20.9*	*16.9–22.0*	*21.2–26.6*	*24.0–30.9*
Female	18.1	14.0	17.0	17.5	21.8	19.9
	16.7–19.5	*11.9–16.5*	*14.6–19.7*	*15.0–20.3*	*19.4–24.3*	*17.5–22.6*
Indigenous identity						
Non-Indigenous	18.6	14.3	16.6	17.1	21.7	23.1
	17.3–19.9	*12.4–16.3*	*14.6–18.8*	*15.2–19.3*	*19.7–23.8*	*21.0–25.3*
Indigenous	37.3	32.5	33.6	38.6	43.2	39.0
	31.7–43.3	*23.4–43.2*	*23.7–45.1*	*30.0–48.0*	*33.8–53.2*	*28.2–51.0*
Parents' country of birth						
Australian born	16.6	12.6	13.4	15.9	20.5	20.7
	15.4–17.9	*10.7–14.8*	*11.4–15.7*	*13.9–18.0*	*18.3–22.9*	*18.3–23.2*
Overseas born	24.5	20.2	24.3	22.4	26.6	28.9
	22.4–26.7	*17.0–23.8*	*21.0–28.0*	*19.2–26.1*	*23.5–29.9*	*25.2–32.9*
Parental education						
School	31.4	27.2	30.3	30.7	34.6	33.8
	29.1–33.7	*23.3–31.4*	*26.1–34.8*	*26.3–35.4*	*30.7–38.7*	*29.7–38.0*
Vocational training	16.9	12.6	14.5	17.0	18.4	21.1
	15.3–18.6	*9.8–16.1*	*11.1–18.6*	*13.7–20.9*	*15.1–22.2*	*17.2–25.6*
Tertiary education	12.9	8.6	11.0	11.0	16.3	17.8
	11.7–14.1	*7.1–10.4*	*9.1–13.4*	*9.2–13.0*	*14.1–18.8*	*15.2–20.8*
Household income						
Low	31.0	26.0	30.2	31.8	35.7	31.2
	29.0–33.1	*22.7–29.6*	*26.2–34.6*	*28.3–35.7*	*32.0–39.5*	*27.5–35.2*
Medium	15.3	11.3	13.7	12.9	18.0	20.5
	14.0–16.6	*9.5–13.5*	*11.5–16.1*	*10.7–15.5*	*15.5–20.9*	*17.6–23.9*
High	10.0	5.7	7.3	7.7	12.4	17.4
	8.8–11.5	*4.2–7.7*	*5.3–9.9*	*5.8–10.0*	*10.1–15.3*	*13.7–21.7*
Residential location						
Major city	19.4	14.7	17.8	18.3	22.3	24.1
	17.7–21.2	*12.4–17.3*	*15.1–20.8*	*15.8–21.1*	*19.8–25.1*	*21.3–27.1*
Inner regional	18.9	15.0	16.1	20.0	21.9	21.1
	17.1–20.9	*11.7–18.9*	*12.8–20.1*	*16.5–24.1*	*18.5–25.7*	*18.1–24.5*
Outer regional	20.0	18.3	16.9	15.8	24.7	23.9
	16.6–24.0	*13.3–24.8*	*12.6–22.3*	*12.0–20.6*	*18.8–31.7*	*20.3–27.8*
Remote/Very remote	27.1	24.1	23.3	19.7	37.0	33.1
	18.9–37.2	*11.3–44.2*	*12.1–40.2*	*9.5–36.2*	*26.3–49.1*	*21.8–46.6*
Reason for last dental visit						
Check-up	16.4	10.1	12.7	14.9	19.4	21.9
	15.1–17.7	*8.5–12.0*	*10.9–14.7*	*12.9–17.1*	*17.3–21.6*	*19.7–24.2*
Dental problem	26.6	24.6	23.9	22.7	32.1	30.1
	24.2–29.1	*19.3–30.9*	*19.8–28.5*	*19.0–26.8*	*27.7–36.8*	*24.2–36.8*

Row 1: Proportions were computed using weighted data.
Row 2: 95% CI: Confidence intervals for estimates were computed using weighted data.
Columns are arranged by age at time of Survey.

Average number of drinks containing free sugar consumed a in a day provides population level indicators of sugar consumption from drinks. Australian children usually drank an average of 2.3 glasses of drinks containing free sugar each day (Table 8-8). This amount varied with age, and children aged 11–14 years drank 30% more drinks containing free sugar than children aged 5–6 years.

For all ages, Indigenous children had the highest average number of glasses of drinks containing sugar (3.4) while children from the highest income group consumed the fewest (1.6). Significant gradients were observed across groups by Indigenous identity, parent's country of birth, parental education, household income and reason for last dental visit.

Children with a parent born overseas and children whose last dental visit was for a problem drank around 1.3 times more than their counterparts. Indigenous children and children of a parent with a school-only education drank 1.6 times that of non-Indigenous children and children of tertiary-educated parents. The largest differences were evident for parental education where children from low income households drank almost twice as much as children from high income households.

In all cases where differences between groups were evident, relative differences were largest at age 5–6 years and decreased with age. However, in most cases, the absolute differences in average number of glasses of drinks containing sugar remained stable. Children aged 13–14 years whose parents had school-only education and children from households with low income still consumed a glass more a day than their counterparts in the tertiary education and high income groups, respectively.

In summary, a considerable amount of drinks containing free sugars was reportedly consumed by Australian children daily. This amount was higher among those of lower socioeconomic background and those whose last dental visit was associated with a dental problem.

Table 8-8: Average number of glasses of sugar-containing drinks per day in a usual day among the Australian child population (includes SSB, fruit juice, flavoured milk)

	Population: children aged 5–14 years					
	All ages	5–6	7–8	9–10	11–12	13–14
All	**2.3**	**2.0**	**2.2**	**2.2**	**2.6**	**2.6**
	2.2–2.4	*1.9–2.1*	*2.0–2.3*	*2.1–2.4*	*2.4–2.7*	*2.5–2.8*
Sex						
Male	2.4	2.1	2.2	2.4	2.6	2.8
	2.3–2.5	*1.9–2.3*	*2.0–2.4*	*2.2–2.5*	*2.5–2.8*	*2.7–3.1*
Female	2.2	1.9	2.1	2.1	2.5	2.4
	2.1–2.3	*1.7–2.0*	*1.9–2.2*	*2.0–2.3*	*2.3–2.6*	*2.2–2.6*
Indigenous identity						
Non-Indigenous	2.3	1.9	2.1	2.2	2.5	2.6
	2.2–2.3	*1.8–2.1*	*1.9–2.2*	*2.1–2.3*	*2.4–2.6*	*2.5–2.8*
Indigenous	3.4	3.1	3.2	3.4	3.9	3.4
	3.1–3.8	*2.5–3.7*	*2.7–3.8*	*2.8–4.0*	*3.3–4.6*	*2.9–4.0*
Parents' country of birth						
Australian born	2.1	1.8	1.9	2.0	2.3	2.4
	2.0–2.1	*1.7–1.9*	*1.8–2.0*	*1.9–2.1*	*2.2–2.5*	*2.3–2.5*
Overseas born	2.7	2.3	2.6	2.6	2.9	3.0
	2.5–2.9	*2.1–2.6*	*2.3–2.9*	*2.4–2.8*	*2.7–3.1*	*2.7–3.3*
Parental education						
School	3.1	2.8	3.0	3.1	3.3	3.3
	3.0–3.3	*2.6–3.1*	*2.8–3.3*	*2.8–3.4*	*3.0–3.5*	*3.0–3.6*
Vocational training	2.2	1.8	2.0	2.1	2.4	2.5
	2.1–2.3	*1.7–2.0*	*1.8–2.3*	*2.0–2.3*	*2.2–2.6*	*2.2–2.9*
Tertiary education	1.9	1.5	1.7	1.8	2.1	2.2
	1.8–1.9	*1.4–1.6*	*1.6–1.8*	*1.7–1.9*	*2.0–2.3*	*2.1–2.4*
Household income						
Low	3.0	2.8	3.0	3.0	3.3	3.1
	2.9–3.2	*2.5–3.0*	*2.7–3.3*	*2.8–3.3*	*3.1–3.5*	*2.8–3.4*
Medium	2.0	1.7	1.8	2.0	2.3	2.4
	2.0–2.1	*1.6–1.9*	*1.7–2.0*	*1.8–2.1*	*2.2–2.4*	*2.2–2.6*
High	1.6	1.2	1.5	1.5	1.8	2.1
	1.6–1.7	*1.1–1.4*	*1.4–1.6*	*1.4–1.6*	*1.7–2.0*	*1.9–2.4*
Residential location						
Major city	2.3	2.0	2.2	2.3	2.6	2.7
	2.2–2.5	*1.8–2.2*	*2.0–2.4*	*2.1–2.4*	*2.4–2.8*	*2.5–2.9*
Inner regional	2.2	1.9	2.0	2.2	2.5	2.4
	2.1–2.3	*1.7–2.1*	*1.8–2.2*	*2.0–2.3*	*2.3–2.7*	*2.2–2.5*
Outer regional	2.2	2.0	2.0	2.1	2.4	2.6
	2.1–2.4	*1.8–2.3*	*1.8–2.1*	*1.9–2.3*	*2.2–2.6*	*2.5–2.8*
Remote/Very remote	2.8	2.5	3.0	2.7	2.8	2.9
	2.3–3.3	*1.8–3.2*	*2.3–3.8*	*2.0–3.4*	*2.2–3.5*	*2.4–3.4*
Reason for last dental visit						
Check-up	2.1	1.6	1.8	2.0	2.4	2.5
	2.0–2.2	*1.5–1.7*	*1.7–1.9*	*1.9–2.1*	*2.2–2.5*	*2.4–2.7*
Dental problem	2.7	2.5	2.6	2.5	2.9	3.1
	2.6–2.9	*2.2–2.9*	*2.3–2.9*	*2.3–2.8*	*2.7–3.2*	*2.6–3.6*

Row 1: Means were computed using weighted data.
Row 2: 95% CI: Confidence intervals for estimates were computed using weighted data.
Columns are arranged by age at time of Survey.

8.3 Patterns of other dietary sugar consumption

Historically, sugar in food was consumed either as added table sugar (into drinks etc.) or added by the home cook. Increasingly, sugar consumed in foods is likely to be found in processed foods (Williams 2001). Sugary foods, including sweetened dairy products, biscuits, cakes, puddings, chocolate, lollies, jams, sweet spreads and muesli bars, all add to children's sugar consumption.

Almost half of all children usually consumed at least four serves of various sugary foods on a usual day (Table 8-9). This proportion increased with age. Older children were around 1.2 times more likely to do so than younger children.

At all ages, Indigenous children were most likely to consume four or more serves of sugary foods a day (60%) while children form the high income households were least likely to do so (40%). Gradients were evident for Indigenous identity, parent's country of birth, parental education, household income and reason for last dental visit.

Children with a parent born overseas and those who last visited for a check-up were 10% more likely to consume four or more serves of sugary food a day while Indigenous children were 20% more likely than non-Indigenous children to do so. Children of a parent with school-only education and children from low income households were 1.4 times more likely than children of tertiary-educated parents and children from high income households to usually consume at least four serves of sugary foods on a usual day.

While differences persisted across age groups for both of these characteristics, the differences were smaller in the older age groups, due mainly to a greater increase in consumption at higher ages in the lower risk groups.

In summary, half of Australian children consumed a large quantity of sugary foods per day. This pattern was established early among children from low socioeconomic backgrounds. Socioeconomic gradients existed in this dietary pattern.

Table 8-9: Percentage of children who had four or more serves of sugar-containing snacks in a usual day in the Australian child population (includes sweetened dairy, biscuits, cake, pudding, chocolate, lollies, jams, sweet spreads, muesli bars)

| | Population: children aged 5–14 years | | | | | |
	All ages	5–6	7–8	9–10	11–12	13–14
All	49.8	45.1	47.2	48.9	53.6	54.2
	48.4–51.1	*42.5–47.7*	*44.9–49.5*	*46.7–51.1*	*51.4–55.7*	*51.9–56.4*
Sex						
Male	50.5	46.7	47.9	49.3	53.3	55.5
	48.9–52.1	*43.3–50.2*	*44.8–51.1*	*46.2–52.3*	*50.3–56.2*	*52.3–58.7*
Female	49.0	43.3	46.4	48.5	53.8	52.8
	47.3–50.7	*40.3–46.4*	*43.4–49.6*	*45.7–51.3*	*51.1–56.6*	*49.4–56.2*
Indigenous identity						
Non-Indigenous	49.2	44.1	46.8	48.4	53.2	53.8
	47.9–50.6	*41.5–46.7*	*44.4–49.2*	*46.1–50.7*	*51.0–55.4*	*51.5–56.0*
Indigenous	59.6	60.3	52.9	58.1	61.8	66.9
	54.3–64.8	*51.7–68.4*	*43.2–62.5*	*48.9–66.7*	*51.3–71.3*	*56.6–75.8*
Parents' country of birth						
Australian born	48.2	43.2	44.6	48.4	52.9	51.8
	46.8–49.5	*40.6–45.8*	*42.0–47.3*	*45.7–51.0*	*50.4–55.4*	*49.2–54.5*
Overseas born	52.8	48.7	51.8	49.9	54.9	58.6
	50.5–55.1	*44.1–53.4*	*48.1–55.5*	*46.4–53.4*	*51.2–58.6*	*54.8–62.2*
Parental education						
School	59.9	57.4	60.5	60.3	59.9	61.3
	57.7–62.0	*53.2–61.5*	*56.2–64.6*	*55.7–64.7*	*55.7–63.9*	*56.9–65.6*
Vocational training	51.2	47.4	46.9	48.4	55.3	57.1
	48.9–53.4	*42.6–52.2*	*42.3–51.6*	*43.6–53.1*	*50.3–60.2*	*51.8–62.1*
Tertiary education	43.0	36.6	39.8	42.0	49.0	48.3
	41.3–44.6	*33.6–39.6*	*36.9–42.7*	*39.2–44.9*	*46.1–51.9*	*45.4–51.2*
Household income						
Low	58.7	58.1	58.1	56.3	60.6	60.4
	56.8–60.7	*53.7–62.4*	*54.1–62.0*	*52.5–60.0*	*56.9–64.2*	*56.4–64.4*
Medium	48.4	42.0	45.6	49.0	52.5	52.8
	46.7–50.1	*38.8–45.3*	*42.5–48.7*	*45.5–52.5*	*49.1–56.0*	*49.1–56.6*
High	40.9	32.5	38.5	39.4	46.7	48.2
	38.8–43.0	*28.6–36.6*	*34.3–42.9*	*35.4–43.6*	*42.8–50.6*	*44.1–52.4*
Residential location						
Major city	49.0	44.1	47.1	46.6	53.4	53.8
	47.2–50.7	*40.8–47.5*	*44.0–50.2*	*43.7–49.6*	*50.7–56.1*	*50.8–56.9*
Inner regional	49.0	43.9	44.1	52.5	52.2	51.8
	46.7–51.3	*39.5–48.5*	*40.1–48.1*	*49.0–56.0*	*47.2–57.1*	*48.0–55.7*
Outer regional	56.3	51.9	54.1	57.4	58.6	59.1
	53.5–59.1	*46.6–57.2*	*49.8–58.4*	*53.0–61.6*	*53.2–63.8*	*54.0–63.9*
Remote/Very remote	52.4	56.1	48.1	48.5	48.7	61.2
	46.6–58.1	*45.9–65.8*	*37.8–58.5*	*39.3–57.9*	*39.4–58.2*	*50.2–71.1*
Reason for last dental visit						
Check-up	47.9	39.5	44.0	47.8	52.0	53.1
	46.4–49.4	*36.7–42.4*	*41.3–46.6*	*45.1–50.5*	*49.7–54.3*	*50.5–55.8*
Dental problem	54.0	52.3	51.9	51.2	57.5	57.4
	51.4–56.5	*46.5–58.0*	*46.8–56.9*	*47.1–55.4*	*52.5–62.4*	*51.0–63.6*

Row 1: Proportions were computed using weighted data.
Row 2: 95% CI: Confidence intervals for estimates were computed using weighted data.
Columns are arranged by age at time of Survey.

Average number of serves of sugary foods consumed indicates the total amount of population level consumption of sugary foods. On average, children consumed just over four servings of sugary foods on a usual day (Table 8-10). There was some variation with age with older children consuming about 10% more than the youngest age group.

For all ages, Indigenous children and children whose parents had school-only education consumed the largest number of serves of sugary foods a day (4.8 serves) while children from the high income households had the lowest consumption (3.5). Significant gradients existed across groups by Indigenous identity, parent's country of birth, parental education, household income and reason for last dental visit.

Children who had a parent born overseas and children whose last visit was for a problem, consumed around 10% more serves than those with Australian-born parents or who last visited for a check-up. Indigenous children consumed around 20% more serves of sugary food than non-Indigenous children. Children of a parent with a school-only education and those from the lowest income households consumed 30% and 40% more sugary snacks than children of tertiary-educated parents or from high income households, respectively. Children whose last dental visit was because of a dental problem had a significantly higher than average amount of serves of sugary foods than those who last visited for a check-up. There was a slight attenuation of the difference across age groups, reflecting a larger increase in consumption with higher ages in the lower risk groups.

In summary, the average daily amount of sugary foods consumed by Australian children varied across socioeconomic groups and reason for last dental visit.

Table 8-10: Average number of serves of sugar containing snacks in the Australian child population consumed in a usual day (includes sweetened dairy, biscuits, cake, pudding, chocolate, lollies, jams, sweet spreads, muesli bars)

	Population: children aged 5–14 years					
	All ages	5–6	7–8	9–10	11–12	13–14
All	4.1	3.9	3.9	4.0	4.3	4.4
	4.0–4.2	3.8–4.1	3.8–4.1	3.9–4.1	4.2–4.5	4.2–4.5
Sex						
Male	4.2	3.9	4.0	4.1	4.3	4.4
	4.1–4.3	3.8–4.1	3.8–4.2	3.9–4.2	4.1–4.5	4.3–4.6
Female	4.1	3.9	3.9	4.0	4.4	4.4
	4.0–4.2	3.7–4.1	3.7–4.0	3.8–4.1	4.2–4.5	4.1–4.6
Indigenous identity						
Non-Indigenous	4.1	3.8	3.9	4.0	4.3	4.4
	4.0–4.2	3.7–4.0	3.8–4.1	3.9–4.1	4.2–4.4	4.2–4.5
Indigenous	4.8	4.8	4.3	4.6	5.1	5.4
	4.4–5.2	4.1–5.5	3.7–4.9	4.0–5.2	4.4–5.8	4.7–6.1
Parents' country of birth						
Australian born	3.9	3.8	3.7	3.9	4.2	4.2
	3.9–4.0	3.6–3.9	3.6–3.8	3.8–4.0	4.0–4.3	4.0–4.3
Overseas born	4.4	4.2	4.3	4.2	4.6	4.8
	4.3–4.6	3.9–4.5	4.0–4.6	4.0–4.5	4.4–4.9	4.5–5.2
Parental education						
School	4.8	4.6	4.7	4.7	4.9	4.9
	4.6–4.9	4.3–4.9	4.4–5.0	4.4–5.0	4.6–5.2	4.6–5.3
Vocational training	4.1	3.9	3.8	3.9	4.2	4.4
	3.9–4.2	3.7–4.1	3.6–4.1	3.7–4.1	4.0–4.5	4.1–4.7
Tertiary education	3.7	3.5	3.5	3.6	4.0	4.0
	3.6–3.8	3.3–3.6	3.4–3.7	3.5–3.8	3.9–4.2	3.9–4.2
Household income						
Low	4.8	4.8	4.7	4.7	5.0	4.9
	4.7–4.9	4.5–5.0	4.4–5.0	4.4–4.9	4.7–5.2	4.6–5.1
Medium	3.9	3.7	3.8	3.9	4.1	4.2
	3.8–4.0	3.5–3.9	3.6–3.9	3.7–4.0	4.0–4.3	4.0–4.4
High	3.5	3.1	3.4	3.4	3.9	4.0
	3.4–3.7	3.0–3.3	3.2–3.6	3.2–3.6	3.6–4.1	3.7–4.3
Residential location						
Major city	4.1	3.8	3.9	3.9	4.4	4.4
	4.0–4.2	3.6–4.0	3.7–4.1	3.8–4.1	4.2–4.5	4.2–4.6
Inner regional	4.1	3.9	3.8	4.2	4.2	4.3
	3.9–4.2	3.6–4.2	3.6–4.0	4.0–4.4	3.9–4.4	4.1–4.5
Outer regional	4.4	4.4	4.2	4.2	4.5	4.6
	4.2–4.6	4.0–4.8	3.9–4.6	4.0–4.5	4.2–4.9	4.2–4.9
Remote/Very remote	4.4	4.3	4.1	4.4	4.5	4.6
	4.0–4.8	3.9–4.7	3.6–4.7	3.5–5.3	3.7–5.3	3.8–5.3
Reason for last dental visit						
Check-up	4.0	3.5	3.7	3.9	4.2	4.3
	3.9–4.0	3.4–3.7	3.5–3.8	3.7–4.0	4.1–4.3	4.2–4.5
Dental problem	4.5	4.4	4.4	4.3	4.7	4.7
	4.3–4.7	4.1–4.7	4.1–4.8	4.0–4.6	4.4–5.0	4.2–5.2

Row 1: Means were computed using weighted data.
Row 2: 95% CI: Confidence intervals for estimates were computed using weighted data.
Columns are arranged by age at time of Survey.

Table sugar is a common source of sugar consumed daily by the population. Almost half (44%) of Australian children added one or more teaspoons of table sugar to their food or drink in a usual day (Table 8-11). The prevalence of this behaviour increased as age increased with the oldest children 1.6 times more likely to add sugar to food or drink than the youngest children.

For all ages, over 60% of Indigenous children consumed table sugar daily while just over 35% of children from high income households did so. Significant gradients were observed across groups by Indigenous identity, parental education, household income, residential location and reason for last dental visit.

Children living in Inner Regional and Outer regional areas were 1.1 and 1.2 times more likely than children living in Major city areas to add sugar to food or drinks. Children of a parent with a school–only education and children living in low income households were 1.4 times more likely than children of a tertiary-educated parent or those living in high income households to do so.

The socioeconomic gradients in consumption of table sugar remained consistent across age groups. Over three-quarters of Indigenous children aged 13–14 years had added table sugar while just over half of non-Indigenous children of the same age did so. Children of that same age group whose parent had school-only education and children from low income households were 1.3 times more likely to consume table sugar than children of parents with a tertiary education and children from high income households.

In summary, the use of table sugar was high among Australian children. Significant socioeconomic gradients existed in the use of table sugar.

Table 8-11: Percentage of children who added one or more teaspoon(s) of table sugar (for example, in tea, Milo or cereal) in a usual day in the Australian child population

	Population: children aged 5–14 years					
	All ages	5–6	7–8	9–10	11–12	13–14
All	**44.0**	**33.4**	**41.2**	**43.4**	**49.5**	**52.4**
	42.4–45.5	*30.9–36.0*	*38.7–43.7*	*40.7–46.1*	*47.1–51.9*	*49.8–55.1*
Sex						
Male	44.4	32.2	41.3	45.3	48.8	55.1
	42.4–46.4	*29.0–35.5*	*38.0–44.7*	*41.8–48.7*	*45.7–52.0*	*51.0–59.1*
Female	43.5	34.8	41.1	41.5	50.2	49.9
	41.7–45.4	*31.5–38.1*	*38.0–44.2*	*38.2–44.9*	*47.0–53.4*	*46.3–53.5*
Indigenous identity						
Non-Indigenous	43.0	31.8	39.7	43.1	48.8	51.4
	41.4–44.5	*29.4–34.4*	*37.3–42.2*	*40.4–45.9*	*46.4–51.3*	*48.7–54.1*
Indigenous	61.5	58.9	63.2	50.1	60.9	76.7
	56.2–66.5	*49.1–68.0*	*53.5–72.0*	*39.4–60.8*	*51.1–69.8*	*66.7–84.4*
Parents' country of birth						
Australian born	42.5	32.7	39.1	42.3	47.8	50.9
	40.8–44.2	*29.9–35.6*	*36.1–42.1*	*39.3–45.4*	*45.1–50.5*	*47.7–54.1*
Overseas born	46.5	34.8	44.7	45.3	52.5	55.1
	44.2–48.8	*30.9–38.9*	*41.0–48.4*	*41.1–49.6*	*48.5–56.4*	*50.5–59.6*
Parental education						
School	53.9	44.6	53.8	53.6	56.4	61.0
	51.5–56.4	*40.4–48.9*	*49.2–58.4*	*48.6–58.4*	*52.1–60.6*	*55.4–66.3*
Vocational training	43.5	33.3	41.4	42.6	48.0	51.1
	40.9–46.1	*29.1–37.8*	*36.3–46.7*	*37.8–47.6*	*43.3–52.7*	*45.3–56.9*
Tertiary education	37.7	26.8	33.6	37.5	45.0	46.9
	35.9–39.5	*23.7–30.2*	*31.0–36.3*	*34.2–40.8*	*41.9–48.2*	*43.7–50.2*
Household income						
Low	53.3	42.1	52.0	53.3	58.3	60.5
	51.1–55.4	*38.1–46.3*	*47.4–56.6*	*49.0–57.6*	*54.3–62.2*	*55.5–65.4*
Medium	41.6	31.1	39.2	40.8	48.9	48.1
	39.7–43.5	*27.8–34.6*	*36.0–42.6*	*37.2–44.5*	*45.1–52.7*	*44.1–52.1*
High	35.9	25.3	32.3	35.4	39.7	47.5
	33.7–38.2	*21.1–30.0*	*28.4–36.4*	*30.8–40.2*	*35.4–44.2*	*42.7–52.2*
Residential location						
Major city	41.7	31.8	40.2	39.8	47.1	50.1
	39.7–43.7	*28.8–35.0*	*37.0–43.5*	*36.5–43.2*	*44.2–50.2*	*46.5–53.7*
Inner regional	46.7	34.3	40.0	51.7	53.7	53.0
	43.9–49.4	*29.9–38.9*	*35.5–44.6*	*46.8–56.5*	*48.7–58.6*	*48.3–57.7*
Outer regional	51.5	41.9	46.0	49.0	54.2	64.1
	47.8–55.2	*35.3–48.9*	*41.0–51.0*	*43.7–54.4*	*47.9–60.3*	*58.3–69.6*
Remote/Very remote	54.0	41.4	57.0	52.5	61.1	57.5
	43.2–64.5	*25.4–59.5*	*41.6–71.2*	*31.3–72.8*	*50.0–71.1*	*40.5–72.9*
Reason for last dental visit						
Check-up	42.3	29.1	37.2	41.9	47.6	50.8
	40.6–44.0	*26.1–32.2*	*34.3–40.3*	*39.0–44.9*	*45.0–50.2*	*47.8–53.8*
Dental problem	48.3	42.0	46.9	42.8	53.0	58.5
	45.6–51.1	*35.6–48.6*	*41.8–52.0*	*38.0–47.7*	*47.7–58.2*	*51.6–65.1*

Row 1: Proportions were computed using weighted data.
Row 2: 95% CI: Confidence intervals for estimates were computed using weighted data.
Columns are arranged by age at time of Survey.

Summary

The majority of Australian children consumed at least one glass of tap or mains water, and at least 60% consumed 80% or more of their drinking water from tap or mains. Importantly, the consistently high proportion of children consuming fluoridated water reinforces both the effectiveness and equity of water fluoridation. There were, however, significant variations with children living outside of Major city areas less likely to consume tap or mains water, as were Indigenous children, children whose parents had school-only education, those from lower income households and children who made their last dental visit for a dental problem. These children were also more likely to consume bottled water. The gradients were established from a young age and continued through to older age (13–14 years). These patterns of water consumption may contribute to a widening of social inequalities in child oral health.

Australian dietary guidelines advise that sweetened beverages and snacks are 'discretionary choices' because they are not an essential or necessary part of healthy dietary patterns. As such they should be consumed 'only sometimes and in small amounts' (National Health and Medical Research Council 2013). Around half of all children consumed at least one discretionary drink on a usual day and one in five drank four or more glasses of these sugary drinks. Further, half of all children consumed at least four serves of sugary foods on a usual day. These findings indicate that a significant proportion of Australian children exceeded the daily recommended sugar intake.

With the exception of water consumption and one measure of sugary drink consumption, there were few variations according to remoteness location and there were few differences between males and females. Where differences between males and females were evident, they tended to be largest in the older age groups and consistently showed males consuming more sugary drinks than females.

There were consistent differences in consumption of sugary drinks and food by parental education and household income. The inequalities between groups by parental education and household income attenuated somewhat as age increased for a number of the consumption items examined. However, when they did so, it was because the children of more highly educated parents or from higher income households increased their consumption more rapidly than the children of less highly educated parents or from lower income households. The fact that children in the less well educated and lower income groups have a higher level of exposure to sugary drinks and food for a longer period of time means that their permanent teeth are at higher risk of developing caries early in life. However, the 'catch-up' in high levels of consumption by children from more highly educated or higher income households suggests that the benefits of lower levels of risk behaviours will be lost over time.

To conclude, the results from this chapter demonstrated that a large proportion of Australian children consume large amounts of sugar which can contribute to population burden of oral diseases. The socioeconomic gradients in general health behaviours are likely to be a strong contributor to socioeconomic inequality in child oral health. The health promotion challenge that these patterns of water and sugar consumption pose is complex. Health promotion efforts are needed to promote consumption of tap/public water and prevent uptake of sugar consumption in the whole population. While these efforts must be universal, their scale and intensity should be proportionate to the level of exposure experienced by children in various socioeconomic groups. That is, strategies should be selected to have their largest impact on children with the highest risk of having the health damaging behaviours. Finally, efforts to promote tap/public water consumption and prevent uptake of sugar will need to be in operation from early life and throughout childhood. Given that oral diseases are more immediate outcomes related to sugar consumption, timely prevention of oral diseases through general health promotion will also lead to prevention of later onset general health conditions such as obesity/overweight and diabetes.

References

Armfield JM & Spencer AJ 2004. Consumption of nonpublic water: implications for children's caries experience. Community Dent Oral Epidemiol 32(4):283–96.

Australian Bureau of Statistics 2015. Australian Health Survey: Nutrition First Results — Food and Nutrients, 2011–12. Canberra: Australian Bureau of Statistics.

Burt BA 2002. Fluoridation and social equity. J Public Health Dent 62(4):195–200.

Iheozor-Ejiofor Z, Worthington HV, Walsh T, O'Malley L, Clarkson JE, Macey R, Alam R, Tugwell P, Welch V & Glenny AM 2015. Water fluoridation for the prevention of dental caries. Cochrane Database Syst Rev (6):CD010856.

Moynihan PJ & Kelly SA 2014. Effect on caries of restricting sugars intake: systematic review to inform WHO guidelines. J Dent Res 93(1):8–18.

National Health and Medical Research Council 2007. A systematic review of the efficacy and safety of fluoridation. Canberra: National Health and Medical Research Council.

National Health and Medical Research Council 2013. Eat for health. Australian dietary guidelines. NHMRC. Canberra: Australian Government.

Rugg-Gunn AJ & Do L 2012. Effectiveness of water fluoridation in caries prevention. Community Dent Oral Epidemiol 40 Suppl 2:55–64.

Sheiham A & James WP 2014. A reappraisal of the quantitative relationship between sugar intake and dental caries: the need for new criteria for developing goals for sugar intake. BMC Public Health 14:863.

Slade GD, Spencer AJ, Davies MJ & Stewart JF 1995. Influence of exposure to fluoridated water on socioeconomic inequalities in children's caries experience. Community Dent Oral Epidemiol 24:89–100.

Spencer AJ, Slade GD & Davies M 1996. Water fluoridation in Australia. Community Dent Health 13 Suppl 2:27–37.

Williams P 2001. Sugar: Is there a need for a dietary guideline in Australia. Australian Journal of Nutrition and Dietetics. 58(1):26–31.

World Health Organization 2015. Guideline: Sugars intake for adults and children. Geneva: World Health Organization.

9 Social gradients in child oral health

MA Peres, X Ju and AJ Spencer

Introduction

Health and behaviours are determined above all by social conditions (Sheiham et al. 2014) and for this reason social conditions in which people live have been considered as the cause of causes of diseases and health disorders (Braveman & Gottlieb 2014).

Differences in levels of oral health that disproportionally affect socially disadvantaged members of society and that are avoidable, unfair and unjust are defined as oral health inequalities. It is not only the difference between the rich and the poor but a consistent gradient across the social economic ladder that exists and is universally found (Watt et al. 2016). The huge extent of contemporary health inequalities has led to be termed as the plague of our era (Farmer 2001). Therefore, it is important to document and understand oral health inequalities in order to allow the implementation of the most appropriate oral health interventions.

There are several individual and area-based measures of socioeconomic position. This chapter presents Australia's child oral health outcomes according to parents' educational level, household income, Index of Relative Socio-economic Advantage and Disadvantage (IRSAD) and Index of Community Socio-Educational Advantage (ICSEA).

Among several individual measures of socioeconomic position, income and education are most widely used. Education usually results from an individual's schooling until the beginning of the third decade of life, and has little variation from then on. Its impact can occur either in the increase of knowledge and ability to take on healthy habits or in their insertion in the job market, in better positions and with higher incomes (Lynch & Kaplan 2000).

Income is a useful measure of socioeconomic position because it is related directly to the material circumstances that may influence health and health-related behaviours (Lynch & Kaplan 2000).

The IRSAD summarises information about the economic and social conditions of people and households within an area, including both relative advantage and disadvantage measures. The average IRSAD value is 1000. A lower score indicates that an area is relatively disadvantaged compared to an area with a higher score (Australian Bureau of Statistics 2014).

The ICSEA is an index which combines students' characteristics (such as parental occupation and level of education) and school's area characteristics such as proportion of Indigenous children and geographical location. The lower the ICSEA value, the lower the level of educational advantage of students who attend this school.

ICSEA is set at an average of 1000 (Australian Curriculum, Assessment and Reporting Authority 2013).

9.1 Socioeconomic aspects of child oral health

Table 9-1 presents the percentage of children according to parental education, household income and area (IRSAD) and school levels (ICSEA) of relative socioeconomic disadvantage.

Overall, the highest proportion of children (48.6%) had parents with a tertiary education, the lowest proportion (22.5%) had parents with vocational training, while the remaining children (28.9%) had parents with school-only education. Very little variation was seen when comparing children aged 5–8 years and those aged 9–14 years.

More children (38.4%) were from households with a medium income, followed by those from low income households (32.5%) and those from high income households (29.1%). Again, little differences were observed between age groups.

Overall, slightly over one-third of children are placed in the highest IRSAD group (IRSAD score >1026), 28.4% of children are from the lowest IRSAD group (IRSAD<948), while 37.0% are in the medium IRSAD group (ISRAD 948–1044). The proportion distribution of children aged 5–8 and 9-14 years across IRSAD groups is almost identical.

Overall, nearly one-third of the sampled children were allocated in one of the three ICSEA groups (lowest, medium and highest scores).

Oral health of Australian children

Table 9-1: Estimated percentages of children by selected socioeconomic characteristics in the Australian child population

Age (years)	Population: children aged 5–14 years		
	All ages	5–8	9–14
All	–	**40.2**	**59.8**
	–	*39.3–41.1*	*58.9–60.7*
Parental education			
EDU1 (Lowest: School)	28.9	27.8	29.6
	28.0–29.8	*26.4–29.2*	*28.4–30.8*
EDU2 (Medium: Vocational training)	22.5	21.5	23.1
	21.7–23.3	*20.3–22.8*	*22.1–24.2*
EDU3 (Highest: Tertiary)	48.6	50.6	47.3
	47.7–49.6	*49.2–52.1*	*46.0–48.5*
Household income			
Income1 (Lowest: <$60,000)	32.5	31.6	33.1
	31.6–33.4	*30.3–33.0*	*31.9–34.3*
Income2 (Medium: $60,000 to $120,000)	38.4	37.8	38.8
	37.5–39.3	*36.4–39.2*	*37.6–40.0*
Income3 (Highest: >$120,000)	29.1	30.6	28.1
	28.2–30.0	*29.1–32.0*	*27.0–29.3*
Area level (IRSAD)			
IRSAD1 (Lowest: IRSAD score<948)	28.4	28.8	28.1
	27.6–29.2	*27.5–30.0*	*27.1–29.2*
IRSAD2 (Medium: IRSAD score 948–1026)	37.6	38.2	37.3
	36.7–38.5	*36.8–39.5*	*36.1–38.4*
IRSAD3 (Highest: IRSAD score >1026)	34.0	33.1	34.6
	33.1–34.9	*31.7–34.5*	*33.4–35.8*
School level (ICSEA)			
ICSEA1 (Lowest: ICSEA score<986)	34.0	33.6	34.3
	33.1–34.9	*32.3–34.9*	*33.1–35.4*
ICSEA2 (Medium: ICSEA score 986–1044)	30.9	31.3	30.7
	30.1–31.8	*30.0–32.6*	*29.6–31.8*
ICSEA3 (Highest: ICSEA score >1044)	35.1	35.2	35.0
	34.2–36.0	*33.8–36.6*	*33.9–36.2*

Row 1: Proportions were computed using weighted data.
Row 2: 95% CI: Confidence intervals for estimates were computed using weighted data.
Columns are arranged by age at time of Survey.

Caries prevalence in the primary dentition

The prevalence of dental caries in the primary dentition was expressed as the percentage of children with dmfs>0.

Table 9-2 displays the prevalence of dental caries in the primary dentition according to parental education, household income and area and school socioeconomic indicators. Overall, the prevalence of dental caries in the primary dentition was 39.5% varying from 34.3% among children aged 5–6 years to 45.1% among children aged 7–8 years.

A higher proportion of children whose parents had school-only education had dental caries compared to children of parents who had vocational education and tertiary education (50.0%, 37.5% and 33.2%, respectively). The highest prevalence of dental caries in the primary dentition was 54.4% among children aged 7–8 years of parents who had school-only education, while the lowest prevalence was 27.5% among children aged 5–6 years whose parents were tertiary educated.

The lower the household income the higher prevalence there was of dental caries in the primary dentition. Overall, half of children from the lowest household income group had dental caries in their primary dentition, a prevalence of 40% and 66% higher than among children from medium and high income households, respectively. The highest prevalence (53.4%) was among children aged 7–8 years from the lowest household income group and the lowest prevalence (22.8%) was among children aged 5–6 years from the highest household income group.

A clear distinction in the prevalence of dental caries in the primary dentition across IRSAD groups was identified. The highest prevalence (53.7%) was among children aged 7–8 years living in the most disadvantaged areas while the lowest prevalence (24.8%) was among children aged 5–6 years from less disadvantaged areas.

Prevalence of dental caries in the primary dentition varied across levels of ICSEA from 30.6% among children from the highest ISCEA group to 51.1% among those children from the lowest ICSEA group. The ratio between dental caries prevalence in the primary dentition in children aged 5–6 years from low and high ICSEA groups was 1.9 and 1.4 between low and medium ICSEA groups, respectively. Children aged 7–8 years from the lowest ICSEA group had 52% and 36% higher prevalence of dental caries compared to high and medium ICSEA groups, respectively.

There was a clear gradient in the percentage of children with dental caries in the primary dentition across parental education, household income, IRSAD and ICSEA groups.

Table 9-2: Prevalence of dental caries experience (dmfs>0) in the primary dentition in the Australian child population

Age (years)	Population: children aged 5—8 years		
	All ages	5—6	7—8
All	**39.5**	**34.3**	**45.1**
	38.2–40.9	*32.3–36.2*	*43.1–47.0*
Parental education			
EDU1 (Lowest: School)	50.0	45.9	54.4
	47.0–53.0	41.7–50.2	50.1–58.7
EDU2 (Medium: Vocational training)	37.5	32.6	42.5
	34.4–40.6	28.4–36.8	38.0–47.1
EDU3 (Highest: Tertiary)	33.2	27.5	39.1
	31.4 – 35.0	*25.0 - 30.0*	*36.4–41.7*
Household income			
Income1 (Lowest)	50.2	47.4	53.4
	47.46–52.8	*43.6–51.2*	*49.7–57.0*
Income2 (Medium)	35.8	30.7	41.0
	33.7–37.9	*27.9–33.6*	*37.9–44.1*
Income3 (Highest)	30.3	22.8	38.0
	27.7–33.0	*19.4–26.3*	*34.0–42.0*
Area level (IRSAD)			
IRSAD1 (Lowest)	48.4	43.0	53.7
	45.9–51.0	*39.2–46.7*	*50.2–57.2*
IRSAD2	40.8	36.1	46.0
	38.6–43.0	*33.1–39.2*	*42.8–49.2*
IRSAD3 (Highest)	30.4	24.8	36.2
	28.0–32.7	*21.7–27.9*	*32.7–39.7*
School level (ICSEA)			
ICSEA 1(Lowest)	51.1	45.6	56.7
	48.7–53.4	*42.2–49.0*	*53.5–60.0*
ICSEA 2	37.3	33.5	41.5
	34.8–39.7	*30.1–36.8*	*38.0–45.0*
ICSEA 3 (Highest)	30.6	24.0	37.1
	28.3–32.9	*20.9–27.1*	*33.7–40.5*

Row 1: Proportions were computed using weighted data.
Row 2: 95% CI: Confidence intervals for estimates were computed using weighted data.
Columns are arranged by age at time of Survey.

Caries experience in the primary dentition

Caries experience in the primary dentition is presented by the average number of decayed, missing and filled surfaces due to dental caries (dmfs).

Table 9-3 shows the average dmfs across parental education, household income, area and school socioeconomic indicators. Overall, children aged 5–8 years had an average of 3.1 surfaces affected by dental caries in the primary dentition ranging from 2.7 surfaces among children aged 5–6 years to 3.6 surfaces among children aged 7–8 years.

Children of less educated parents had a higher average of caries experience than those children of more educated parents. The highest average of dmfs was 5.0 among children aged 7–8 years whose parents had school-only education while the lowest dmfs was 1.7 among children aged 5–6 years whose parents were tertiary educated.

There was a gradient in dental caries experience in the primary dentition across household income groups. The highest average dmfs was among children from low income households (4.6). Children from the lowest household income group had 2.4 times and 1.8 times higher average dmfs than children from high and medium income households, respectively. The highest ratio in average dmfs was 3.3 between children aged 5–6 years from the lowest and the highest household income groups.

Overall, children from the lowest IRSAD group had an average dmfs of 95% and a 38% higher score than those children from the highest and intermediate IRSAD groups respectively. The highest dental caries experience ratio was 2.2 between children aged 5–6 years from the lowest and the highest IRSAD groups.

Caries experience was 2.4 times higher among children from the lowest ICSEA group than among children of the highest ICSEA group. The highest average dmfs across ICSEA groups was 5.2 among children aged 7–8 years from the lowest ICSEA group and the lowest average dmfs was 1.5 among children from the highest ICSEA group.

Oral health of Australian children

Table 9-3: Average number of decayed, missing or filled primary tooth surfaces (dmfs) per child in the Australian child population

Age (years)	Population: children aged 5—8 years		
	All ages	5—6	7—8
All	3.1	2.7	3.6
	3.0 –3.3	*2.5 –2.9*	*3.4–3.8*
Parental education			
EDU1 (Lowest)	4.8	4.5	5.0
	4.4–5.1	*4.0–5.1*	*4.5–5.5*
EDU2	2.7	2.2	3.3
	2.4–3.0	*1.8–2.5*	*2.9–3.7*
EDU3 (Highest)	2.2	1.7	2.7
	2.1–2.3	*1.5–1.9*	*2.5–2.9*
Household income			
Income1(Lowest)	4.6	4.3	5.0
	4.3–4.9	*3.9–4.7*	*4.6–5.4*
Income2	2.6	2.2	2.9
	2.4–2.7	*1.9–2.5*	*2.7–3.2*
Income3 (Highest)	1.9	1.3	2.5
	1.7–2.1	*1.1–1.6*	*2.2–2.8*
Area level (IRSAD)			
IRSAD1(Lowest)	4.3	3.7	4.8
	4.0–4.5	*3.3–4.1*	*4.5–5.2*
IRSAD2	3.1	2.8	3.4
	2.9–3.3	*2.5–3.1*	*3.1–3.6*
IRSAD3 (Highest)	2.2	1.7	2.7
	2.0–2.4	*1.5–2.0*	*2.4–3.0*
School level (ICSEA)			
ICSEA 1(Lowest)	4.7	4.2	5.2
	4.4–5.0	*3.8–4.6*	*4.9–5.6*
ICSEA 2	2.7	2.4	3.1
	2.6–2.9	*2.2–2.7*	*2.8–3.4*
ICSEA 3 (Highest)	2.0	1.5	2.5
	1.8–2.2	*1.3–1.7*	*2.2–2.7*

Row 1: Proportions were computed using weighted data.
Row 2: 95% CI: Confidence intervals for estimates were computed using weighted data.
Columns are arranged by age at time of Survey.

Untreated dental caries in the primary dentition

The experience of untreated dental caries in the primary dentition across socioeconomic groups is presented in Table 9-4. Overall, children had, on average, 1.4 surfaces with untreated dental caries with very small to no statistically significant differences between age groups.

The higher the average number of untreated dental caries surfaces the lower the level of parental education. Children whose parents had school-only education had 2.8 and 2.3 times higher the average number of surfaces with untreated dental caries than children whose parents had a tertiary education and vocational education, respectively.

There was a gradient in the average number of untreated surfaces across household income groups. Children in the highest income group had an average of 0.7 untreated surfaces compared to 1.0 among those with medium income and 2.4 among children from the lowest income group. There was a 2.4-fold ratio in the average number of surfaces with untreated dental caries between the lowest and highest income groups and a 1.6-fold ratio between the lowest and medium income groups. This pattern was seen across all age groups.

A very similar pattern is observed for household income when area (IRSAD) and school (ISCEA) indicators are compared.

Among all children, the highest average number of untreated dental caries (2.4) was among those children from the lowest ICSEA. This average was 1.8 and 3.4 times higher than among children from the medium and high ICSEA groups, respectively.

In summary, there was a consistent gradient in the average number of untreated surfaces with dental caries in the permanent dentition across parental education, household income, IRSAD and ICSEA groups.

Table 9-4: Average number of untreated decayed tooth surfaces (ds) in the primary dentition in the Australian child population

Age (years)	Population: children aged 5–8 years		
	All ages	5–6	7–8
All	**1.4**	**1.5**	**1.4**
	1.4–1.5	*1.4–1.6*	*1.3–1.5*
Parental education			
EDU1 (Lowest)	2.5	2.7	2.3
	2.3–2.8	*2.3–3.1*	*2.0–2.6*
EDU2	1.1	1.2	1.0
	0.9–1.3	*0.9–1.5*	*0.8–1.2*
EDU3 (Highest)	0.9	0.8	0.9
	0.8–0.9	*0.7–0.9*	*0.8–1.0*
Household income			
Income1 (Lowest)	2.4	2.6	2.1
	2.2–2.6	*2.3–2.9*	*1.9–2.4*
Income2	1.0	1.1	1.0
	0.9–1.2	*0.9–1.3*	*0.9–1.1*
Income3 (Highest)	0.7	0.6	0.7
	0.6–0.7	*0.5–0.7*	*0.6–0.8*
Area level (IRSAD)			
IRSAD1 (Lowest)	2.2	2.2	2.2
	2.0–2.4	*1.9–2.5*	*2.0–2.4*
IRSAD2	1.4	1.5	1.3
	1.3–1.5	*1.3–1.7*	*1.2–1.5*
IRSAD3 (Highest)	0.9	1.0	0.8
	0.8–1.0	*0.8–1.1*	*0.6–0.9*
School level (ICSEA)			
ICSEA 1 (Lowest)	2.4	2.4	2.3
	2.2–2.5	*2.2–2.7*	*2.1–2.5*
ICSEA 2	1.3	1.3	1.2
	1.1–1.4	*1.1–1.5*	*1.0–1.3*
ICSEA 3 (Highest)	0.7	0.8	0.7
	0.7–0.8	*0.6–0.9*	*0.6–0.8*

Row 1: Proportions were computed using weighted data.
Row 2: 95% CI: Confidence intervals for estimates were computed using weighted data.
Columns are arranged by age at time of Survey.

Caries prevalence in the permanent dentition

The prevalence of dental caries in the permanent dentition was expressed as the percentage of children with DMFS>0.

Table 9-5 reports the prevalence of dental caries in the permanent dentition according to parental education, household income, area and school socioeconomic indicators. Overall, the prevalence of dental caries in the permanent dentition was 30.6%, increasing with age from 20.6% among children aged 9–10 years, 30.0% among those aged 11–12 years and reaching 40.9% among children aged 13–14 years.

A higher proportion of children whose parents had school-only education had dental caries compared to children of parents who had vocational education and tertiary education (36.1%, 30.2% and 26.6%, respectively). The highest prevalence of dental caries in the permanent dentition was 46.7% among children aged 13–14 years of parents who had school-only education while the lowest prevalence was 17.4% among children aged 9–10 years whose parents had vocational education.

The lower the household income the higher the prevalence of dental caries in the permanent dentition. Overall, 35.7% of children from the lowest household income group had dental caries in the permanent dentition, a prevalence of 22% and 39% higher than among children from the medium and high income household groups, respectively. The highest prevalence (45.5%) was among children aged 13–14 years from the lowest household income group and the lowest prevalence (14.5%) was among children aged 9–10 years from the highest household income group.

A wide difference in the prevalence of dental caries in the permanent dentition across IRSAD groups was found. The highest prevalence (43.7%) was among children aged 13–14 years living in the medium IRSAD areas while the lowest prevalence (16.5%) was among children aged 9–10 years from less disadvantaged areas.

Overall, the prevalence of dental caries in the permanent dentition varied across school levels of ICSEA from 24.0% among children from the highest ISCEA group to 37.3% among those children of the lowest ICSEA group. The ratio between dental caries prevalence in the permanent dentition in children aged 9–10 years from low and high ICSEA groups was 1.9 and 1.5 between low and medium ICSEA groups. Children aged 11–12 years from the low ICSEA group had 7% and 50% higher prevalence of dental caries compared to medium and high ICSEA groups, respectively. The prevalence of dental caries in children aged 13–14 years varied from 34.2% in the highest ICSEA group, 41.6% in the medium group and 46.6% in the lowest ICSEA group.

There was a clear gradient in the percentage of children with dental caries in the permanent dentition across parental education, household income, IRSAD and ICSEA groups.

Table 9-5: Prevalence of dental caries experience in the permanent dentition (DMFS>0) in the Australian child population

Age (years)	Population: children aged 9–14 years			
	All ages	9–10	11–12	13–14
All	30.6	20.6	30.0	40.9
	29.4–31.7	*19.0–22.1*	*28.2–31.8*	*38.6–43.2*
Parental education				
EDU1 (Lowest)	36.1	25.8	34.9	46.7
	33.8–38.5	*22.1–29.4*	*31.3–38.6*	*40.2–51.4*
EDU2	30.2	17.4	28.9	43.1
	27.7–32.8	*14.3–20.6*	*24.8–32.9*	*38.1–48.1*
EDU3 (Highest)	26.6	18.3	26.7	34.9
	25.1–28.1	*16.2–20.4*	*24.4–29.1*	*31.9–37.9*
Household income				
Income1 (Lowest)	35.7	26.3	34.8	45.5
	33.6–37.8	*23.1–29.5*	*31.5–38.1*	*41.3–49.7*
Income2	29.2	19.2	28.1	40.0
	27.4–31.0	*16.8–21.5*	*25.2–31.0*	*36.4–43.6*
Income3 (Highest)	25.6	14.5	25.7	36.0
	23.4–27.7	*11.8–17.3*	*22.2–29.3*	*31.6–40.4*
Area level (IRSAD)				
IRSAD1 (Lowest)	33.9	26.1	32.9	43.6
	31.8–36.0	*22.9–29.3*	*29.5–36.2*	*39.3–47.9*
IRSAD2	32.1	19.9	32.4	43.7
	30.2–33.9	*17.5–22.4*	*29.5–35.3*	*40.0–47.4*
IRSAD3 (Highest)	26.2	16.5	25.0	36.0
	24.3–28.1	*13.9–19.1*	*22.0–27.9*	*32.2–39.9*
School level (ICSEA)				
ICSEA 1 (Lowest)	37.3	28.3	35.3	46.6
	35.3–39.2	*25.3–31.3*	*32.2–38.4*	*42.8–50.4*
ICSEA 2	30.6	19.2	32.8	41.6
	28.6–32.6	*16.5–21.8*	*29.5–36.1*	*37.4–45.8*
ICSEA 3 (Highest)	24.0	14.6	22.8	34.2
	22.1–25.8	*12.2–17.0*	*20.0–25.7*	*30.3–38.0*

Row 1: Proportions were computed using weighted data.
Row 2: 95% CI: Confidence intervals for estimates were computed using weighted data.
Columns are arranged by age at time of Survey.

Caries experience in the permanent dentition

Caries experience in the permanent dentition is presented by the average number of decayed, missing and filled surfaces due to dental caries (DMFS).

Table 9-6 shows the average DMFS across household area and school socioeconomic indicators. Overall, children had, on average, 1.0 surface affected by dental caries in their permanent dentition varying from 0.5 among children aged 9–10 years to 1.5 among children aged 13–14 years.

Children of less educated parents had a higher average of caries experience than those children of more educated parents. The highest average of DMFS was 2.0 among children aged 13–14 years whose parents had school-only education while the lowest DMFS was 0.4 among children aged 9–10 years whose parents had tertiary education.

There was a gradient in dental caries experience in the permanent dentition across household income groups. The highest average DMFS was among children from the lowest household income group (1.8). Overall, children from the lowest household income group had 1.5 times and 1.3 times higher average DMFS than children from the high and medium household income groups. The highest ratio in average DMFS was 2.3 between children aged 9–10 years from the lowest and the highest household income groups.

Overall, children from the lowest and medium IRSAD groups had an average DMFS 40% higher than those children from the highest IRSAD group. The highest dental caries experience ratio was 1.7 between children aged 9–10 years from the lowest and the highest IRSAD groups.

Caries experience was 1.9 times higher among children from the lowest ICSEA group than among children of the highest ICSEA group. The highest average DMFS across ICSEA groups was 1.8 among children aged 13–14 years from the lowest ICSEA group and the lowest average DMFS was 0.4 among children aged 9–10 years from the highest ICSEA group.

Table 9-6: Average number of decayed, missing or filled permanent tooth surfaces per child (DMFS) in the Australian child population

Age (years)	Population: children aged 9–14 years			
	All ages	9–10	11–12	13–14
All	1.0	0.5	0.9	1.5
	0.9–1.0	*0.5–0.6*	*0.9–1.0*	*1.4–1.6*
Parental education				
EDU1 (Lowest)	1.3	0.7	1.1	2.0
	1.2–1.4	*0.6–0.8*	*1.0–1.3*	*1.8–2.3*
EDU2	0.9	0.4	0.9	13
	0.8–1.0	*0.3–0.5*	*0.8–1.1*	*1.2–1.5*
EDU3 (Highest)	0.8	0.4	0.8	1.1
	0.7–0.8	*0.4–0.5*	*0.7–0.9*	*1.0–1.2*
Household income				
Income1 (Lowest)	1.2	0.7	1.1	1.8
	1.1–1.3	*0.6–0.8*	*1.0–1.2*	*1.6–2.0*
Income2	0.9	0.5	0.8	1.4
	0.8–0.9	*0.4– 0.5*	*0.7–0.9*	*1.2–1.5*
Income3 (Highest)	0.8	0.3	0.8	1.2
	0.7–0.8	*0.3–0.4*	*0.7–0.9*	*1.0–1.3*
Area level (IRSAD)				
IRSAD1 (Lowest)	1.1	0.7	1.0	1.5
	1.0–1.2	*0.6 –0.8*	*0.9–1.1*	*1.4–1.7*
IRSAD2	1.1	0.5	1.0	1.7
	1.0–1.1	*0.4–0.6*	*0.9–1.2*	*1.5–1.8*
IRSAD3 (Highest)	0.8	0.4	0.7	1.3
	0.7–0.9	*0.3–0.4*	*0.6–0.8*	*1.1–1.4*
School level (ICSEA)				
ICSEA 1 (Lowest)	1.3	0.7	1.2	1.8
	1.2–1.3	*0.7–0.8*	*1.0–1.3*	*1.6–2.0*
ICSEA 2	1.0	0.5	1.0	1.5
	0.9–1.0	*0.4–0.5*	*0.9–1.1*	*1.3–1.7*
ICSEA 3 (Highest)	0.7	0.4	0.7	1.1
	0.7–0.8	*0.3–0.4*	*0.6–0.8*	*1.0–1.2*

Row 1: Proportions were computed using weighted data.
Row 2: 95% CI: Confidence intervals for estimates were computed using weighted data.
Columns are arranged by age at time of Survey.

Untreated dental caries in the permanent dentition

The experience of untreated dental caries in the permanent dentition across socioeconomic groups is presented in Table 9-7. Overall, children had an average of 0.3 untreated dental caries surfaces in their permanent teeth and it increased with age.

Children whose parents had school-only education had 2.5 times higher average number of untreated dental caries surfaces than children whose parents had vocational education and tertiary education. The highest average of untreated surfaces was 0.7 among children aged 13–14 years whose parents had school-only education while the lowest was 0.1 among children aged 9–10 years whose parents had a tertiary education.

There was a gradient in the average number of untreated surfaces across household income groups. Children from high income households had an average of 0.1 untreated surfaces compared to 0.2 among those from medium income households and 0.5 among children from the lowest income households.

A very similar pattern observed for household income is seen when area and school indicators are compared. There was a 2.5-fold ratio in the average of untreated dental caries between the lowest and highest income groups and a 1.6-fold ratio between the low and medium income groups. This pattern was seen across all age groups.

Among all children, the highest average number of untreated caries (0.6) was among those children from the lowest ICSEA. This average was 6.0 and 3.0 times higher than among children from the highest and medium ICSEA groups respectively.

In summary, there was a consistent gradient in the average number of untreated dental caries in the permanent dentition across parental education, household income, IRSAD and ICSEA groups.

Table 9-7: Number of untreated decayed tooth surfaces (DS) of the permanent dentition in the Australian child population

Age (years)	Population: children aged 9–14 years			
	All ages	9–10	11–12	13–14
All	0.3	0.2	0.3	0.4
	0.3–0.3	*0.2–0.2*	*0.3–0.3*	*0.4–0.5*
Parental education				
EDU1 (Lowest)	0.5	0.3	0.5	0.7
	0.5–0.6	*0.3–0.4*	*0.4–0.5*	*0.6–0.9*
EDU2	0.2	0.1	0.2	0.3
	0.2–0.3	*0.1–0.2*	*0.2–0.3*	*0.2–0.4*
EDU3 (Highest)	0.2	0.1	0.2	0.2
	0.2 - 0.2	*0.1–0.2*	*0.1–0.2*	*0.2–0.3*
Household income				
Income1(Lowest)	0.5	0.3	0.5	0.6
	0.4–0.5	*0.3–0.4*	*0.4–0.5*	*0.5–0.7*
Income2	0.2	0.1	0.2	0.4
	0.2–0.3	*0.1–0.2*	*0.2–0.3*	*0.3–0.4*
Income3 (Highest)	0.1	0.1	0.1	0.2
	0.1–0.2	*0.0–0.1*	*0.1–0.1*	*0.2–0.3*
Area level (IRSAD)				
IRSAD1 (Lowest)	0.5	0.4	0.5	0.5
	0.4–0.5	*0.3–0.4*	*0.4–0.6*	*0.4–0.6*
IRSAD2	0.3	0.2	0.3	0.5
	0.3–0.4	*0.1–0.2*	*0.2–0.3*	*0.5–0.6*
IRSAD3 (Highest)	0.2	0.1	0.2	0.3
	0.2–0.2	*0.1–0.1*	*0.1–0.2*	*0.2–0.3*
School level (ICSEA)				
ICSEA 1 (Lowest)	0.6	0.4	0.5	0.7
	0.5–0.6	*0.3–0.5*	*0.4–0.6*	*0.6–0.8*
ICSEA 2	0.2	0.1	0.3	0.3
	0.2–0.3	*0.1–0.2*	*0.2–0.3*	*0.3–0.4*
ICSEA 3 (Highest)	0.1	0.1	0.1	0.2
	0.1–0.2	*0.1–0.1*	*0.1–0.2*	*0.2–0.3*

Row 1: Proportions were computed using weighted data.
Row 2: 95% CI: Confidence intervals for estimates were computed using weighted data.
Columns are arranged by age at time of Survey.

Toothbrushing at age 2–3 years

Table 9-8 describes the proportion of children aged 5–14 years according to their toothbrushing habits at the age of 2–3 years across parental education, household income, area and school socioeconomic indicators.

Overall, nearly half of the studied population brushed their teeth more than once a day at the age of 2–3 years. This proportion was higher (52.5%) for children aged 9–14 years than for those aged 5–8 years (45.6%).

A higher proportion of children whose parents were tertiary educated (52.9%) brushed their teeth more than once a day at age 2-3 years compared to children of parents who had vocational education (50.8%) and those whose parents had school-only education (43.6%). The proportion of children who brushed their teeth was higher among children aged 9–14 years than those aged 5–8 years across all parental education groups.

There was a gradient in the percentage of children who brushed their teeth more than once a day at age 2–3 years across household income groups with 42.7% of children from low income households compared to 50.3% from medium income households and 55.4% from high income households. The highest proportion was among children aged 9–14 years from high income households (59.4%) while the lowest proportion was among children aged 5–8 years from low income households (38.0%).

Overall, children from the lowest IRSAD group had the lowest proportion of toothbrushing more than once a day at age 2–3 years (45.6%), children from the medium IRSAD group had a proportion of 47.9% while the highest proportion was among children from the highest IRSAD group (54.7%).

Toothbrushing behaviour varied across level of ICSEA. Toothbrushing more than once a day at age 2-3 years was 30% and 13% higher among children from the highest ICSEA group than among those from the lowest and medium ICSEA groups, respectively.

In summary, nearly half of children brushed their teeth more than once a day at age 2–3 years and this was positively associated with age and negatively associated with parental education, household income, area and school socioeconomic indicators.

Table 9-8: Proportion of toothbrushing with toothpaste >1/day at age 2-3 years in the Australian child population

Age (years)	Population: children aged 5–14 years		
	All ages	5–8	9–14
All	49.7	45.6	52.5
	48.7–50.7	*44.2–47.1*	*51.2–53.8*
Parental education			
EDU1 (Lowest)	43.6	38.0	47.2
	41.6–45.7	*34.9–41.0*	*44.5–49.9*
EDU2	50.8	47.8	52.7
	48.7–53.0	*44.5–51.2*	*49.9–55.5*
EDU3 (Highest)	52.9	48.9	55.8
	51.5–54.2	*46.9–50.9*	*54.0–57.5*
Household income			
Income1 (Lowest)	42.7	38.0	45.8
	40.9–44.5	*35.4–40.6*	*43.5–48.2*
Income2	50.3	48.5	51.6
	48.8–51.8	*46.2–50.7*	*49.5–53.6*
Income3 (Highest)	55.4	50.0	59.4
	53.4–57.3	*47.0–53.0*	*56.9–61.9*
Area level (IRSAD)			
IRSAD1 (Lowest)	45.6	43.0	47.4
	43.9–47.4	*40.4–45.7*	*45.1–49.8*
IRSAD2	47.9	42.7	51.5
	46.4–49.5	*40.4–45.0*	*49.5–53.6*
IRSAD3 (Highest)	54.7	50.9	57.3
	53.0–56.5	*48.2–53.5*	*55.1–59.5*
School level (ICSEA)			
ICSEA 1 (Lowest)	43.8	38.5	47.2
	42.1–45.4	*36.1–40.9*	*45.0–49.3*
ICSEA 2	49.2	46.2	51.4
	47.5–50.9	*43.6–48.8*	*49.1–53.7*
ICSEA 3 (Highest)	55.6	51.5	58.5
	53.9–57.3	*48.9–54.1*	*56.3–60.6*

Row 1: Proportions were computed using weighted data.
Row 2: 95% CI: Confidence intervals for estimates were computed using weighted data.
Columns are arranged by age at time of Survey.

Current toothbrushing

Table 9-9 shows the proportion of children aged 5–14 years according to their current toothbrushing habits across parental education, household income, area and school socioeconomic indicators.

Overall, 68.5% of children currently brush their teeth more than once a day with no variation across age groups.

A higher proportion of children whose parents were tertiary educated (75.0%) brush their teeth more than once a day compared to children of parents who had vocational education (67.0%) and those whose parents had school-only education (59.6%).

There was a gradient in the percentage of children who brush their teeth more than once a day across household income groups with 58.7% of children from low income households compared to 69.6% from medium income and 78.0% from high income households. The highest proportion was among children aged 9–14 years from high income households (79.8%) while the lowest proportion was among children aged 5–8 years from low income households (59.1%).

Overall, children from the lowest IRSAD group had the lowest proportion of children who brush their teeth more than once a day (62.9%), 66.3% among children from the medium IRSAD group, and the highest proportion was among children from the highest IRSAD group (75.4%).

Current toothbrushing behaviour varied across level of ICSEA. Current toothbrushing more than once a day was 25% and 11% higher among children from the highest ICSEA group than among those from the lowest and medium ICSEA groups respectively.

In summary, nearly 70% of children currently brush their teeth more than once a day. Current toothbrushing was not associated with age and it was positively associated with parental education, household income, area and school socioeconomic indicators.

Table 9-9: Proportion of toothbrushing with toothpaste >1/day currently in the Australian child population

Age (years)	Population: children aged 5–14 years		
	All ages	5–8	9–14
All	68.5	67.4	69.2
	67.6–69.4	66.0–68.8	68.1–70.4
Parental education			
EDU1 (Lowest)	59.6	58.3	60.5
	57.7–61.5	55.2–61.3	58.0–62.9
EDU2	67.0	66.7	67.1
	65.0–68.9	63.7–69.8	64.5–69.7
EDU3 (Highest)	75.0	73.2	76.2
	73.9–76.1	71.5–75.0	74.8–77.7
Household income			
Income1 (Lowest)	58.7	59.1	58.5
	57.0 – 60.4	56.4 – 61.7	56.3 – 60.7
Income2	69.6	68.7	70.2
	68.2–71.0	66.6–70.9	68.3–72.0
Income3 (Highest)	78.0	75.6	79.8
	76.4–79.6	73.0–78.1	77.8–81.8
Area level (IRSAD)			
IRSAD1 (Lowest)	62.9	63.4	62.6
	61.2–64.6	60.8–65.9	60.4–64.8
IRSAD2	66.3	64.8	67.3
	64.8–67.7	62.6–67.1	65.4–69.2
IRSAD3 (Highest)	75.4	73.6	76.6
	73.9–76.8	71.2–75.9	74.7–78.4
School level (ICSEA)			
ICSEA 1 (Lowest)	60.9	60.1	61.4
	59.3–62.4	57.7–62.4	59.4–63.4
ICSEA 2	68.2	67.6	68.7
	66.7–69.8	65.1–70.0	66.6–70.7
ICSEA 3 (Highest)	76.1	74.2	77.4
	74.7–77.5	71.9–76.4	75.6–79.2

Row 1: Proportions were computed using weighted data.
Row 2: 95% CI: Confidence intervals for estimates were computed using weighted data.
Columns are arranged by age at time of Survey.

First dental visit for a check-up

Table 9-10 presents the proportion of children who had their first dental visit for a check-up according to parental education, household income, area and school socioeconomic indicators.

Overall, more than 85% of the studied children had a first dental visit for a check-up with no difference across age groups.

Parental education was positively associated with the proportion of the first dental visit for a check-up. A higher proportion of children whose parents were tertiary educated (89.6%) had their first dental visit for a check-up followed by those of parents who had a vocational education (87.6%) and fro those children whose parents had school-level education (81.2%).

There was a gradient in the proportion of children who had their first dental visit for a check-up. Children from high income households had 20% and 3% higher proportion of first dental visit for a check-up than children from low and medium household income groups respectively. This pattern was seen across all age groups.

A difference in the proportion of children who had their first dental visit for a check-up across IRSAD groups was found. The highest prevalence (91.0%) was among children from the most advantaged areas while the lowest prevalence (81.4%) was among children from less advantaged areas.

The proportion of children who had their first dental visit for a check-up varied across school levels and ICSEA groups. The proportion was higher among children from the highest ICSEA group (91.4%), intermediate among children from the medium ICSEA group (86.3%) and lower among children from the lowest ICSEA group (81.3%).

Table 9-10: Proportion of first dental visit for a check-up in the Australian child population

Age (years)	Population: children aged 5–14 years		
	All ages	5–8	9–14
All	**86.7**	**85.0**	**87.6**
	86.0–87.4	*83.9–86.2*	*86.8–88.5*
Parental education			
EDU1 (Lowest)	81.2	77.4	82.9
	79.5–82.8	*74.4–80.4*	*80.9–84.9*
EDU2	87.6	84.8	89.0
	86.2–89.1	*82.1–87.5*	*87.3–90.8*
EDU3 (Highest)	89.6	88.9	89.9
	88.8–90.4	*87.6–90.3*	*88.9–91.0*
Household income			
Income1 (Lowest)	78.5	75.7	79.8
	76.9–80.1	*72.9–78.6*	*77.8–81.8*
Income2	89.1	86.7	90.4
	88.1–90.0	*85.0–88.3*	*89.2–91.5*
Income3 (Highest)	92.4	91.5	93.0
	91.4–93.4	*89.7–93.2*	*91.8–94.2*
Area level (IRSAD)			
IRSAD1 (Lowest)	81.4	78.8	82.7
	79.8–83.0	*76.1–81.6*	*80.8–84.6*
IRSAD2	86.2	83.3	87.7
	85.0–87.3	*81.3–85.3*	*86.3–89.2*
IRSAD3 (Highest)	91.0	91.0	91.1
	90.1–92.0	*89.5–92.4*	*89.9–92.3*
School level (ICSEA)			
ICSEA 1 (Lowest)	81.3	76.8	83.5
	79.9–82.8	*74.2–79.4*	*81.8–85.2*
ICSEA 2	86.3	85.5	86.8
	85.1–87.6	*83.5–87.5*	*85.2–88.3*
ICSEA 3 (Highest)	91.4	90.6	91.9
	90.5–92.4	*89.1–92.1*	*90.8–93.1*

Row 1: Proportions were computed using weighted data.
Row 2: 95% CI: Confidence intervals for estimates were computed using weighted data.
Columns are arranged by age at time of Survey.

Last dental visit for a check-up

Table 9-11 shows the proportion of children who had their last dental visit for a check-up according to parental education, household income, area and school socioeconomic indicators.

Overall, eight in ten children last visited for a dental check-up with difference across age groups. Children aged 9–14 years had a higher proportion (81.1%) of their last dental visit for a check-up than younger children (78.5%)

Parental education was positively associated with the proportion of the last dental visit for a check-up. A higher proportion of children whose parents had a tertiary education (83.6%) had their last dental visit for a check-up followed by children of parents who had a vocational education (80.3%) and from those whose parents had school-level education (74.1%). The highest proportion was among children aged 9–14 years whose parents were tertiary educated (83.8%) while the lowest was among children aged 5–8 years of parents with school-level education (69.7%).

There was a gradient in the proportion of children who had their last dental visit for a check-up. Children from the highest household income group had 23% and 7% higher proportion of the last dental visit for a check-up than children from the lowest and medium household income groups, respectively. This pattern was seen across all age groups.

A difference in the proportion of children who had their last dental visit for a check-up across IRSAD groups was identified. The highest prevalence (85.0%) was among children from the most advantaged areas while the lowest prevalence (74.9%) was among children from less advantaged areas.

The proportion of children who had their last dental visit for a check-up ranged across ICSEA groups. The proportion was higher among children from the highest ICSEA group (85.4%), intermediate among children from the medium ICSEA group (78.9%) and lower among children from the lowest ICSEA group (74.9%).

In short, 80% of children had their last dental visit for a check-up and the proportion was higher among older than younger children. A wide socioeconomic gradient was identified in the proportion of children who had their last dental visit for a check-up.

Table 9-11: Proportion of last dental visit for a check-up in the Australian child population

Age (years)	Population: children aged 5–14 years		
	All ages	5–8	9–14
All	80.2	78.5	81.1
	79.4–81.0	*77.1–79.8*	*80.1–82.1*
Parental education			
EDU1 (Lowest)	74.1	69.7	76.2
	72.3–76.0	*66.4–73.0*	*74.0–78.4*
EDU2	80.3	77.1	81.8
	78.5–82.1	*74.0–80.3*	*79.7–83.9*
EDU3 (Highest)	83.6	83.1	83.8
	82.6–84.5	*81.6–84.7*	*82.6–85.1*
Household income			
Income1 (Lowest)	71.0	67.9	72.5
	69.3–72.8	*64.8–70.9*	*70.3–74.6*
Income2	81.3	79.6	82.2
	80.1–82.5	*77.7–81.6*	*80.7–83.7*
Income3 (Highest)	87.5	86.4	88.2
	86.2–88.8	*84.3–88.6*	*86.6–89.8*
Area level (IRSAD)			
IRSAD1 (Lowest)	74.9	71.4	76.7
	73.2–76.6	*68.5–74.4*	*74.7–78.7*
IRSAD2	79.1	77.4	80.0
	77.8–80.4	*75.1–79.5*	*78.4– - 81.7*
IRSAD3 (Highest)	85.0	84.5	85.2
	83.7–86.2	*82.5–86.4*	*83.7–86.8*
School level (ICSEA)			
ICSEA 1 (Lowest)	74.9	69.3	77.7
	73.4–76.5	*66.5–72.1*	*75.9–79.5*
ICSEA 2	78.9	78.2	79.3
	77.4–80.3	*75.8–80.6*	*77.4–81.1*
ICSEA 3 (Highest)	85.4	85.3	85.5
	84.2–86.6	*83.4– – 87.2*	*84.0–87.1*

Row 1: Proportions were computed using weighted data.
Row 2: 95% CI: Confidence intervals for estimates were computed using weighted data.
Columns are arranged by age at time of Survey.

9.2 Impact reported by parents of survey participants

Table 9-12 presents the proportion of parents who reported child's fair/poor oral health. One in eight parents reported that their child had fair/poor oral health and this proportion was higher among children aged 9–14 years than among children aged 5–8 years.

Parents reporting of child's fair/poor oral health varied across parent education groups and children's age. Overall, the highest proportion was among children whose parents had school-level education (18.4%) followed by those whose parents had vocational education (11.8%) and by children of parents who had a tertiary education (9.3%). Children aged 9–14 years of parents who had school-level education presented the highest proportion of fair/poor oral health (19.1%) while the lowest proportion was among children aged 5–8 years whose parents were tertiary educated (8.0%).

The higher the household income the lower the proportion of rating child's fair/poor oral health. There was a 2.8-fold ratio in the proportion of parents reporting their child as having fair/poor oral health between children whose parents' highest education was school-level and children of tertiary-educated parents. This pattern was seen across all age groups.

A clear distinction in the proportion of child's fair/poor oral health across IRSAD groups was identified. Overall, the highest prevalence (16.5%) was among children living in the most disadvantaged areas while the lowest prevalence (9.8%) was among children from less disadvantaged areas.

Proportion of child's fair/poor oral health varied across levels of ICSEA from 9.0% among children from the highest ISCEA group to 17.4% among children of the lowest ICSEA group. The ratio between child's fair/poor oral health in children aged 5–8 years from low and high ICSEA groups was 2.2 and 1.5 between low and medium ICSEA groups, respectively. Children aged 9–14 years from the lowest ICSEA group had 84% and 43% higher proportion of child's fair/poor oral health compared to medium and high ICSEA groups, respectively.

There was a clear gradient in the proportion of child's fair/poor oral health across parental education, household income, IRSAD and ICSEA groups.

Table 9-12: Proportion of parents reporting child's fair/poor oral health in the Australian child population

Age (years)	Population: children aged 5–14 years		
	All ages	5–8	9–14
All	12.6	10.9	13.8
	12.0–13.3	*10.0–11.9*	*12.9–14.7*
Parental education			
EDU1 (Lowest)	18.4	17.2	19.1
	16.8–19.9	*14.8–19.5*	*17.0–21.1*
EDU2	11.8	9.0	13.5
	10.4–13.2	*7.1–10.8*	*11.6–15.4*
EDU3 (Highest)	9.3	8.0	10.3
	8.6 –10.1	*6.9–9.1*	*9.3–11.3*
Household income			
Income1 (Lowest)	19.8	16.5	21.9
	18.3–21.3	*14.3–18.7*	*19.9–23.9*
Income2	10.7	9.3	11.6
	9.7–11.6	*8.0–10.5*	*10.3–12.8*
Income3 (Highest)	7.0	5.9	7.7
	6.0–8.0	*4.6–7.3*	*6.3–9.1*
Area level (IRSAD)			
IRSAD1 (Lowest)	16.5	14.7	17.7
	15.1– 17.9	*12.5 –16.8*	*15.8–19.6*
IRSAD2	12.6	10.7	14.0
	11.6–13.7	*9.2–12.1*	*12.5 - 15.4*
IRSAD3 (Highest)	9.8	8.3	10.7
	8.7–10.8	*6.8–9.7*	*9.3–12.1*
School level (ICSEA)			
ICSEA 1 (Lowest)	17.4	15.5	18.6
	16.1–18.7	*13.5–17.5*	*16.8–20.3*
ICSEA 2	12.0	10.6	13.0
	10.9–13.1	*9.0–12.2*	*11.5–14.5*
ICSEA 3 (Highest)	9.0	7.2	10.1
	8.0–9.9	*5.9–8.6*	*8.7–11.5*

Row 1: Proportions were computed using weighted data.
Row 2: 95% CI: Confidence intervals for estimates were computed using weighted data.
Columns are arranged by age at time of Survey.

Summary

Findings in this chapter indicate that there is a clear gradient in children's dental caries prevalence and experience in the primary and permanent dentitions across parental education, household income, area and school socioeconomic indicators. The worse the socioeconomic indicator the greater the level of disease. The same pattern is found for dental health related behaviours and parents' perception of child's fair/poor oral health even when the overall figures are fairly positive, such as the proportion of current regular toothbrushing and last dental visit for a check-up.

The magnitude of socioeconomic inequalities in child oral health varies across age groups and socioeconomic indicators. The highest ratio in average dmfs was 3.3 between children aged 5–6 years from the lowest and the highest income households. Children from the lowest ICSEA group had 3.4 times higher average number of untreated primary teeth than among children from the highest ICSEA group. Caries experience in the permanent dentition was 1.9 times higher among children from the lowest ICSEA group than among children of the highest ICSEA group.

Inequalities in dental caries experience was similar among the four socioeconomic indicators. Inequalities in dental caries experience was more pronounced in the primary than in the permanent dentition. Untreated dental caries presents higher socioeconomic inequalities when compared with dental caries experience in the primary and permanent dentition.

The magnitude of socioeconomic inequalities on oral-health-related behaviours are less pronounced than those identified for dental caries and similar across all four socioeconomic indicators. The higher relative inequalities were found for toothbrushing habits between the extremes of household income groups. The lower socioeconomic inequalities were identified for pattern of last dental visit and it was similar across all socioeconomic indicators.

Access and utilisation of dental care, as indicated by untreated dental caries, should not only be dependent on individual's socioeconomic circumstances and where they live. Research in oral health inequalities should continue to inform policy makers and health providers on the best way of delivering oral health services to reduce socioeconomic inequalities.

References

Australian Curriculum Assessment and Reporting Authority (ACARA) 2013. Guide to understanding 2013 Index of Community Socio-educational Advantage (ICSEA) values. Available at: http://www.myschool.edu.au.

Australia Bureau of Statistics 2014. Socio-Economic Indexes for Areas (SEIFA). Canberra: Australia Bureau of Statistics.

Braveman P & Gottlieb L 2014. The social determinants of health: it's time to consider the causes of the causes. Public Health Rep 129 Suppl 2:19–31.

Farmer P 2011. Infections and inequalities: the modern plagues. Berkeley: University of California Press.

Lynch J & Kaplan G 2000. Socioeconomic position. Pp. 13–35. In: Berkman LF, Kawachi I (Editors). Social Epidemiology. Oxford: Oxford University Press.

Sheiham A, Moyses S, Watt R & Bonecker M 2014. Introduction. Promoting the oral health of children. Second edition. Sao Paulo: Quintessence Editorial.

Watt RG, Heilmann A, Listl S & Peres MA 2016. London Charter on Oral Health Inequalities. J Dent Res 95(3):245–7.

10 Oral health status and behaviours of Indigenous Australian children

KF Roberts-Thomson, K Kapellas, DH Ha, LM Jamieson, P Arrow and LG Do

Chapter 10 compares the oral health and behaviours of various groupings within the population of Indigenous children. Differences are examined by sex, parental education, household income, residential location and reason for last dental visit.

Indigenous people in Australia have the poorest health outcomes. Indigenous children also have poorer health outcomes than their non-Indigenous counterparts (Australian Bureau of Statistics 2014). These have been related to social disadvantage. However, within the Indigenous population there is variation in social status. This chapter explores that social variation in relation to oral health status and oral health behaviours.

Indigenous identity data was collected using the Australian Bureau of Statistics (ABS) question 'Are you of Aboriginal or Torres Strait Islander origin?' Responses that the child was 'Yes, Aboriginal', 'Yes, Torres Strait Islander' or Yes, Torres Strait Islander and Aboriginal' meant the child was classified as Indigenous.

10.1 Oral health status of Indigenous children

Oral health status was measured using both the prevalence in the population and the average number of tooth surfaces with dental decay experience. This was categorised into the following elements: untreated decayed surfaces, missing surfaces due to decay and surfaces filled due to decay. Both the primary and secondary dentitions were examined and are reported separately.

In this chapter on the oral health of Indigenous children, the age groups on which data are reported differ from those in Chapter 5. This difference was due to the insufficient numbers of Indigenous children in the study to report on two-year age groups. For caries experience in the primary dentition the tables report on children aged 5–9 years and for the permanent dentition 9–14 years.

Caries experience in the primary dentition

Table 10-1 shows the average number of tooth surfaces with untreated decay, missing due to decay and filled surfaces and the average total number of affected surfaces (dmfs) by sociodemographic factors for Indigenous children aged 5–8 years. The average number of tooth surfaces decayed, missing or filled gives an indication of the severity of the disease, the burden it makes for the child and reflects access to timely dental care. Each tooth was divided into five surfaces and each surface decayed or filled was counted, but each missing tooth was counted as three surfaces. Untreated decay was defined as a cavity in the surface enamel caused by the caries process, a missing surface if the tooth had been extracted because of decay and a filled surface when the filling had been placed due to decay.

Among all Indigenous children aged 5–8 years, there were an average 3.7 surfaces with untreated decay, 0.8 missing surfaces and 1.8 filled surfaces, leading to an average total dmfs score of 6.3 surfaces with caries experience.

Indigenous children who last made a dental visit because of a problem had the highest average number of untreated decayed tooth surfaces (7.5 surfaces) and children in high income households had the lowest (0.2 surfaces). Children of parents with school-level education had, on average, more decayed surfaces (5.7 surfaces) than children of parents with vocational education (0.6 surfaces) and with tertiary education (1.5 surfaces). There was a 20-fold relative difference in average decayed surfaces between children from low and high income households (4.0 versus 0.2 surfaces). The relative difference in average number of decayed surfaces between children who made their last dental visit for a problem compared with those who visited for a check-up was 4.2-fold (7.5 versus 1.8 surfaces).

A similar pattern was seen in missing tooth surfaces. Children of school educated parents had more missing surfaces (1.5 surfaces) than children of parents with vocational (0.3 surfaces) and tertiary education (0.2 surfaces). Children from low income households had more missing surfaces (1.3 surfaces) compared to children from medium (0.4 surfaces) and high income households (0.0 surfaces). There were few differences in average filled surfaces between population groups among Indigenous children aged 5–8 years. Children from low income households had, on average, more filled surfaces than children from medium income households.

The highest average dmfs score was found in children who last made a dental visit for a problem (13.0 surfaces) and the lowest among Indigenous children from high income households (0.8 surfaces). There was almost a three-fold relative difference in the average number of tooth surfaces affected by caries between children of parents with school-level education and children of vocationally and tertiary-educated parents (9.1 versus 3.3 and 3.2 surfaces, respectively). Indigenous children from low income households had 2.6 times the number of affected surfaces relative to children from medium income households (8.1 versus 3.1 surfaces) and 10.0 times the average number of children from high income households (8.1 versus 0.8 surfaces).

The relative difference in average number of caries affected surfaces between children who made their last dental visit for a problem compared with those who visited for a check-up was 2.8-fold (13.0 versus 4.6 surfaces).

In summary, differences in average number of untreated decayed tooth surfaces and dmfs score were seen between groups of children of parents with varying levels of education and household incomes and with different reason for making a dental visit. Average number of missing surfaces were related to parental education and household income. Filled surfaces were related to household income. Some of the differences seen between population groups were large.

Table 10-1: Average number of decayed, missing and filled primary tooth surfaces among Australian Indigenous children in the Australian child population

	Population: children aged 5–8 years			
	Decayed	Missing	Filled	dmfs
All	**3.7**	**0.8**	**1.8**	**6.3**
	2.5–4.9	*0.4–1.2*	*1.2–2.4*	*4.8–7.7*
Sex				
Male	4.0	0.9	1.5	6.3
	2.3–5.7	*0.3–1.5*	*1.0–1.9*	*4.3–8.3*
Female	3.4	0.7	2.2	6.2
	2.0–4.8	*0.3–1.1*	*1.0–3.4*	*4.3–8.2*
Parental education				
School	5.7	1.5	1.8	9.1
	3.4–8.0	*0.7–2.4*	*1.2–2.5*	*6.3–11.8*
Vocational training	0.6	0.3	2.5	3.3
	0.2–0.9	*0.1–0.6*	*0.1–5.1*	*0.7–6.0*
Tertiary education	1.5	0.2	1.5	3.2
	0.6–2.5	*0.0–0.3*	*0.4–2.7*	*1.5–4.9*
Household income				
Low	4.0	1.3	2.7	8.1
	2.5–5.6	*0.5–2.1*	*1.4–4.1*	*5.8–10.4*
Medium	1.8	0.4	0.9	3.1
	0.3–3.9	*0.2–1.0*	*0.5–1.3*	*0.8–5.3*
High	0.2	0.0	0.6	0.8
	0.0–0.4	*0.0–0.1*	*0.2–1.4*	*0.1–1.8*
Residential location				
Major city	3.4	0.4	1.1	4.9
	1.0–5.7	*0.1–0.7*	*0.5–1.7*	*2.3–7.4*
Inner regional	3.4	1.5	3.6	8.4
	1.5–5.1	*0.1–2.9*	*1.3–5.8*	*5.1–11.6*
Outer regional	3.1	0.4	1.7	5.2
	0.8–5.4	*0.1–0.8*	*0.7–2.7*	*2.8–7.6*
Remote/Very remote	5.0	1.0	1.3	7.3
	2.8–7.3	*0.4–1.6*	*0.9–1.6*	*4.8–9.9*
Reason for last dental visit				
Check-up	1.8	0.8	2.0	4.6
	1.0–2.5	*0.2–1.4*	*0.7–3.4*	*2.9–6.4*
Dental problem	7.5	2.0	3.4	13.0
	3.8–11.3	*0.7–3.4*	*1.8–4.9*	*9.2–16.7*

Row 1: Means were computed using weighted data.
Row 2: 95% CI: Confidence intervals for estimates were computed using weighted data.
Columns are arranged by age at time of Survey.

Prevalence of caries experience in primary dentition

The percentage of all Indigenous children aged 5–8 years who had at least one tooth surface with caries experience in the primary dentition was 59.4% (Table 10-2). Over 47% had at least one untreated decayed tooth surface, 10.4% had at least one primary tooth missing due to caries and nearly one-third (31.7%) had at least one filled tooth surface.

Among all Indigenous children aged 5-8 years, the lowest proportion with untreated caries were those in households with a high income (16.5%) and the highest proportion was among children who last made a dental visit because of a problem (60.6%). More Indigenous children of parents whose highest level of education was school only (58.7%) had untreated decay than children of parents with vocational education (20.6%). Indigenous children from low income households had a higher prevalence of untreated decay than children from medium and high income households (50.7% versus 29.0% and 16.5%, respectively). A higher proportion of children who last visited for a dental problem had untreated decay (60.6%) compared to children who visited for a check-up (37.1%).

The proportion of Indigenous children with at least one tooth missing due to decay was lowest in children from high income households (0.4%) and highest among children who last made a dental visit for a problem (28.1%). Children whose parents had school-level education had a substantially higher prevalence of missing teeth (16.2%) than children with vocationally educated (3.4%) and tertiary-educated parents (3.3%). More Indigenous children from households with low income had at least one missing tooth (16.4%) compared to those from medium income (2.1%) and high income households (0.4%). Over four times more children who last made a dental visit because of a problem had a missing tooth compared to children who last visited for a check-up (28.1% versus 7.8%).

There were no differences between population groups for prevalence of filled tooth surfaces.

Four out of five Indigenous children who made their last dental visit for a problem had caries experience in the primary dentition, whereas only 28.8% of children who were from high income households had caries experience. Greater proportion of children of parents with school-level education had caries experience (69.9%) compared to children of parents with vocational education (37.9%). There was a 1.5-fold relative difference in the prevalence of children with caries experience between those who last visited for a problem and those who visited for a check-up (80.0% versus 52.0%).

In summary, the prevalence of untreated caries and missing teeth in the primary dentition in Indigenous children was related to parental education, household income and reason for last dental visit. Caries experience was related to parental education and reason for last dental visit.

Table 10-2: Percentage of Australian Indigenous children with decayed, missing and filled primary tooth surfaces in the Australian child population

	Population: children aged 5–8 years			
	Decayed	Missing	Filled	dmfs >0
All	47.1	10.4	31.7	59.4
	39.5–54.9	*7.4-14.4*	*26.1-37.8*	*51.9-63.4*
Sex				
Male	46.3	10.9	28.2	56.8
	37.4–54.4	*6.7.17.2*	*22.1-35.1*	*48.0-65.1*
Female	48.2	9.7	35.8	62.4
	37.7–58.7	*5.7-15.9*	*27.6-45.0*	*51.8-71.8*
Parental education				
School	58.7	16.2	40.9	69.9
	48.5–68.2	*10.8-23.6*	*32.1-50.4*	*60.5-77.8*
Vocational training	20.6	3.4	23.4	37.9
	11.5–34.0	*1.2-9.0*	*12.8-38.9*	*23.7-54.4*
Tertiary education	38.9	3.3	25.2	51.3
	26.9–52.3	*1.0-10.3*	*15.9-37.5*	*38.1-64.2*
Household income				
Low	50.7	16.4	36.3	63.7
	41.5–59.8	*10.6-24.5*	*28.1-45.3*	*54.2-72.1*
Medium	29.0	2.1	28.4	44.5
	19.5–40.8	*0.6-7.1*	*18.2-41.3*	*31.9-57.8*
High	16.5	0.4	18.3	28.8
	5.5–40.0	*0.1-2.9*	*6.0-44.3*	*12.0-54.5*
Residential location				
Major city	37.4	7.4	26.8	50.2
	26.4–49.8	*3.6-14.8*	*18.0-37.9*	*37.3-63.0*
Inner regional	46.8	18.0	42.5	63.6
	32.3–61.8	*9.7-30.8*	*31.1-54.8*	*49.7-75.4*
Outer regional	55.8	6.4	28.2	67.2
	38.7–71.6	*3.4-11.7*	*18.7-39.9*	*52.4-79.2*
Remote/Very remote	58.5	10.9	31.2	63.6
	47.3–68.8	*6.9-16.8*	*19.7-45.4*	*52.7-73.1*
Reason for last dental visit				
Check-up	37.1	7.8	32.0	52.0
	27.4–48.0	*4.2-14.1*	*22.5-43.4*	*40.0-63.7*
Dental problem	60.6	28.1	52.4	80.0
	46.9–72.7	*18.6-39.9*	*41.2-63.4*	*68.7-87.9*

Row 1: Proportions were computed using weighted data.
Row 2: 95% CI: Confidence intervals for estimates were computed using weighted data.
Columns are arranged by age at time of Survey.

Caries experience in the permanent dentition

Permanent teeth (adult or secondary teeth) begin to erupt about 6 years of age and continue until the late teens. By about age 13 years all the primary teeth have been replaced. Caries experience in the permanent dentition was measured by the DMFS index. This index counts surfaces with untreated decay (D), surfaces missing due to caries (M) and surfaces filled because of caries (F). The number of missing surfaces counted for each missing tooth was three.

The average number of permanent tooth surfaces in Indigenous children aged 9–14 years with untreated decay, missing due to caries and filled because of caries and the total DMFS score are shown in Table 10-3. On average, each Indigenous child had 0.9 surfaces with untreated decay, 0.1 missing surfaces and 0.8 filled surfaces, leading to an average DMFS score of 1.8.

There were few differences between population groups. Indigenous children who lived in Remote or Very remote areas had 4.3 times the number of untreated decayed surfaces than Indigenous children in Major cities (1.7 versus 0.4 surfaces).

Table 10-3: Average number of permanent decayed, missing and filled surfaces among Australian Indigenous children in the Australian child population

	Population: children aged 9–14 years			
	Decayed	Missing	Filled	DMFS
All	0.9	0.1	0.8	1.8
	0.6–1.3	*0.0-0.1*	*0.6–0.9*	*1.3–2.3*
Sex				
Male	0.8	0.1	0.7	1.6
	0.5–1.1	*0.0-0.1*	*0.5–1.0*	*1.2–2.0*
Female	1.1	0.1	0.8	2.0
	0.6–1.6	*0.0-0.2*	*0.6–1.1*	*1.3–2.7*
Parental education				
School	1.0	0.1	0.9	2.1
	0.5–1.5	*0.0-0.2*	*0.6–1.2*	*1.3–2.8*
Vocational training	0.4	0.1	0.6	1.1
	0.2–0.6	*0.0-0.1*	*0.3–1.0*	*0.7–1.5*
Tertiary education	0.4	0.1	0.8	1.2
	0.2–0.6	*0.0-0.1*	*0.5–1.1*	*0.9–1.6*
Household income				
Low	1.0	0.1	0.9	2.0
	0.6–1.4	*0.0-0.2*	*0.6–1.1*	*1.5–2.5*
Medium	0.5	0.0	0.7	1.2
	0.2–0.8	*0.0-0.1*	*0.3–1.0*	*0.7–1.8*
High	0.3	0.1	0.9	1.3
	0.0–0.6	*0.1-0.3*	*0.3–1.5*	*0.5–2.1*
Residential location				
Major city	0.4	0.0	0.8	1.3
	0.2–0.7	*0.0-0.0*	*0.6–1.1*	*0.9–1.6*
Inner regional	0.9	0.1	0.7	1.7
	0.4–1.4	*0.0-0.2*	*0.4–0.9*	*1.0–2.3*
Outer regional	1.3	0.2	0.9	2.4
	0.3–2.4	*0.0-0.3*	*0.6–1.2*	*1.1–3.8*
Remote/Very remote	1.7	0.1	0.7	2.5
	0.8–2.6	*0.1-0.2*	*0.4–1.0*	*1.5–3.5*
Reason for last dental visit				
Check-up	0.7	0.1	0.8	1.6
	0.3–1.2	*0.0-0.1*	*0.6–1.0*	*1.0–2.1*
Dental problem	0.9	0.1	1.0	2.1
	0.5–1.4	*0.0-0.3*	*0.7–1.3*	*1.5–2.8*

Row 1: Means were computed using weighted data.
Row 2: 95% CI: Confidence intervals for estimates were computed using weighted data.
Columns are arranged by age at time of Survey.

Prevalence of caries experience in permanent dentition

The percentages of Indigenous children with untreated decay, a missing tooth due to caries and a filling due to caries as well as the percentage with any decay experience at all, are shown in Table 10-4.

Over one-quarter of Indigenous children aged 9–14 years (28.4%) had untreated decay, only 2.0% had a missing tooth and 28.4% had a filling for decay. In all, nearly half of all Indigenous children had experience of caries in their permanent dentition (46.2%).

There were differences by residential location. Indigenous children in Remote or Very remote areas had more than twice the prevalence of untreated decay compared to children in Major cities (47.8% versus 20.3%). More than 30 times more children from Inner and Outer regional areas had at least one missing tooth compared to those in Major cities (3.3% and 3.6% versus 0.1%).

Table 10-4: Percentage of Australian Indigenous children with decayed, missing and filled permanent tooth surfaces in the Australian child population

| | Population: children aged 9–14 years | | | |
	Decayed	Missing	Filled	DMFS >0
All	**28.4**	**2.0**	**28.4**	**46.2**
	22.8-34.6	*1.1-3.8*	*24.1-33.0*	*40.5–51.9*
Sex				
Male	28.2	1.4	27.8	47.9
	21.5-35.8	*0.5-3.7*	*21.9-34.4*	*39.7–56.2*
Female	28.6	2.6	28.9	44.6
	20.8-37.7	*1.2-5.5*	*22.2-36.6*	*36.4–53.2*
Parental education				
School	27.3	2.4	29.6	43.2
	19.6-36.7	*0.9-6.3*	*22.4-37.9*	*34.8–52.1*
Vocational training	20.5	1.7	26.3	41.3
	12.2-32.2	*0.2-10.8*	*16.3-39.5*	*28.5–55.3*
Tertiary education	20.7	1.7	31.5	42.2
	13.5-30.3	*0.6-4.5*	*23.8-40.3*	*31.9–53.2*
Household income				
Low	32.5	2.1	32.6	50.6
	25.2-40.8	*1.0-4.7*	*26.3-39.6*	*42.8–58.3*
Medium	16.9	1.7	22.3	32.6
	10.8-25.4	*0.5-5.7*	*15.4-31.2*	*23.4–43.4*
High	16.6	3.4	26.1	40.5
	5.6-40.0	*0.5-20.8*	*12.6-46.3*	*22.5–61.4*
Residential location				
Major city	20.3	0.1	30.4	38.5
	13.8-28.9	*0.0-0.7*	*22.8-39.3*	*29.4–48.4*
Inner regional	25.8	3.3	28.1	47.7
	18.6-34.7	*1.2-8.3*	*21.2-36.2*	*37.0–58.6*
Outer regional	32.1	3.6	29.0	47.7
	19.0-48.8	*1.5-8.3*	*20.6-39.2*	*36.4–59.2*
Remote/Very remote	47.8	2.4	22.1	58.5
	34.0-61.9	*0.4-13.7*	*15.0-31.2*	*43.4–72.2*
Reason for last dental visit				
Check-up	21.3	1.2	31.6	43.0
	14.7-29.8	*0.3-4.6*	*25.3-38.5*	*35.6–50.6*
Dental problem	31.3	4.0	30.6	48.1
	23.5-40.3	*1.6-10.0*	*23.8-38.3*	*38.9–57.4*

Row 1: Proportions were computed using weighted data.
Row 2: 95% CI: Confidence intervals for estimates were computed using weighted data.
Columns are arranged by age at time of Survey.

Other oral health conditions

Table 10-5 shows the proportion of Indigenous children aged 5–14 years with dental fluorosis, dental trauma, non-fluorotic dental opacities and oral mucosal lesions.

Dental fluorosis is a developmental condition of dental enamel which reflects higher intake of fluoride during tooth development. In the Survey, dental fluorosis was distinguished from other non-fluorotic conditions using Russell's criteria for differential diagnosis (Russell 1961). Fluorosis was measured using the Thylstrup & Fejerskov Index for fluorosis (Fejerskov et al. 1988) on the two permanent maxillary incisors. Any level of fluorosis present was used in determining the prevalence of dental fluorosis. The prevalence of dental fluorosis was found to be 13.6%. There were no differences between population groups.

The percentage of children with dental trauma in their permanent dentition was 14.6%. Over three times more males than females had experienced dental trauma (22.1% versus 7.3%).

The presence of non-fluorotic enamel lesions in their maxillary incisors was found in 6.9% of Indigenous children aged 5–14 years.

The prevalence of oral mucosal lesions was 7.1%. There were no differences between population groups.

Table 10-5: Percentage of Australian Indigenous children aged 5–14 years with dental fluorotic lesions, dental trauma, enamel opacities and oral mucosal lesions in the Australian child population

| | Population: children aged 5–14 years | | | |
	Presence of dental fluorosis	Presence of dental trauma	Presence of non-fluorotic enamel opacities	Presence of oral mucosal lesions
All	13.6	14.6	6.9	7.1
	10.2–17.9	*11.7–18.1*	*4.9–9.6*	*5.5–9.2*
Sex				
Male	11.7	22.1	6.5	7.7
	7.7–17.3	*17.3–27.9*	*4.2–10.1*	*5.4–10.9*
Female	15.5	7.3	7.3	6.6
	11.0–21.2	*4.8–11.0*	*4.7–11.1*	*4.6–9.3*
Parental education				
School	12.8	15.4	7.2	5.5
	7.7–20.5	*10.6–21.9*	*4.4–11.7*	*3.4–8.6*
Vocational training	17.6	15.8	5.8	9.6
	10.1–28.8	*9.5–25.2*	*2.4–13.4*	*5.9–15.1*
Tertiary education	10.7	14.7	10.3	9.9
	7.0–16.2	*8.9–23.3*	*5.8–17.6*	*6.1–15.5*
Household income				
Low	12.6	17.0	8.5	7.7
	8.5–18.5	*12.6–22.5*	*5.2–13.5*	*5.2–11.2*
Medium	13.8	16.0	7.9	7.8
	8.3–21.9	*10.2–24.1*	*4.6–13.2*	*4.7–12.7*
High	16.6	9.7	6.9	7.4
	6.3–37.0	*4.1–21.1*	*2.8–16.0*	*3.0–17.1*
Residential location				
Major city	18.1	15.9	7.6	5.6
	11.4–27.6	*10.8–22.8*	*4.7–12.2*	*3.3–9.4*
Inner regional	10.6	19.0	11.7	9.1
	6.4–17.0	*12.8–27.4*	*6.6–19.7*	*5.6–14.6*
Outer regional	8.3	14.1	5.5	6.7
	4.2–15.9	*10.0–19.5*	*3.1–9.6*	*4.1–10.8*
Remote/Very remote	14.5	8.8	2.3	7.8
	8.1–24.5	*4.7–16.0*	*0.4–11.5*	*4.8–12.3*
Reason for last dental visit				
Check-up	13.6	13.7	7.5	6.9
	9.5–19.2	*10.0–18.4*	*4.8–11.4*	*4.9–9.7*
Dental problem	11.1	17.4	9.2	7.0
	6.4–18.6	*12.0–24.5*	*5.4–15.2*	*4.1–11.8*

Row 1: Proportions were computed using weighted data.
Row 2: 95% CI: Confidence intervals for estimates were computed using weighted data.
Columns are arranged by age at time of Survey.

10.2 Oral health behaviours of Indigenous children

The oral health behaviours of Indigenous children described in this section include patterns of dental attendance, toothbrushing behaviours and intake of sugar-sweetened beverages. The tables refer to children aged 5–14 years unless specified.

Dental attendance pattern

Patterns of dental attendance have an influence on the type of dental care a child receives. Visits for a check-up are more likely to result in a child receiving timely treatment and preventive care.

Dental attendance patterns of Indigenous children were assessed using the proportion making one or more dental visits per year, making the first dental visit for a check-up rather than because of a problem, and making the last dental visit for a check-up (Table 10-6).

The proportion of Indigenous children aged 5–14 years who usually make one or more dental visits a year was 61.8%. More children who made their last dental visit for a check-up usually visited at least once a year (67.3%) than children who last made a dental visit for a problem (50.4%).

Over three-quarters of Indigenous children made their first dental visit for a check-up (77.6%). Nearly 90% of children who last visited for a check-up had made their first visit for a dental check-up (87.7%) compared to 56.1% of children who last made a dental visit for a problem.

More than two-thirds of Indigenous children aged 5–14 years (68.8%) made their last dental visit for a check-up.

Table 10-6: Dental attendance patterns among Australian Indigenous children aged 5–14 years in the Australian child population

	Population: children aged 5–14 years		
	Making 1+ dental visits per year	Making the first dental visit for a check-up	Making the last dental visit for a check-up
All	61.8	77.6	68.8
	56.9–66.5	*73.5–81.2*	*63.4–73.7*
Sex			
Male	60.4	77.6	66.0
	53.7–66.7	*72.0–82.4*	*58.0–73.2*
Female	63.1	77.6	71.3
	56.7–69.0	*71.8–82.5*	*65.5–76.5*
Parental education			
School	53.9	75.2	64.1
	46.9–60.8	*68.2–81.2*	*56.4–71.1*
Vocational training	69.0	78.8	73.6
	57.7–78.5	*68.2–86.6*	*62.8–82.1*
Tertiary education	67.5	82.1	71.3
	57.9–75.8	*75.2–87.3*	*61.2–79.7*
Household income			
Low	58.0	75.6	63.8
	50.6–65.1	*69.5–80.8*	*56.4–70.6*
Medium	66.7	83.6	76.5
	58.2–74.1	*76.8–88.7*	*68.5–83.0*
High	66.2	83.2	72.4
	50.2–79.2	*70.0–91.3*	*57.3–83.7*
Residential location			
Major city	61.4	80.6	69.0
	52.2–69.8	*74.6–85.5*	*57.9–78.2*
Inner regional	60.7	70.0	70.7
	51.2–69.4	*61.4–77.3*	*61.7–78.4*
Outer regional	63.7	83.6	66.9
	53.4–72.8	*75.1–89.6*	*58.8–74.1*
Remote/Very remote	62.5	72.7	67.9
	56.2–68.4	*59.8–82.7*	*56.1–77.8*
Reason for last dental visit			
Check-up	67.3	87.7	100.0
	62.0–72.2	*84.1–90.7*	—
Dental problem	50.4	56.1	0.0
	40.9–59.9	*48.6–63.3*	—

Row 1: Proportions were computed using weighted data.
Row 2: 95% CI: Confidence intervals for estimates were computed using weighted data.
Columns are arranged by age at time of Survey.

Overall, the attendance of Indigenous children for public dental-service-provided care was high (Table 10-7); approximately 91% of Indigenous children aged 5–14 years had usually attended a public dental clinic when aged 1–4 years (90.7%), and three-quarters of Indigenous children aged 5–14 years reported visiting a public dental clinic at their last dental visit (75.4%). When considering 'usually attended a public dental clinic when aged 1–4 years', there were no differences observed by sex, level of parental education or residential location. However, the proportion of children who usually attended a public dental clinic when aged 1–4 years was significantly higher in households with low income (94.3%) relative to their counterparts residing in households with high income (67.4%).

When considering 'attending public dental clinic at last dental visit', there were no differences observed by sex or reason for last dental visit. However, a higher proportion of children who attended a public dental clinic at their last dental visit had parents with school-only educational attainment relative to children of tertiary-educated parents (83.3% versus 61.9%). More Indigenous children from low income households made their last dental visit at a public clinic than children from households with medium or high income (88.1% versus 59.5% and 49.1%, respectively).

A higher proportion of children in Remote or Very remote (94.6%) and in Outer regional areas (83.9%) attended a public clinic for their last dental visit than metropolitan children (66.7%). More children in remote areas also last visited a public dental clinic compared to children in Inner regional areas (94.6% versus 71.8%).

In summary, use of a public dental clinic was related to parental education, household income and residential location.

Table 10-7: Use of a public dental clinic among Australian Indigenous children aged 5–14 years in the Australian child population

| | Population: children aged 5–14 years | |
	Usually attend public dental clinic at aged 1–4 year old	Attend public dental clinic at last dental visit
All	90.7	75.4
	86.2–93.9	*69.7–80.4*
Sex		
Male	91.1	73.9
	83.0–95.5	*65.8–80.7*
Female	90.4	76.8
	83.9–94.4	*70.0–82.5*
Parental education		
School	89.8	83.3
	81.6–94.6	*76.0–88.8*
Vocational training	91.5	73.9
	80.3–96.6	*61.3–83.5*
Tertiary education	91.6	61.9
	84.2–95.7	*52.1–70.8*
Household income		
Low	94.3	88.1
	89.0–97.1	*81.9–92.4*
Medium	92.1	59.5
	82.6–96.6	*49.6–68.7*
High	67.4	49.1
	41.6–85.7	*33.7–64.5*
Residential location		
Major city	89.7	66.7
	79.7–95.1	*57.3–74.9*
Inner regional	90.2	71.8
	80.4–95.4	*60.3–81.0*
Outer regional	93.7	83.9
	86.5–97.2	*75.7–89.8*
Remote/Very remote	89.6	94.6
	75.8–95.9	*86.8–98.0*
Reason for last dental visit		
Check-up	0.0	71.9
	—	*64.9–78.0*
Dental problem	76.7	83.0
	67.5–83.9	*75.3–88.6*

Row 1: Proportions were computed using weighted data.
Row 2: 95% CI: Confidence intervals for estimates were computed using weighted data.
Columns are arranged by age at time of Survey.

The proportion of children who make a dental visit because of pain gives an indication of access to timely and preventive care and severity of disease.

Approximately 10% of Indigenous children across all age groups from 5–14 years had last received dental care due to pain (Table 10-8). This ranged from 6.9% of children aged 7–8 years to 14.3% of children aged 11–12 years. When considering all age groups, there were no significant differences by sex, parental education, household income or residential location. Differences were noted, however, when more narrow age-groups were considered. A higher proportion of children aged 7–8 years who resided in Remote/Very remote locations had last received dental care due to pain compared with their 7–8-year old counterparts residing in Major cities (13.0% versus 0.4%). Similarly, a higher proportion of children aged 11–12 years with parents whose highest educational attainment was school only had last received dental care due to pain relative to those with tertiary-educated parents (22.1% versus 3.1%). Finally, a higher proportion of children aged 13–14 years with low household income had last received dental care due to pain (12.6%) than children aged 13–14 years in households with medium income (0.5%).

Table 10-8: Percentage of Indigenous children who had last dental visit due to dental pain

	Population: children aged 5–14 years					
	All ages	**5–6**	**7–8**	**9–10**	**11–12**	**13–14**
All	10.6	9.0	6.9	13.2	14.3	8.2
	7.8–14.2	*4.0–19.2*	*3.4–13.5*	*7.5–22.2*	*8.2–23.7*	*3.8–16.8*
Sex						
Male	11.7	8.4	10.7	5.8	21.0	9.7
	7.7–17.4	*2.5–24.9*	*4.5–23.4*	*1.9–16.0*	*11.1–36.2*	*2.9–27.4*
Female	9.6	9.7	3.4	18.7	7.3	6.8
	6.4–14.2	*3.4–24.4*	*1.5–7.7*	*9.9–32.4*	*3.2–15.8*	*2.5–17.5*
Parental education						
School	14.6	12.7	11.4	11.9	22.1	11.0
	9.9–21.0	*4.6–30.8*	*4.5–26.0*	*4.8–26.6*	*11.3–38.6*	*2.7–35.4*
Vocational training	8.1	2.8	4.4	17.8	9.7	9.0
	4.4–14.5	*0.5–13.3*	*1.0–17.0*	*4.7–48.5*	*2.9–28.0*	*3.2–22.6*
Tertiary education	6.3	2.4	3.4	14.5	3.1	3.9
	3.7–10.4	*0.3–15.5*	*1.3–8.9*	*7.1–27.4*	*1.0–9.4*	*1.4–10.7*
Household income						
Low	11.9	7.4	6.8	15.5	15.3	12.6
	7.9–17.7	*1.1–37.1*	*2.7–16.2*	*7.8–28.6*	*6.6–31.7*	*5.2–27.6*
Medium	6.0	8.4	2.5	12.8	6.5	0.6
	3.3–10.7	*2.1–27.7*	*0.6–10.4*	*5.2–28.4*	*2.3–17.3*	*0.1–4.0*
High	15.5	1.8	4.4	20.7	29.4	2.9
	6.9–31.3	*0.2–13.3*	*0.7–22.0*	*6.2–50.8*	*9.9–61.3*	*0.4–19.5*
Residential location						
Major city	10.2	10.3	0.4	21.3	13.7	1.1
	5.6–17.9	*3.2–28.6*	*0.1–2.5*	*9.5–41.2*	*4.9–33.2*	*0.1–7.8*
Inner regional	8.7	0.0	17.0	5.2	18.6	0.0
	5.0–14.5	—	*6.3–38.3*	*1.3–18.4*	*9.4–33.5*	—
Outer regional	11.7	0.0	3.3	15.2	14.0	17.7
	6.5–20.1	—	*1.3–8.5*	*6.3–32.5*	*5.6–30.8*	*6.1–41.4*
Remote/Very remote	13.6	23.1	13.0	3.1	11.1	21.0
	8.2–21.7	*11.3–41.4*	*5.2–28.7*	*0.5–17.0*	*2.3–39.8*	*7.7–45.9*
Reason for last dental visit						
Check-up	0.0	0.0	0.0	0.0	0.0	0.0
	—	—	—	—	—	—
Dental problem	34.0	28.6	23.3	36.3	40.2	40.3
	26.8–42.0	*15.8–46.2*	*12.0–40.2*	*21.6–54.0*	*26.7–55.3*	*21.3–62.6*

Row 1: Proportions were computed using weighted data.
Row 2: 95% CI: Confidence intervals for estimates were computed using weighted data.
Columns are arranged by age at time of Survey.

Toothbrushing behaviour

The toothbrushing behaviour of Australian Indigenous children is shown in Table 10-9. A little over half the children reported brushing at least twice a day (54.4%) whilst nearly one-third of the children (30.2%) had late commencement of toothbrushing with toothpaste.

There was more than a two-fold difference in the percentage of Australian Indigenous children who had late commencement of toothbrushing with toothpaste among children whose parents had school-only education (38.0%) compared with children whose parents had either vocational (15.8%) or tertiary (18.7%) level education.

A higher percentage of Australian Indigenous children who are from a low-income household reported never brushing their teeth or brushing less than once a day (9.1%) than children from medium income households (2.9%). A higher percentage of Australian Indigenous children who lived in Remote or Very remote locations reported never brushing or brushing less than once a day (17.1%) compared with children in Outer regional (3.2%) or Major city locations (4.0%).

A higher percentage of children whose parents had tertiary level education brushed at least twice a day (66.0%) compared with children whose parents had school-only education (45.6%). The percentage of children who brushed at least twice a day was greater among children from medium income households (66.4%) than among children from low-income households (48.9%). While 61.3% of children who had a check-up at their last dental visit brushed their teeth at least twice a day, a lower percentage (45.1%) of children who attended for a dental problem at their last visit brushed their teeth at least twice a day.

Overall, toothbrushing behaviours among Indigenous Australians were associated with parent education level, household income and residential location.

Table 10-9: Toothbrushing among Australian Indigenous children

	Population: children aged 5–14 years		
	Late commencement of toothbrushing with toothpaste (after 30 months of age)	Per cent of children who never brush or brush less than once a day	Per cent of children who brush twice or more a day
All	30.2	7.9	54.4
	25.7–35.2	*5.9–10.6*	*49.5–59.1*
Sex			
Male	31.7	9.3	51.2
	26.4–37.7	*6.5–13.2*	*44.8–57.5*
Female	28.6	6.5	57.7
	22.8–35.3	*4.2–9.9*	*51.6–63.5*
Parental education			
School	38.0	9.4	45.6
	30.3–46.4	*5.9–14.7*	*38.5–53.0*
Vocational training	15.8	3.9	63.4
	10.1–23.9	*1.9–8.1*	*52.9–72.8*
Tertiary education	18.7	5.2	66.0
	13.3–25.6	*2.4–11.2*	*56.7–74.2*
Household income			
Low	30.0	9.1	48.9
	24.3–36.5	*6.0–13.7*	*42.2–55.5*
Medium	23.0	2.9	66.4
	16.8–30.6	*1.5–5.8*	*58.5–73.4*
High	12.4	2.5	64.8
	4.6–29.1	*0.9–7.1*	*48.1–78.5*
Residential location			
Major city	27.1	4.0	55.6
	20.1–35.5	*2.0–8.1*	*45.5–65.2*
Inner regional	26.7	9.9	54.9
	20.1–34.6	*5.8–16.4*	*46.3–63.3*
Outer regional	28.7	3.2	58.1
	21.8–36.7	*1.6–6.4*	*49.9–65.9*
Remote/Very remote	41.7	17.1	47.7
	30.2–54.1	*12.4–23.1*	*40.0–55.5*
Reason for last dental visit			
Check-up	28.5	4.5	61.3
	22.9–34.9	*2.7–7.4*	*54.9–67.3*
Dental problem	26.2	11.6	45.1
	18.9–35.0	*7.4–17.9*	*36.1–54.3*

Row 1: Proportions were computed using weighted data.
Row 2: 95% CI: Confidence intervals for estimates were computed using weighted data.
Columns are arranged by age at time of Survey.

Sugar consumption among Indigenous children

Sugar intake is strongly correlated to experience of dental decay. One measure of sugar intake is the number of sugar-sweetened drinks consumed per day. Table 10-10 describes the proportion of Indigenous children who consume at least one sugar-sweetened drink on a usual day and the average number of drinks consumed.

Australian Indigenous children, on average, consumed two sugar-sweetened beverages (SSBs) in a day and 72% of children consumed one or more cups of SSB in a usual day.

Australian Indigenous children whose parents had school-only education consumed nearly twice as much SSB in a usual day compared with children whose parents had tertiary-level education (2.2 versus 1.2). Australian Indigenous children in Remote/Very remote locations, on average, consumed a higher number of SSBs in a usual day than children in Inner regional locations (2.4 versus 1.5).

A higher percentage of children whose parents had school-only education drank at least one cup of SSB in a usual day than children whose parents had tertiary level education (79.5% versus 57.2%). A higher percentage of Australian Indigenous children from low income households drank at least one cup of SSB in a usual day than children from medium income households (76.3% versus 58.8%).

Overall, the consumption of SSBs by Australian Indigenous children is associated with parental education level, household income and residential location.

Table 10-10: Sugar-sweetened beverage (SSB) consumption among Australian Indigenous children in the Australian child population

	Population: children aged 5–14 years	
	Mean number of SSB consumption in usual day	Per cent of children drink one or more cups of SSB in usual day
All	1.8	71.7
	1.6–2.1	*66.4–76.5*
Sex		
Male	1.8	71.4
	1.5–2.0	*64.8–77.2*
Female	1.9	72.0
	1.6–2.2	*65.1–78.0*
Parental education		
School	2.2	79.5
	1.9–2.5	*72.0–85.4*
Vocational training	1.3	62.0
	1.0–1.6	*50.6–72.3*
Tertiary education	1.2	57.2
	0.9–1.5	*48.2–65.8*
Household income		
Low	2.0	76.3
	1.7–2.3	*69.2–82.2*
Medium	1.2	58.8
	1.0–1.5	*49.7–67.3*
High	1.1	59.7
	0.5–1.7	*43.3–74.2*
Residential location		
Major city	1.7	71.1
	1.3–2.1	*62.2–78.6*
Inner regional	1.5	61.7
	1.1–1.8	*52.1–70.5*
Outer regional	1.9	72.8
	1.6–2.2	*63.9–80.2*
Remote/Very remote	2.4	81.1
	1.9–2.9	*69.2–89.2*
Reason for last dental visit		
Check-up	1.6	67.8
	1.3–1.9	*60.8–74.0*
Dental problem	2.0	75.2
	1.7–2.3	*65.5–82.9*

Row 1: Proportions/Means were computed using weighted data.
Row 2: 95% CI: Confidence intervals for estimates were computed using weighted data.
Columns are arranged by age at time of Survey.
SSB include: Sweetened fruit drinks/juices, sweetened (non-diet) soft drinks, mineral waters, cordials, sports and isotonic drinks (e.g. Gatorade and Powerade) or energy drinks (e.g. Red Bull, V, Mother).

Summary

Nearly 60% of Indigenous children aged 5–9 years had experience of dental caries in the primary dentition and this varied by parental education, household income and reason for last dental visit. The average number of primary surfaces with caries experience was 6.3, and children of parents with school-only education and children from low income households had higher numbers of caries affected surfaces and decayed and missing surfaces.

There were lower levels of disease in the permanent dentition with an average of 1.8 surfaces affected. Children in Major cities had few surfaces with untreated decay than those in Remote or Very remote areas. Just less than half of Indigenous children (46.8%) aged 9–14 years had experienced caries in the permanent dentition. This was related to residential location with more children from Remote areas having untreated caries and children in regional areas having more missing teeth than children in Major cities.

There were no differences between groups of Indigenous children for fluorosis, non-fluorotic lesions and oral mucosal lesions, but more males had experienced dental trauma than females.

Over 60% of Indigenous children made one or more dental visits per year, over three-quarters made their first visit for a check-up and two thirds made their last dental visit for a check-up. Fewer children who last visited for a dental problem made one or more visits per year or made their first visit for a check-up compared to children who last visited for a check-up.

Over 90% of Indigenous children usually attended a public clinic in preschool years but about three-quarters made their last dental visit at a public clinic. More children from low income households usually attended a public clinic at age 1–4 years than children from high income households. More children of parents with school-only education, more children from low income households and more children in Outer regional and Remote areas made their last dental visit at a public clinic.

About 10% of Indigenous children made their last dental visit because of pain. Among those aged 7–8 years, more remote children than city children visited for pain; among those aged 11–12 years, more children of parents with school-only education than children of tertiary-educated parents and in the oldest age group, more children from low income households than medium income households.

Almost 8% of Indigenous children brushed their teeth less than once a day and just over half brushed at least twice a day. Brushing less than once a day was associated with low income and remote location, while brushing at least twice a day was associated with last visiting for a check-up.

Nearly three-quarters of Indigenous children had one or more sugar-sweetened drinks a day with an average of nearly two drinks. This was associated with parental education and household income.

Differences were seen between sub-population groups within the population of Indigenous children in both oral health status and oral health behaviours.

References

Australian Bureau of Statistics 2014. Australian Aboriginal and Torres Strait Islander Health Survey: Updated Results, 2012–13. Canberra: Australian Bureau of Statistics.

Fejerskov O, Manji F & Baelum V 1988. Dental fluorosis: a handbook for health workers. Copenhagen: Munksgaard.

Russell AL 1961. The differential diagnosis of fluoride and nonfluoride enamel opacities. J Public Health Dent 21:143-6.

11 Trends in child oral health in Australia

LG Do, L Luzzi, DH Ha, KF Roberts-Thomson, S Chrisopoulos, JM Armfield and AJ Spencer

Assessing time trend in health and health-related factors is important in monitoring population health and its determinants. The social and economic changes have been at a fast pace in recent times. However, the rate of change is not similar for every population subgroup. There were also different changes in policies and practices related to dental service delivery for children between states and territories. All these differences can have an effect on child oral health.

This chapter presents an analysis of trends between the current Survey and several existing surveys of child oral health in Australia. Australia's previous national survey among children, the National Oral Health Survey of Australia (NOHSA) was conducted in 1987–88. Dental caries experience was collected for samples of children across Australia. The National Survey of Adult Oral Health (NSAOH) 2004-06 collected dental fluorosis experience that allows for analysing time trend of fluorosis by year of birth (Slade et al. 2007).

The other available surveys are a series of the National Dental Telephone Interview Surveys (NDTIS) 1994–2013 and the Child Dental Health Surveys (CDHS) series. Dental service use by Australian children has been routinely collected in the NDTIS. The CDHS series collects administrative data on the oral health status of children attending school dental services in Australian states and territories. Therefore, those surveys covered just a proportion of the child population within each state/territory. This difference should be taken into account in interpreting results of this analysis. The CDHS data have been presented for age groups 6 years and 12 years. The presented data had been collected in Australia for the CDHS series from 1989 to 2010.

Two other oral epidemiological studies conducted among children attending school dental services were the Child Fluoride Study (CFS) Mark I 1992–93 and the Child Fluoride Study Mark II 2002–03. The CFS Mark I was conducted in Queensland and South Australia while the CFS Mark II was conducted in four states: Queensland, South Australia, Victoria and Tasmania. Information on child oral health behaviours was collected.

11.1 Trends in oral health status

Trend in dental caries experience

Time trend in dental caries experience was assessed using the NOHSA 1987–88, the CDHS series and the NCOHS 2012-14. Data of caries experience in NCOHS are presented for all children and separately for children who attended public dental services or private dental services at their last dental visit.

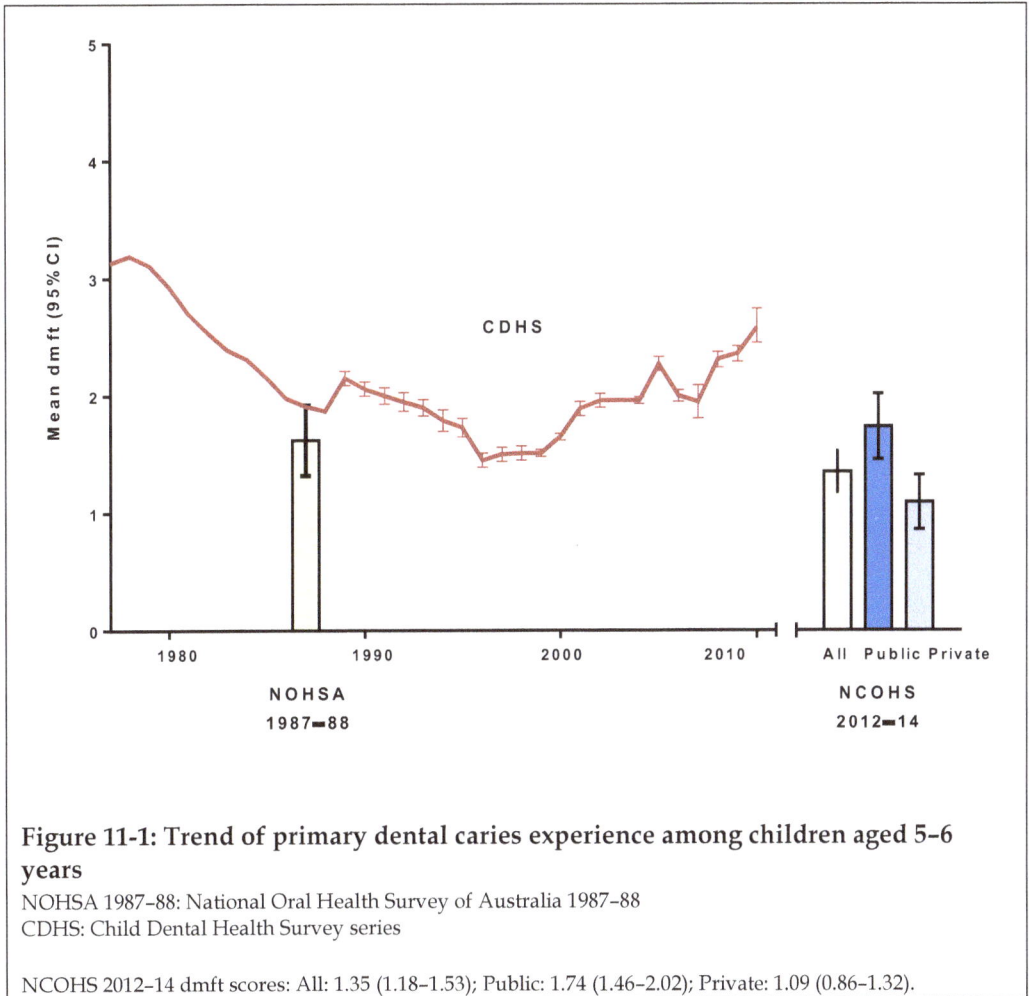

Figure 11-1: Trend of primary dental caries experience among children aged 5–6 years

NOHSA 1987–88: National Oral Health Survey of Australia 1987–88
CDHS: Child Dental Health Survey series

NCOHS 2012–14 dmft scores: All: 1.35 (1.18–1.53); Public: 1.74 (1.46–2.02); Private: 1.09 (0.86–1.32).

The experience of dental caries in children aged 5-6 years attending school dental services in Australia, captured in the CDHS series, varied over the last two decades (Mejia et al. 2012). There was a decline in child dental caries experience since the 1970s to late the 1980s that was captured by both CDHS and NOHSA 1987–88. Children aged 5-6 years who were examined in this Survey (NCOHS) had an average mean number of primary teeth with dental caries experience slightly lower than that reported in the NOHSA 1987–88. The CDHS series captured the variations in dental caries experience during the period between these two national surveys. There was a further decline after NOHSA until the 2000s followed by an increase until 2010. It should be noted that the CDHS series since the early 2000s did not have data from NSW and Victoria. NSW contributed data in 2007. The dental caries experience reported for NCOHS public children was comparable to that reported by the CDHS during late 1990s. It appears that the dental caries experience has not improved since the year 2000 until the NCOHS in 2012–14.

There was a sharp decline in the mean dental caries experience in the permanent dentition since the 1970s until the late 1990s as captured by the CDHS series. Cross-sectional findings of the NOHSA were comparable to that reported by the CDHS. Since the year 2000, dental caries experience of the permanent dentition in the Australian child population fluctuated with an increase toward 2010. The findings of NCOHS 2012–14 were comparable to the level reported by the CDHS during the late 1990s. It is summarised that the dental caries experience of the permanent dentition of Australian children improved significantly. However, such improvement has plateaued since the year 2000.

Oral health of Australian children

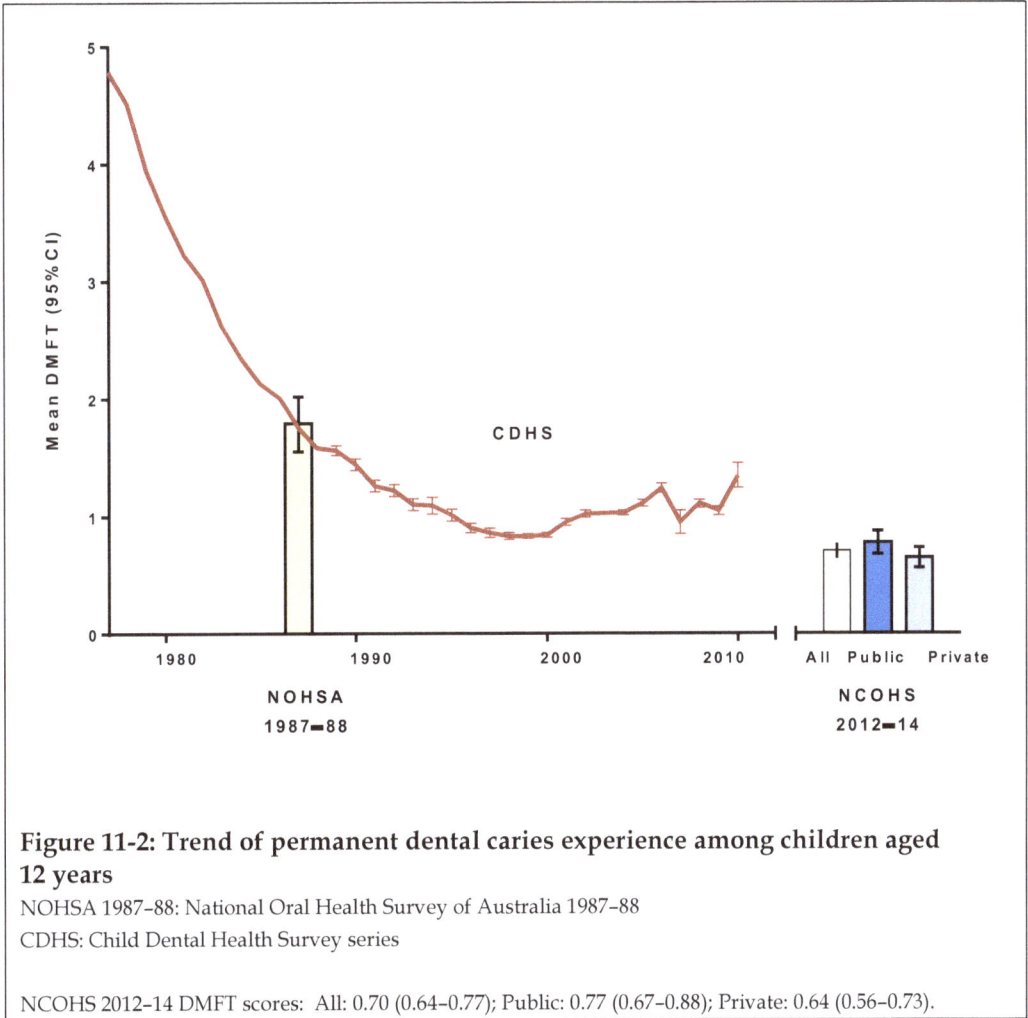

Figure 11-2: Trend of permanent dental caries experience among children aged 12 years

NOHSA 1987–88: National Oral Health Survey of Australia 1987–88

CDHS: Child Dental Health Survey series

NCOHS 2012–14 DMFT scores: All: 0.70 (0.64–0.77); Public: 0.77 (0.67–0.88); Private: 0.64 (0.56–0.73).

Trend in components of the decayed, missing and filled index of the primary dentition

The components of the decayed, missing or filled index may change over time dependent on the overall disease levels as well as dental care availability and treatment philosophy which may change with time. The NOHSA 1987–88 and NCOHS 2012-14 offer an opportunity to examine over time changes in the prevalence of children with different components of dental caries measures.

The prevalence of total caries experience, decayed, missing or filled primary teeth within three age groups (5–6 years, 7–8 years and 9–10 years) were compared between the two national surveys, NOHSA 1987–88 and NCOHS 2012–14 (Figure 11-3). The prevalence of dental caries in the primary dentition was slightly lower among the NCOHS children than their same age counterparts two decades earlier. The only significant difference was observed in the 5-6-year age group. The proportions with decayed teeth were comparable across times and age groups. The proportion of children with at least one missing primary tooth were relatively low and varied between the two surveys. Such proportions were higher among children aged 9–10 years in NCOHS than that in the earlier survey. The proportions with filled teeth were slightly lower in the more recent survey. Such proportions were lowest in the 5-6-years age group in either survey.

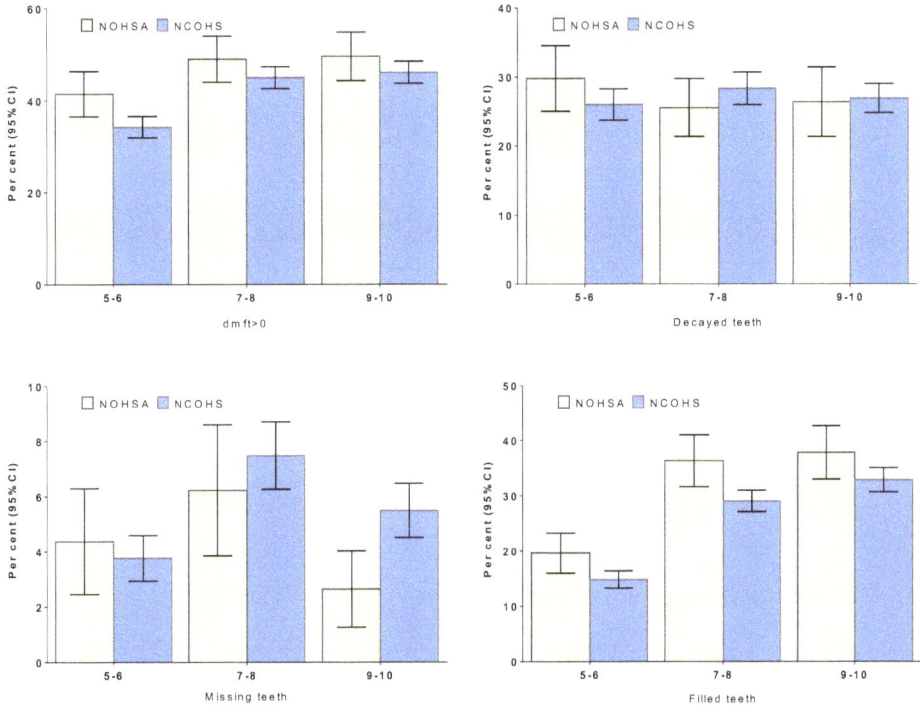

Figure 11-3: Age-group changes in proportions of children with total dental caries, decayed, missing or filled primary teeth

(The vertical axes differ in scale).

Trend in components of the decayed, missing and filled index of the permanent dentition

The proportions of Australian children with total dental caries experience, decayed, missing or filled permanent teeth in three age groups (6–8 years, 9–11 years and 12–14 years) were compared between the two national surveys (Figure 11-4). As expected, the prevalence of dental caries in the permanent dentition increased with age at either time. However, such age-related changes differed between the two surveys. A higher proportion of Australian children in late 1980s had dental caries at a young age of 6–8 years than those in the NCOHS. Some 67% of children aged 12–14 years in the 1980s had dental caries in their permanent dentition compared with some 37% of the same age group in the recent Survey.

Age-related increases were also observed in the three components of the DMFT index. A common finding across the three components is that Australian children in the early 2010 decade were less likely to have decayed, missing or filled permanent teeth than children of the same age in the late 1980s. Some 11% of children aged 6–8 years and 27% of those aged 12–14 years had untreated decay in the late 1980s compared with 5% and 15% in the recent Survey. Over 56% of children aged 12–14 years had filled teeth in the early survey compared with 27% in the later Survey.

Oral health of Australian children

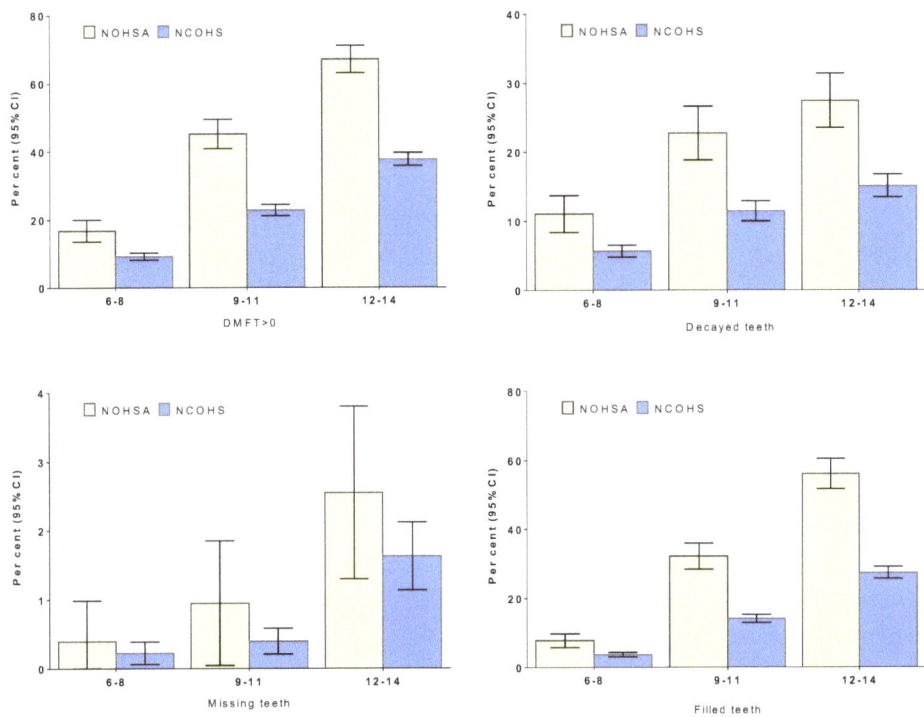

Figure 11-4: Age-group changes in proportions of children with total dental caries, decayed, missing or filled permanent teeth

(The vertical axes differ in scale).

Trend in dental fluorosis experience

Dental fluorosis is a developmental condition of tooth enamel that can be resulted from high intake of fluoride during enamel development period (Fejerskov 1988). The susceptible window for dental fluorosis on maxillary central incisors is the first three years of life. Although mild dental fluorosis diminishes over time with age (Do et al. 2016), it is still possible to assess time trend of dental fluorosis in a population by evaluating trend by years of birth. The availability of oral epidemiological data on dental fluorosis of different birth cohorts in Australia allows for such evaluation.

The National Survey of Adult Oral Health (NSAOH) 2004–06 collected dental fluorosis data on 15+-year old adults who were born from 1961 to 1990. This period included a number of significant changes in policies and practices using fluoride. Water fluoridation was introduced in Australia in the early 1960s reaching 70% of the population by the late 1970s (Spencer et al. 1996). Dietary fluoride supplements and fluoridated toothpaste were introduced in 1970s. The latter reached almost universal coverage by the 1980s in Australia. The time trend of dental fluorosis in Australia reflected those increases in availability of fluoride. There was a significant increase in the prevalence of dental fluorosis among those who were born in the 1970s. More notably, compared to those born in the previous decades, the prevalence of moderate to severe dental fluorosis (TF score of 3+) was triple among the 1980 birth cohort who were born when discretionary fluorides were universal.

Several other studies were conducted among cohorts born in 1990s, the South Australian Dental Fluorosis study (Do & Spencer 2007) and the NSW CDHS (Do et al. 2014). This period was characterised with an introduction of measures limiting exposure by young children to discretionary fluorides (Riordan 2002). These measures included introduction of low concentration fluoride toothpaste for young children, elimination of fluoride in infant formula powder, restriction of dietary fluoride supplements only to children living in non-fluoridated areas and recommendations to spit out toothpaste after brushing. The coverage of water fluoridation remained at 80% of the total population during this period. The abovementioned two studies reported significantly lower prevalence of moderate to severe dental fluorosis compared with the previous birth cohorts.

Children who were examined in NCOHS 2012–14 were born from the late 1990s to mid-2000s. The prevalence of the three levels of fluorosis were lower than the cohorts born since the 1970s. The prevalence of mild (TF score of 2) and moderate to severe (TF score of 3+) fluorosis observed in NCOHS were similar with the 1960s birth cohort. The prevalence of TF score of 1 (very mild fluorosis) was significantly higher than that observed in the 1960s birth cohort. This comparison might be hampered by the fact that very mild dental fluorosis diminished with age (Do et al. 2016).

To conclude, the time trend of dental fluorosis changed according to changes in population level availability of fluoride, especially of discretionary fluorides. While the coverage of water fluoridation has been maintained at a high level and has even expanded, the introduction of measures limiting exposure to discretionary fluorides by young children in early 1990s in Australia had reduced the prevalence and severity of dental fluorosis to the levels observed among those born before universal availability of fluorides in Australia. Most importantly, the prevalence of potential aesthetically objectionable fluorosis (TF score of 3+) has returned to a low level.

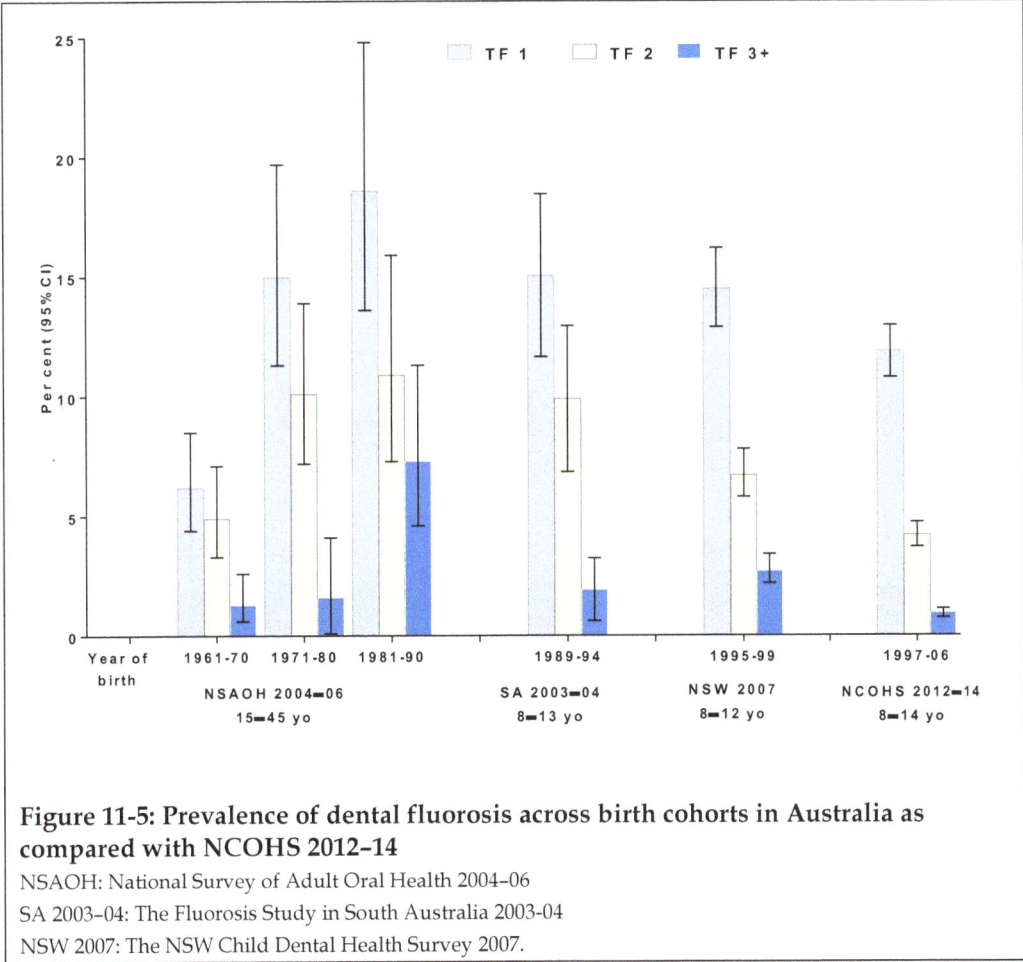

Figure 11-5: Prevalence of dental fluorosis across birth cohorts in Australia as compared with NCOHS 2012–14

NSAOH: National Survey of Adult Oral Health 2004–06
SA 2003–04: The Fluorosis Study in South Australia 2003-04
NSW 2007: The NSW Child Dental Health Survey 2007.

11.2 Trends in oral health behaviours

Frequency of toothbrushing

Health behaviours are considered immediate sources of variance in health outcomes. Oral health behaviours such as toothbrushing are associated with different levels of dental health. Such oral health behaviours are largely controllable by individuals. However, it is also dependent on availability of relevant information about such behaviours and practice.

Frequency of toothbrushing is important to maintain low levels of fluoride in the oral environment. It is also important in controlling plaque levels in the mouth. It is often recommended to brush teeth at least twice daily.

Time trend of the frequency of toothbrushing was assessed using three studies: the Child Fluoride Study (CFS) Mark I (1992–93), the CFS Mark II (2002–03) and the NCOHS. Similar questions were used in each of the studies.

Within each study, there were only little variations across age groups. This is some evidence that this important oral health behaviour is established before the start of school. Across age groups, there were significantly lower proportions of children in the CFS Mark I who reportedly brushed their teeth at least twice daily than the CFS Mark II and the NCOHS. The latter two studies had similar proportions of children who reportedly followed recommendations about toothbrushing.

Oral health of Australian children

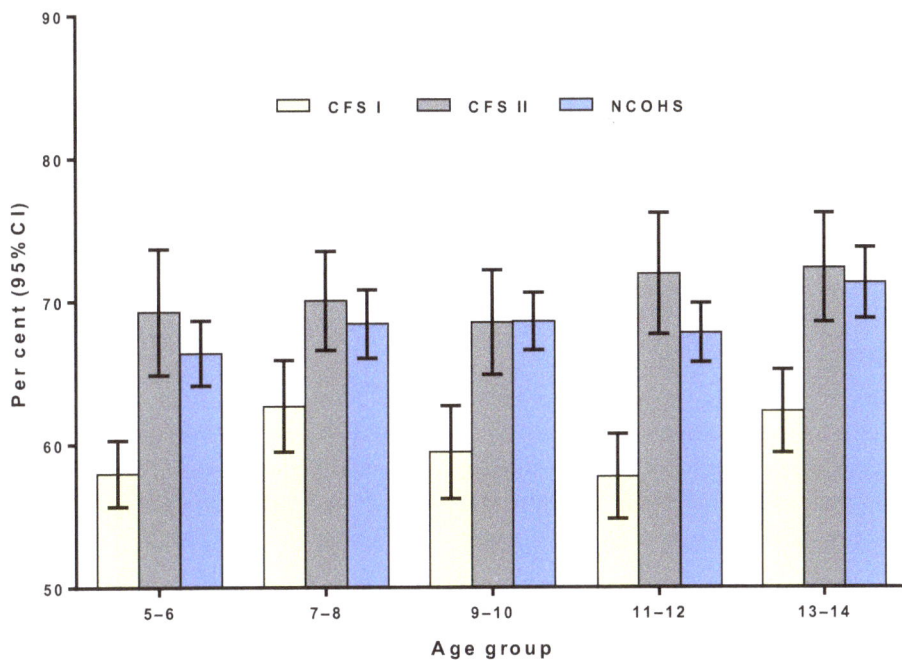

Figure 11-6: Proportions children who brushed at least twice a day in Australia as compared with NCOHS 2012–14

CFS I: Child Fluoride Study Mark I (Qld and SA) 1992-93

CFS II: Child Fluoride Study Mark II (Qld, NSW, Vic, and SA) 2002-03.

11.3 Trends in use of dental services

Evaluation of the time trend in the patterns of use of dental services in Australian children was conducted using data from the National Dental Telephone Interview Surveys (NDTIS), which were conducted periodically across 1994 to 2013 (Harford & Luzzi 2013). The NDTIS is a series of telephone interview surveys conducted by ARCPOH. The NDTIS employs a multi-staged, stratified random sampling selection process. The responses were weighted to adjust for the sampling procedures and different response rates. Children were also randomly selected from households included in the interviews. Therefore, the child sample in NDTIS would reflect the population estimates. Trend of dental service use were reported for the public and private dental care sector.

Two patterns of dental service use were analysed among Australian children aged 5–14 years. The first pattern was the proportion of children whose last dental visit was in the previous 12 months and the second pattern was the percentage of children whose last dental visit was for a check-up. Similar questions were asked in the NCOHS main questionnaire. Data were similarly managed and analysed. The NCOHS data were reported for the whole sample and separately for those children whose last dental visit was to a private or public dental clinic.

Proportion having a dental visit in the previous 12 months

In the early 1990s, the majority of Australian children aged 5–14 years had at least one dental visit in the previous 12 months (Figure 11-7). These proportions were comparable between private and public dental care users. Since then, the difference between the public and private user groups appear to have widened. There were increasingly higher proportions of private dental care users who had a dental visit in the previous 12 month than that of the public dental care users. The differences were largest since the late 2000s.

Similarly, in NCOHS, children whose last visit was to a private dental service were significantly more likely to have a dental visit in the previous 12 months than those who attended a public dental clinic. Overall, there was a declining trend of the proportion making a dental visit in the previous 12 months among those Australian children whose last visit was to a public dental care service.

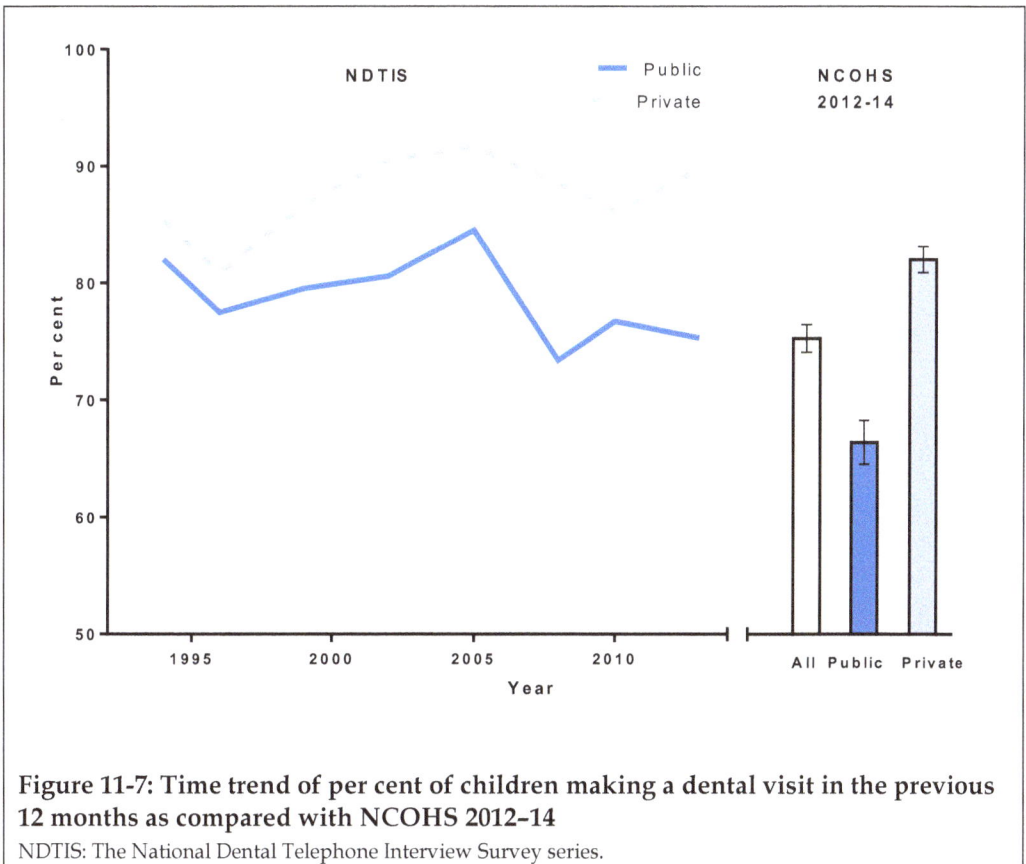

Figure 11-7: Time trend of per cent of children making a dental visit in the previous 12 months as compared with NCOHS 2012–14

NDTIS: The National Dental Telephone Interview Survey series.

Proportion making dental visit for check-up

Having dental service for check-up is an important measure to maintain good oral health. Around 80% of Australian children made their dental visit for a check-up since the early 1990s (Figure 11-8). These proportions fluctuated across times both for those attending private or public care. However, there was a tendency of fewer children whose last visit was to a public dental clinic attended for a check-up. The reverse was true for those who last visited a private dental care.

Some 80% of Australian children observed in the NCOHS visited for a check-up. These proportions differed significantly between children who last visited a private or public dental service. The latter were less likely to visit for a check-up than the former.

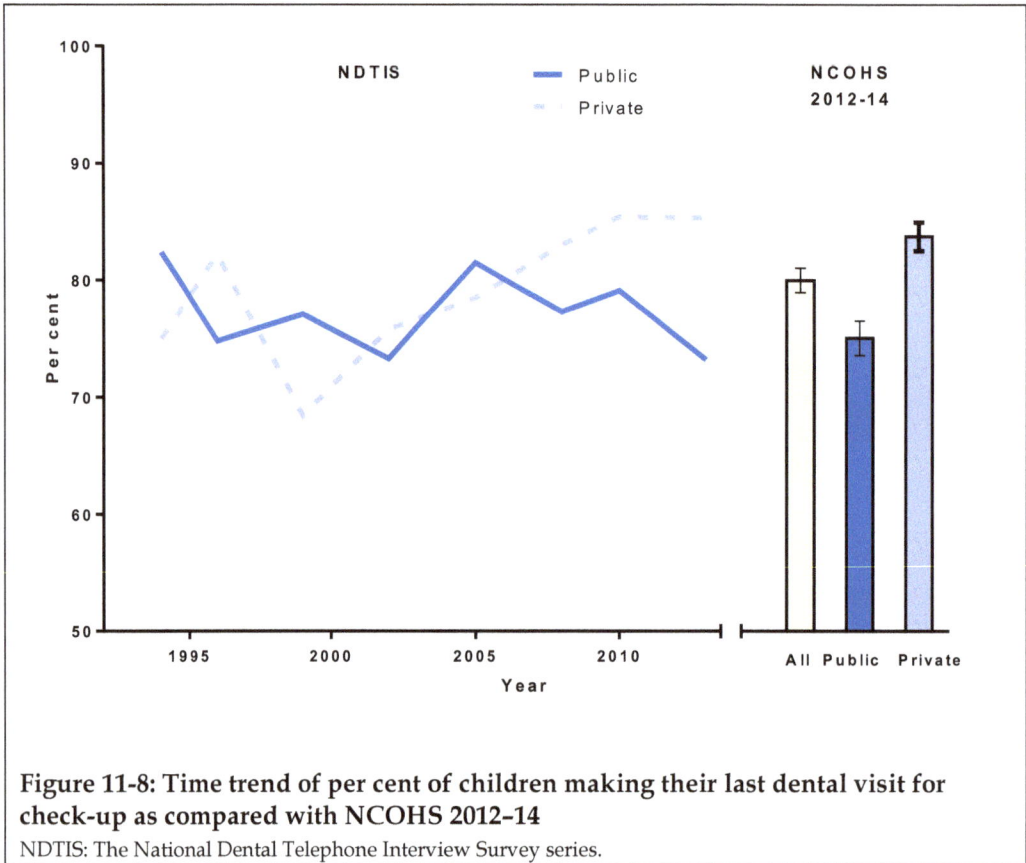

Figure 11-8: Time trend of per cent of children making their last dental visit for check-up as compared with NCOHS 2012–14

NDTIS: The National Dental Telephone Interview Survey series.

Oral health of Australian children

Summaries of trends

This chapter provides a comparison of several indicators collected in NCOHS with comparable indicators collected in other existing studies in Australia. The indicators offer a snapshot of recent changes in child oral health status, dental care use and oral health practices.

Oral health status

Two main child oral health conditions, dental caries and fluorosis, were examined in this chapter. Dental caries is the main oral health condition in children that exerts impact on health and use of healthcare. Dental fluorosis is a possible side effect of the use of fluoride in different forms for preventing dental caries in children.

Assessing time trend of dental caries was possible with the use of data from the only other national survey, the National Oral Health Survey of Australia (NOHSA) 1987–88 and the Child Dental Health Survey (CDHS) series. The latter collected data from children attending public dental services. Due to a high population coverage prior to the year 2000, the CDHS series were representative of the child population. However, there were uncertainties in sample representativeness during the more recent period.

Dental caries experience in the primary dentition did not change markedly between NOHSA 1987–88 and NCOHS 2012–14. There were small reductions in the prevalence of overall dental caries, the prevalence of untreated decay and fillings in the primary dentition between the two surveys. However, the CDHS series reported a fluctuation of dental caries experience between the national surveys.

Dental caries experience in the permanent dentition and its components were markedly lower in the NCOHS child population than that in the NOHSA child population. The reductions were marked across all age groups considered in the two surveys. Combining with the CDHS series, it appeared that the reductions in dental caries in the permanent dentition continued until the year 2000 and then plateaued.

Assessing time trend in dental fluorosis was possible with a number of oral epidemiological surveys conducted in Australia at different times. While post-eruption changes of mild and very mild dental fluorosis are possible (Do et al. 2016), the developmental nature of dental fluorosis allows it to be examined at different ages up to middle age.

The observed time trend of dental fluorosis reflects population exposure to fluoride across time since the 1960s. The sharp increases in the prevalence and severity of dental fluorosis in the Australian cohorts born during the 1970s and 1980s were in accordance with expansion of water fluoridation and, particularly, increase in the use of standard concentration of fluoridated toothpaste and dietary fluoride supplements. While water fluoridation continued to expand during the following decades, the introduction of low-concentration fluoridated toothpaste for children's use, strict regimen of dietary fluoride supplements and elimination of fluoride from infant formulae in Australia brought exposure to discretionary fluorides under control (Riordan 2002; Do and Spencer 2007). The prevalence and severity of dental fluorosis in the Australian cohorts born during the 1990s and 2000s have fallen to the level observed among the cohort born during the

1960s. This is evidence of the contribution of discretionary fluorides to the population burden of dental fluorosis and effectiveness of measures to control those sources.

In summary, dental caries experience in the Australian child population had declined markedly to a low level at the early 2000s and appeared plateaued afterwards. The decline in dental caries experience coincided with a period of expansion of water fluoridation coverage and universal use of fluoride toothpaste. Dental fluorosis, another side of the risk and benefit balance of fluoride use, had been through a period of significant increase but has fallen to a low level after the introduction of measures to control discretionary fluoride sources.

Oral health behaviours

Oral health behaviours of Australian children measured by frequency of toothbrushing improved over time. As it is recommended to brush at least twice a day by the Australian Guidelines on Fluoride Use in 2005 (Australian Research Centre for Population Oral Health 2006) and updated in 2012 (Australian Research Centre for Population Oral Health 2012), the proportion of the population who brushed at least twice a day was used as a measure of oral health behaviours. While the previous data, the Child Fluoride Studies Mark I and II, did not cover the whole Australian child population, the reported results were useable. The improvement in this indicator has plateaued since the CFS Mark II 2002–03 and NCOHS 2012–14. Some 30% of the child population still did not brush their teeth at least twice a day.

Patterns of dental service use

Dental service use was measured by two indicators: per cent of children making a dental visit in the previous 12 months and per cent of children making their last dental visit for a check-up. The time trends were presented separately for children whose last visit was to a public or a private dental service. Comparable national data were used. The two indicators indicate that a high percentage of Australian children demonstrated favourable dental visiting patterns. However, the gap between dental visiting trends of the public and private visiting groups widened in the more recent period. This widening inequality has been confirmed by the NCOHS data. This result is an indicator of increasing hardship borne by children who were from lower socioeconomic backgrounds, the dominant group in the public visiting group.

Oral health of Australian children

References

Australian Research Centre for Population Oral Health 2006. The use of fluorides in Australia: guidelines. Aust Dent J 51(2):195–9.

Australian Research Centre for Population Oral Health 2012. Outcome of fluoride consensus workshop 2012 to review Fluoride Guidelines from 2005. Available at: https://www.adelaide.edu.au/arcpoh/dperu/fluoride/Outcome_of_fluoride_consensus_workshop_2012.pdf.

Do LG & Spencer AJ 2007. Decline in the prevalence of dental fluorosis among South Australian children. Community Dent Oral Epidemiol 35(4):282–91.

Do LG, Miller J, Phelan C, Sivaneswaran S, Spencer AJ & Wright C 2014. Dental caries and fluorosis experience of 8-12-year-old children by early-life exposure to fluoride. Community Dent Oral Epidemiol 42(6):553-62.

Do LG, Spencer AJ & Ha DH 2016. Natural history and impact of dental fluorosis: a prospective cohort study. Med J Aust 204(1):25. DOI: 10.5694/mja15.00703.

Fejerskov O, Manji F & Baelum V 1988. Dental fluorosis: a handbook for health workers. Copenhagen: Munksgaard.

Harford J & Luzzi L 2013. Child and teenager oral health and dental visiting: results from the National Dental Telephone Interview Survey 2010. Dental statistics and research series 64. Canberra: Australian Institute of Health and Welfare.

Mejia G, Amarasena N, Ha D, Roberts-Thomson K & Ellershaw A 2012. Child Dental Health Survey Australia 2007: 30-year trends in child oral health. Canberra: Australian Institute of Health and Welfare.

Riordan PJ 2002. Dental fluorosis decline after changes to supplement and toothpaste regimens. Community Dent Oral Epidemiol 30(3):233-40.

Spencer AJ, Slade GD & Davies M 1996. Water fluoridation in Australia. Community Dent Health 13 Suppl 2:27-37.

12 Interpretation of findings and a way forward to improving oral health and dental care

AJ Spencer and LG Do

The genesis of this research was the need to describe and understand contemporary child oral health in Australia. The population study provided an opportunity to collect detailed information on both oral epidemiological and self-reported oral health indicators on a representative sample of the Australian child population. It also provided the opportunity to accompany those indicators with a rich array of individual, family and community characteristics that positioned every child in terms of their social milieu, behavioural risk and preventive factors and use of dental services for both treatment of existing disease and prevention of future disease.

The sampling strategy for the study was built around the capacity for all states and territories to have sufficient confidence in their estimates of child oral health. As a consequence, the study was really eight separate sub-studies then rolled together to constitute a large national oral epidemiological study. The sampling strategy had as its foundation cluster sampling of children from selected schools across all regions of the country. The probability of every child's selection was known, allowing for each child's contribution to the findings of the study to be weighted to reflect equal probabilities of selection in the sample and the population distribution of children with similar characteristics. The outcome of the complex weighting procedures was a data set that showed negligible bias against the population at large. Therefore, there is confidence in unbiased estimates of child oral health.

Every effort was made to collect high quality oral health information through the use of small teams of calibrated dental examiners, well supported with written and visual materials to aid standardised scoring, and with appropriate refresher activities during the fieldwork. The reliability statistics attest the success in this endeavour at least for the more frequently observed oral health indicators.

The accompanying data from a detailed parental questionnaire was strong in its depth. Yet, parents provided complete data with only a few exceptions. Household income was the item for which there was the most missing data, but even here the level of missing data was relatively low and an alternative marker for social position, highest parental education, was very largely complete.

Therefore, we had a high degree of confidence that the study could document contemporary child oral health in Australia, describe its variation by social milieu and explore associations to help generate hypotheses for future analysis.

Oral health of Australian children

12.1 Child oral health

Dental caries was the dominant oral disease affecting Australian children. Among children aged 5–10 years, the percentage with primary dentition caries experience (dmfs>0) was 41.7% and the average number of decayed (d), missing (m) or filled (f) primary tooth surfaces per child was 3.1 surfaces. Over one-quarter of children (27.1%) had untreated decayed surfaces with an average of 1.3 surfaces presenting as untreated decayed surfaces, about 42% of all surfaces with caries experience. A small percentage of children (5.6%) had one or more surfaces missing due to decay and there was a very low average number of surfaces missing because of caries (0.3). Just over one-quarter of children (26.2%) had filled surfaces, the majority of surfaces with caries experience presented as filled surfaces (1.5 surfaces).

Among children aged 6–14 years the percentage of children with permanent dentition caries experience (DMFS>0) was 23.5% and the average number of Decayed (D), Missing (M) or Filled (F) permanent tooth surfaces was 0.7 surfaces. Just over 1 in 10 children (10.9%) had untreated caries in the permanent dentition with an average number of 0.2 untreated decayed surfaces. A very small percentage of children (0.8%) had one or more missing tooth surfaces due to decay, while about 1 in 6 children (15.6%) had filled tooth surfaces and an average of 0.4 surfaces filled per child. However, components of dental caries experience in the permanent dentition increased with age.

Comparisons: internationally, historically and against other available data

This general picture of child oral health places Australian children at or near the top in good oral health in comparison to OECD countries (OECD 2016). Australian children are in comparatively good oral health. This is recognised by the proportion of parents (87.4%) who rated their child's oral health as better than fair or poor.

This needs to be compared with historical population survey data such as that from the National Oral Health Survey of Australia 1987/88 (Barnard 1993). The caries experience measured by the dmft in children aged 6 years has improved marginally while the DMFT for children aged 12 years has improved more substantially.

The prevalence and severity of caries in the primary dentition for children aged 6 years and the permanent dentition for children aged 12 years were considerably better than that indicated by surveillance among children visiting the school dental services in Australia (Chrisopoulos & Harford 2012). This was true among those who reported a last visit at a school or community dental clinic or a private practice. The difference in the comparison of the surveillance data with those who last visited a private dentist was anticipated. Children captured in the surveillance data use the school or community dental services and are a sub-group of all children with a bias toward lower socioeconomic status households. However, it was anticipated that the comparison of the surveillance data with children who last visited a school or community dental clinic would show greater similarity. The fact that the study findings revealed lower caries experience indicates that the surveillance caries data may be somewhat inflated. There are several possible mechanisms that could contribute. These include (from most to least likely) the inclusion of a higher proportion of high risk children on a more frequent recall cycle than their proportion among all user children, the capturing of data from children seen on an urgent care basis (who might be at higher risk), over-sampling of rural and remote children in the surveillance data, and different diagnostic criteria and limited calibration among staff of the school and community dental services when observing the presence of untreated caries.

Variation in child oral health

Caries in either the primary or the permanent dentition was experienced by a minority of children and average numbers of tooth surfaces involved were low. However, this average was dominated by children who have no caries experience. The distribution of caries experience scores for either the primary dentition of children aged 5–10 years or permanent dentition of children aged 6–14 years was skewed. A small percentage of children had extensive experience of caries, with some 20% of children aged 5–10 years and just over 17% of children aged 11–14 years having around 80% of all tooth surfaces with caries experience in the primary or permanent dentitions, respectively.

Which children are more likely to have caries experience and to have experienced more affected tooth surfaces was indicated by the pattern of caries experience by the suite of sociodemographic, socioeconomic and dental service use characteristics focussed on in earlier chapters. The percentage of children with caries experience in the primary and permanent dentitions was higher in Indigenous than non-Indigenous children, those children from households with lower income and parental education, those children who last visited public rather than private dental services, and whose reason for that last visit was a dental problem rather than a check-up.

All these associations between social characteristics and child caries prevalence and experience point to some social patterning of increased risk of caries. It needs to be pointed out that the associations were not strong. Such social patterning leads to more caries, but not necessarily most caries being experienced in lower socioeconomic status groups. A consequence of this is that targeting of preventive programs to lower socioeconomic groups may not be appropriate. Universal population preventive programs are likely to deliver a greater population preventive benefit.

Prevention of caries among Australian children

Australia's two population preventive programs directly influencing child caries experience are water fluoridation and the use of fluoridated toothpaste. Water fluoridation has wide coverage of the Australian population. Some 90% of Australians live in an area with fluoridated water supplies. However, at the time of the Qld data collection water fluoridation was only just being extended in Qld. Few Qld children were benefiting from a lifetime exposure to fluoridated water. It has been predicted that child caries experience in Qld will improve as successive cohorts are born and develop in largely fluoridated areas (Do & Spencer 2015). The extension of water fluoridation in Qld has still left discrete populations that would benefit from the fluoridation of their water supplies, many in the run of provincial towns on the Queensland central coast.

Oral health of Australian children

Water fluoridation demonstrates effectiveness and is cost-saving to the health care system. It also embodies a proportionate universalism which makes it ideal for population-level prevention of caries (Marmot 2007). This means that whilst the whole population receives a benefit, those population sub-groups who usually experience more caries are likely to gain a greater benefit. This means inequalities in child caries experience could be reduced, but not eliminated.

A great many children in Australia benefit from water fluoridation programs. An emerging concern with the benefit of water fluoridation is the widespread use of water filters which remove fluoride or the drinking of non-fluoridated bottled water. This effectively diminishes the exposure to fluoridated drinking water (Armfield & Spencer 2008). These trends might be countered by new evidence of the effectiveness and safety of fluoride, with households being encouraged to use water filters that don't remove fluoride and bottled water manufacturers voluntarily adding fluoride to bottled water (FSANZ 2009). Further, the drinking of sugar-sweetened beverages like soft drinks that are manufactured with fluoride free water, but contain high levels of sugar both contributes to a reduced exposure to fluoride and a higher intake of sugar. Fortunately, the WHO recommendations on reductions in free sugars as a proportion of energy intake is likely to lead to programs to encourage the drinking of tap water (World Health Organization 2015).

Toothbrushing and the use of fluoridated toothpaste is the important preventive dental behaviour examined in the Study. Toothbrushing is a near universal behaviour (Armfield & Spencer 2012). However, that doesn't mean that it is practised as recommended. There is evidence that children's teeth are not cleaned early enough (Slade et al. 2006). An infant's teeth should be 'cleaned' with tooth wipes or even a small headed toothbrush from the time teeth erupt (approximately 6 months) without the use of toothpaste. Toothpaste should be introduced around 18 months of age, possibly earlier if the child lives in a non-fluoridated area and other family members have a history of caries indicating that the child might be at elevated risk of caries (Australian Research Centre for Population Oral Health 2006). For the majority of Australian children who live in a fluoridated area, a children's low fluoride toothpaste should be used through to around the sixth birthday. Thereafter, a regular or standard toothpaste can be used.

Toothbrushing should be supervised; only a small, pea-sized amount of toothpaste should be applied to the bristles of the toothbrush, toothpaste foam should be spat out and not swallowed, and there is no need to rinse with water. Toothpaste should not be licked or eaten directly from the tube. There is a worrying proportion of families that introduce toothpaste before 18 months of age (33.8%), which is a risk factor for dental fluorosis and equally a worrying proportion of families who introduce toothpaste after 30 months of age (26.4%), which is a risk factor for caries experience (Do & Spencer 2007). Many children are reported to use more than a pea-sized amount of toothpaste when brushing at age 2–3 years. There is a need to continue to promulgate guidance about appropriate toothbrushing behaviour with toothpaste among Australian children. This is a task that falls to dental authorities (public dental services and the organised dental profession) through health promotion programs and to oral health care product manufacturers through labelling and advice on use of their products.

The use of fluoridated toothpaste is attributed with a major role in the prevention of caries. In theory, its action in the prevention of caries is topical and no ingestion of toothpaste is necessary. However, ingestion of toothpaste foam is unavoidable, all the more so in young children (Ophaug et al. 1980). The ingestion of fluoridated toothpaste is a relatively major contributor to total fluoride ingestion in young children in fluoridated and non-fluoridated water supply areas (Zoohouri et al. 2012). As a result, fluoridated toothpaste has been attributed with a sizeable proportion of the occurrence of dental fluorosis in Australian and other children (Do & Spencer 2007; Pendrys 2000). Policy and guidance are required to bring about a balance in the prevention of caries and the occurrence of dental fluorosis as a result of the use of fluoridated toothpaste. Australia has been at the forefront of such activity through the development of guidelines on the use of fluorides (Australian Research Centre for Population Oral Health 2007). The findings of the Study confirm earlier research that much has been achieved (Riordan 2002; Do & Spencer, 2007; Spencer & Do 2008), but that there is still a requirement to extend the proportion of children whose use of fluoridated toothpaste adheres to current guidelines.

Enamel defects: dental fluorosis and enamel hypoplasia

The occurrence of dental fluorosis in the study was reasonably infrequent. Only some 16.8% of children showed any signs of dental fluorosis and nearly all that occurred was at the very mild or mild level, i.e., a TF score of 1 or 2. Only 0.9% had a fluorosis score of 3 or above. There is Australian research that indicates that a TF score of 3 is associated with an oral health rating or oral health related quality of life score no different to a TF score of zero (Do & Spencer 2007). Therefore, the occurrence of dental fluorosis associated with children's fluoride intake (intentional or unintentional) is at a level where it is not a public health concern. The future challenge is to maintain the prevention of caries from the use of fluorides at near maximal levels while minimising the occurrence and severity of dental fluorosis. The study results indicate that still more can be done to optimise the prevention of caries and dental fluorosis.

An important finding of the study was the occurrence of enamel hypoplasia and non-fluorotic enamel defects. Hypoplasia involves a change in the surface contour of the tooth while non-fluorotic enamel defects only involve a change in colour. Both had a prevalence of about 10%. These two conditions are important to distinguish from dental fluorosis through a differential diagnosis applying a set of distinguishing criteria (Russell 1961; Horowitz 1986). Confusion of these other conditions with dental fluorosis has unnecessarily concerned some people about the use of fluorides. However, they are conditions that are important on their own. Both can be associated with a more general developmental condition called molar-incisor hypomineralisation which has been associated with increased caries (Arrow 2008). Both conditions require consideration about the need for treatment.

Oral health of Australian children

Other aspects of child oral health

Challenges also arise from the findings on other aspects of oral health. The accumulation of dental plaque was obvious in nearly half of the children and just over one-fifth had gingivitis, the soft tissue inflammatory response to that plaque. This comments on the effectiveness and frequency of toothbrushing. Both could be improved. A small proportion of children brush less frequently than once a day and poor toothbrushing technique must play a role in the accumulation of dental plaque on easily cleaned areas of teeth. Social marketing is a powerful tool in establishing toothbrushing behaviour and efforts to bring about even better toothbrushing behaviour (separate to the use of fluoridated toothpaste) need to continue.

Dental trauma had a prevalence of just under 10%. Such dental trauma can vary from minor chipping of the enamel of anterior teeth through to crown fractures involving dentine or even exposing pulp. Treatment can likewise vary from simple repairs to endodontics and post supported crowns. While trauma is sometimes associated with sport, especially contact sport, most of the incidents leading to dental trauma occur in everyday life around the home (Dang et al. 2015). As such, prevention relies on safety in design. Mouthguards should continue to be worn in many sports.

Malocclusion was assessed through the collection of ten traits of occlusion. Together these are used to derive a weighted score of the social acceptability of the appearance of the dentition. In this study this was restricted to permanent dentition for children aged 12–14 years, the age group on which the scoring for the Dental Aesthetic Index was developed (Cons et al. 1986). Some 14% of children at that age had a malocclusion with a DAI score of 36+, termed a handicapping malocclusion. This labelling of a malocclusion as handicapping is a social construct. Decisions on whether an individual child needs or desires treatment for such a malocclusion are negotiated either with individuals and their families or are subject to rationing strategies in public dental services. Previous research has identified that many children who receive orthodontic treatment have DAI scores considerably lower than the DAI score of 36 (Spencer et al. 1995; Allister et al. 1996). Therefore, the distribution of DAI scores doesn't readily paint the picture on either the demand or need for orthodontic treatment.

12.2 General health behaviours

Several general health behaviours were observed during the study. These included patterns of water consumption, the drinking of sugar-sweetened beverages and various foods and snacks containing sugar. While tap/public water is the dominant source of drinking water used by children, sizeable proportions (approximately one-quarter) of children consumed other water between birth and 12 months of age. This may have been from the reconstituting of infant formula with bottled or rain water, something that has been recommended if parents were concerned about fluoride intake in infancy (Australian Research Centre for Population Oral Health 2007). The consumption of non-tap water was limited to a minority of children and was not dominant as the source of drinking water from the age of 1 years old onwards.

The consumption of sugar-sweetened beverages at the frequency of one or more glasses a day was the behaviour of most children and increased across children with increasing age. Approximately one-quarter of children consumed a sugar-sweetened beverage two or more times a day, while more than 10% consumed a sugar-sweetened beverage more than three times a day. This more frequent consumption of sugar-sweetened beverages a day was more common and a higher average number of sugar-sweetened beverages were consumed per day among Indigenous children, and children whose parents had lower educational attainment, lower household income, lived in more remote or very remote locations, and usually visited for a dental problem. The pattern of consumption of sugar-sweetened beverages closely resembles that of late commencement of toothbrushing with toothpaste and together these behaviours may contribute to the social pattern of caries in Australian children.

This is exacerbated by the proportion of children with four or more serves of sugar-containing snacks in a usual day, a threshold close to the average number of serves of sugar-containing snacks in a usual day. Further, nearly half of all children used one or more teaspoons of sugar added to foods and drinks. When it is considered that at least 20% of children exceed the WHO recommended sugar intake in drinks alone, the proportion exceeding the WHO recommendation for total free sugar intake would be high (World Health Organization 2015).

There is an opportunity for oral health to be more strongly linked with current interest in reduction in sugar intake. Current public discussion is predominantly about child obesity. Oral health should position itself to be involved in a wider discussion about the consequences of high sugar intake and with a broader array of groups interested in reducing sugar intake to improve population health (Moynihan & Kelly 2014). Oral health has long had an interest in sugar intake. However, it has tended to pursue this in isolation from other health groups. The recent evidence about sugar and obesity provides an entry for oral health to partner with other health professions in developing and implementing health promotion activities leading to a reduction in sugar intake.

12.3 The dental care system

The dental care system is important to further improvements in child oral health. The dental care system should reinforce the messages at an individual level that are bundled together in population oral health promotion. Dentists and other dental providers have high credibility in all aspects of oral health (Roberts-Thomson & Spencer 1999). They also have contact with most individuals in the population. This provides a platform from which visits to a dentist or other dental provider can be an opportunity for raising the level of dental literacy and understanding of the prevention of oral diseases. More purposeful behaviour change strategies are available to work with families or parents to bring about improvements in aspects of preventive dental behaviours (Badri et al. 2014). An obvious example is in toothbrushing practices.

The dental care system can also engage in specific preventive dental services. There is a basket of such dental services to be considered for children. These include some services with stronger evidence of efficacy in caries prevention like fissure sealants (Ahovuo-Saloranta et al. 2013). It is unfortunate that the provision of fissure sealants seems to be at a low level, especially among children aged 6–8 years who have erupted first permanent molars at risk. Only some 12% of children aged 6–8 years have one or more fissure sealant in the permanent dentition. While the proportion of children with one or more fissure sealant increases across older child age groups, their placement at an older age potentially misses out on providing protection to the most caries susceptible tooth surface of the most caries susceptible permanent teeth in children. There needs to be consideration of how to increase the incentive for parents to demand and dentists and others to provide more fissure sealants at appropriate ages in a child's life. This would require strengthening existing and developing new guidelines among public dental providers and the private profession, as well as the removal of any disincentives in the private dental insurance system.

A higher proportion of children have had fluoride professionally applied to their teeth than have one or more fissure sealant. Yet, such professionally applied fluoride gels or solutions are of equivocal efficacy in fluoridated communities (Marinho 2009) and are of low cost effectiveness. This seems to be a spill over from the well documented effectiveness of water fluoridation and the efficacy of fluoridated toothpaste. However, a common feature of these fluoride vehicles is their lower concentration, but frequent availability at the tooth surface. So, whilst it seems sensible to encourage the greater provision of the diagnostic and preventive package of dental services to children, there should be active differentiation about who could or will benefit from these services and at what frequency.

The use of dental services is an essential component in oral health promotion and specific prevention activities. It is also crucial to intervening early in disease and limiting the consequences of that disease. Several conditions observed in the Survey are developmental. They develop and change little over time. For instance, dental fluorosis is a developmental condition which may slowly diminish in its appearance over time (Do & Spencer 2015). Other diseases observed like gingivitis are reversible, and only rarely progress in the child years. In contrast, dental caries is usually a modestly progressive disease, taking several years to progress from a reversible enamel demineralisation through to frank cavitation, destruction of dentine and possible infection of the pulpal tissues. While many children have experience of caries (over 40% in the primary dentition and nearly one-quarter in the permanent dentition), less than 2% have an odontogenic abscess on teeth in either dentition and only 5.6% have a missing primary tooth and 0.8% a missing permanent tooth because of caries. Most caries is diagnosed and treated before progressing to where tooth extraction becomes a treatment option. This may be less so in the primary dentition as evidenced by the higher proportion of children with an extracted primary tooth. However, this rather positive outcome depends on the rate of development of a carious lesion and the child having a favourable visiting pattern.

A favourable visiting pattern

A favourable visiting pattern might be interpreted as having a visit by the age of 2 years, visiting at least every 2 years, visiting for a check-up and seeing the same dentist or another dental provider (Ellershaw & Spencer 2011). Only just under 60% of children have had a first visit by 5 years of age and some 28.9% of children aged 5–6 years have never visited a dentist. Clearly there is a substantial gap between the recommended age for a first visit and the actual visiting behaviour among Australian children. Policy needs to be supported that would encourage parents to arrange their child's first visit at an early age. This is a feature of the Child Dental Benefits Scheme which funded visits down to the age of 2 years. The proportion of children who have not made their first visit rapidly decreases across the ages associated with primary schooling. This may reflect a still common view in the community that a child's first visit should be at the time they begin school or the success of various public dental services in drawing in children to dental visits in association with the schooling.

Most Australian children last visited a dentist for a check-up (80.2%) and most have made a dental visit at or less than 12 months ago (81.1%). Irregular visiting and last visiting for a problem is limited to about one-fifth of children. However, this is the target group in the population to which policy must be directed. This sub-group of the child population is larger among Indigenous children, those whose parents have a lower educational attainment, whose households have a lower income and living in remote or very remote locations. Broad policy needs to be set that supports a favourable pattern of dental visiting. More targeted policy is required to reach out to sub-groups with a higher proportion of children not in a favourable pattern of care. Special arrangements are needed to overcome access barriers (National Advisory Council on Dental Health 2012). Such arrangements might include partnering with other health services (for instance, early childhood clinics), use of mobile dental services, or biasing dental infrastructure to locations considered 'under-serviced'. Structural elements are needed that not only attract children into dental care, but also retain them in a favourable pattern of care after the first visit. This is generally referred to as recall. Recall is a structural element of any dental care system. It needs to be developed to track and retain children whose backgrounds are less stable and location and circumstances are more fluid. It also needs to be recognised that such children are spread through all socioeconomic status levels in society, but may be more common among disadvantaged groups. Management information systems in the public dental services can be centralised and are therefore capable of actively managing recall. While individual dental practices can operate their own recall system, these cannot be integrated across practices. Private dental insurers could offer some level of support to recall though incentives in their reimbursement systems.

Public and private provision of dental services

Policy and programs around dental visiting operate within a pluralistic context of both strong private and public provision of dental services in Australia. A little over half of all children made their last dental visit to a private practice. This proportion remained the same until the oldest age bracket in the study, children aged 13–14 years, where the proportion was a little higher. The remainder of children have last visited a school or community dental service. This seems reasonably close to the reported levels of visiting of each sector across the 2000s (Ellershaw & Spencer 2009). The strong involvement of both sectors in providing care to children underlies the need for policy about dental services to be relevant to both private and public providers.

12.4 Social inequality in oral health and dental care

Special attention has been given to social inequality in oral health and access to dental care. Interest in social inequalities stems from a broader perspective of the determinants of oral health where the social milieu in which a child is born, grows, learns at school and progresses to adulthood shape opportunity for oral health (Marmot 2011). Such a broader view involves not only the family, but also the school and the community in which a child lives. Taking the broader view moves the focus from the individual and their behaviours to what shapes the psychological vulnerability and resilience of a child, and establishes and maintains behaviours that are associated with increased risk or protection from oral disease. Efforts to change individual behaviours must grapple with the social milieu which is ever present in a child's life.

Oral disease offers an early in life indication of the net outcome of the social determinants of health. Social inequality in oral health was marked even at the earliest age. The social inequality in early in childhood and current toothbrushing practices and dental visiting were of a similar magnitude and direction as the outcomes in the prevalence and severity of caries in the primary and the permanent dentition. However, social inequality in oral health outcomes persisted even after adjusting for individual behaviours associated with oral diseases. There is more to inequalities in oral health than variation in individual oral health behaviours (Sanders et al. 2006).

The broader perspective on social determinants and social inequalities provides an avenue into discussion of a wider set of factors that can be modified though policy to improve health. Health is not just the net outcome of possible individual behaviours, but is influenced by the sum of factors in the social milieu of an individual.

12.5 Indigenous child oral health and access to dental services

A population sub-group that suffers social inequality in oral health is Indigenous children. All potential factors that shape social inequality in the broader population apply to Indigenous populations, but they also experience further disadvantage due to race. This is captured in the notions of dispossession of land, discrimination within society, disadvantage in education and resources and finally a higher disease experience.

Indigenous children were captured in sufficient numbers for comparison to be made with non-Indigenous children. Indigenous children had a higher proportion with untreated decayed teeth, missing teeth due to caries, filled teeth and caries experience in the primary and permanent dentitions. The average number of each caries indicator was also higher for all but filled permanent teeth. Ironically, this single non-significant difference could reflect a special lack of access to dental services. A higher proportion of Indigenous children had visible plaque accumulation and gingivitis. A higher proportion had also suffered dental trauma.

Despite a higher disease experience, Indigenous children had a lower proportion with a favourable visiting pattern, starting from a lower proportion who first visited by 5 years of age, a lower proportion who last visited at 12 or less months, and who last visited for a check-up. Interestingly, the same pattern of variation by parental education, household income and residential location was found within the Indigenous population. So even those Indigenous children whose parents were better educated, had higher household income and lived in major city locations had poorer oral health than their counterparts who were non-Indigenous. Indigenous identity was an additional contributor to poorer oral health.

12.6 Oral health across the states and territories

The sampling for the study allowed comparison between states and territories in child oral health and associated factors. The state or territory estimates of most measures of oral health were reasonably similar. Tight confidence intervals meant that some modest differences were significant. In terms of caries, the prevalence of caries and the average number of teeth with caries experience in the primary dentition was significantly higher in NT and Qld. This may be the result of the high proportion of the NT child population being Indigenous and the low proportion of Qld children having had exposure to fluoridated water across their lifetime. A not dissimilar position existed for caries in the permanent dentition. The prevalence of caries in the permanent dentition was higher in NT and Qld, but this was not significantly higher compared to all states. The average number of permanent teeth with caries experience was significantly higher in Qld than all other states and territories.

The data collection in Qld occurred across 2010–12. Coverage by water fluoridation increased from a low of approximately 4% in 2008 to approximately 90% in 2012. However, Qld children in the study will have had little or none of their lifetime spent in areas that were newly fluoridated. Some contraction of coverage has occurred since

2012, so that approximately 78% of Qld children live in an area with fluoridated water. A consequence of this increased coverage by water fluoridation in Qld is a potentially higher prevalence of any dental fluorosis (TF scores 1 or 2, even 3) as new cohorts of children will be exposed to fluoridated water across the years critical for fluorosis development.

Qld also had a low proportion of children with one or more fissure sealant, but not the lowest among the states and territories. More factors could be at play than just Indigenous identity, fluoridation and the provision of fissure sealants. This can only be discerned though more complex analyses.

Most states and territories showed only modest variation around the national estimates for indicators of a favourable visiting pattern. The exception was children in the NT who reported the lowest proportion last visiting at 12 months or less, the lowest proportion last visiting for a check-up and the highest proportion with an irregular usual visiting pattern.

The standout differences between states and territories was the proportion who last visited a private practice (or conversely a school or community dental service). The proportion of children last visiting a private practice was higher in NSW (72.7%) and Vic (65.7%), close to the national estimate (56.8%) in the ACT, Qld, and SA, but considerably lower in NT (21.7%), Tas (25.9%) and WA (28.7%). This groups the states and territories into three groups by relative proportions of private and public provision of dental services to children. Subsequent analyses will explore to what extent this grouping contributes to differences in child oral health outcomes, and for what oral health indicators. Despite the variation in the relative proportions of private and public provision of dental services, a similar proportion of parents rate the dental care their child receives as excellent or good.

12.7 Summary and a way forward

This general picture of child oral health places Australian children at or near the top in good oral health in comparison to other OECD countries. Australian children are in comparatively good oral health. A small percentage of children had extensive experience of caries, with some 20% of children aged 5–10 years and just over 17% of children aged 11–14 years having around 80% of all tooth surfaces with caries experience in the primary or permanent dentitions respectively.

A small proportion of children have experienced other oral diseases or conditions: various defects of enamel (dental fluorosis, other non-fluorotic enamel opacities and hyperplasia), dental trauma and malocclusion. Caries remains the disease with potentially the greatest impact because it accumulates across the life course.

Caries is modestly socially patterned. More caries is found among socioeconomically disadvantaged groups. Indigenous identity was an additional contributor to poorer oral health with Indigenous children in poorer oral health than non-Indigenous children even in similar socioeconomic status households.

The prevalence of caries and the average number of teeth with caries was higher in NT and Qld. This may be the result of the high proportion of the NT child population being

Indigenous and the low proportion of Qld children having had exposure to fluoridated water across their lifetime. The appropriate use of fluorides is an element in prevention of caries in both situations.

Putative risk and preventive behaviours show similar social patterning to caries. There are concerns with adherence to guidelines for toothbrushing practices among Australian children. Too many children begin tooth cleaning too late and introduce fluoridated toothpaste too late into their toothbrushing behaviour. Most children's oral health is challenged by the high frequency of intake of free sugars, especially sugar-sweetened beverages. The recent recommendation from WHO on sugar intake as a proportion of total energy intake may provide impetus for health professionals to tackle this common risk factor in child health.

A favourable dental visiting pattern is important for early detection and prompt treatment of oral disease. It also provides an opportunity for professional preventive services and reinforcing of wider community oral health promotion messages. About 20% of children have an unfavourable visiting pattern. However, these children are not necessarily matched to those with the most experience of caries. Children need to be actively attracted into contact with the dental system in their early pre-school years and better retained in a favourable visiting pattern through recall systems within organisations and individual practices and by policy incentives.

Most states and territories showed only modest variation around the national estimates for indicators of a favourable visiting pattern. The exception was children in the NT. The standout differences between states and territories was the proportion who last visited a private practice. Despite the variation in the relative proportions of private and public provision of dental services, a similar proportion of parents rate the dental care their child receives as excellent or good. More nuanced policy and practice is required for the system performance to be further improved.

Oral health of Australian children

References

Ahovuo-Saloranta A, Forss H, Walsh T, Hiiri A, Nordblad A, Mäkelä M & Worthington H 2013. Sealants for preventing dental decay in the permanent teeth. Cochrane Database of Systematic Reviews (3).

Allister JH, Spencer AJ & Brennan DS 1996. Provision of orthodontic care to adolescents in South Australia: the type, the provider and the place of treatment. Aust Dent J 41:405–10.

Armfield JM & Spencer AJ 2004. Consumption of nonpublic water: implications for children's caries experience. Community Dent Oral Epidemiol 32:283–96.

Armfield JM & Spencer AJ 2012. Dental health behaviours among children 2002-2004: the use of fluoride toothpaste, fluoride tablets and drops, and fluoride mouthrinse. Dental statistics and research series no. 56. Cat. no. DEN 215. Canberra: Australian Institute of Health and Welfare. Accessed 9 August 2016 at: http://www.aihw.gov.au/publication-detail/?id=10737421052.

Arrow P 2008. Prevalence of developmental enamel defects of the first permanent molars among school children in Western Australia. Aust Dent J 53(3):250–9.

Australian Research Centre for Population Oral Health (Spencer AJ) 2006. The use of fluorides in Australia: guidelines. Aust Dent J 5(2):195–9.

Badri P, Saltaji H, Flores-Mir C & Amin M 2014. Factors affecting children's adherence to regular dental attendance: a systematic review. J Am Dent Assoc 145(8): 817–28.

Barnard PD 1993. National Oral Health Survey Australia 1987–88. Canberra: Australian Government Publishing Service.

Chrisopoulos S & Harford J 2013. Oral health and dental care in Australia: key facts and figures 2012. Canberra: Australian Institute of Health and Welfare. Accessed 2 November 2016 at:http://www.aihw.gov.au/WorkArea/DownloadAsset. aspx?id=60129543387.

Cons NC, Jenny J & Kohout F 1986. DAI: the Dental Aesthetic Index. Iowa City: College of Dentistry University of Iowa.

Dang KM, Day PF, Calache H, Tham R & Parashos P 2015. Reporting dental trauma and its inclusion in an injury surveillance system in Victoria, Australia. Aust Dent J 60(1):88–95.

Do LG & Spencer AJ 2007. Risk-benefit balance in the use of fluoride among young children. J Dent Res 86(8):723–8.

Do LG & Spencer AJ 2007. Decline in the prevalence of dental fluorosis among South Australian children. Community Dent Oral Epidemiol 35:282–91.

Do LG & Spencer AJ 2007. Oral health related quality of life of children by caries and fluorosis experience, J Public Health Dent 67(3):132-9.

Do LG & Spencer AJ 2015. Contemporary multilevel analysis of the effectiveness of water fluoridation in Australia. Aust NZ J Public Health 39(1):44–50.

DOI: 10.1111/1753-6405.12299.

Do LG, Spencer AJ & Ha DH 2016. Natural history and impact of dental fluorosis: a prospective cohort study. Med J Aust 204(1):25. DOI: 10.5694/mja15.00703.

Ellershaw AC & Spencer AJ 2009. Trends in access to dental care among Australian children. Cat. no. DEN 198. Dental Statistics and Research Series no. 51. Canberra: Australian Institute of Health and Welfare.

Ellershaw AC & Spencer AJ 2011. Dental attendance patterns and oral health status. Cat. no. DEN 208. Dental Statistics and Research Series no. 57. Canberra: Australian Institute of Health and Welfare.

Food Standards Australia and New Zealand (FSANZ) 2009. Final assessment report application A588: Voluntary addition of fluoride to packaged water. Canberra: Food Standards Australia and New Zealand.

Horowitz HS 1986. Indexes for measuring dental fluorosis, J Pub Health Dent 46(4): 179–83.

Marinho VC 2009. Cochrane reviews of randomized trials of fluoride therapies for preventing dental caries. Eur Arch Paediatr Dent 10(3):183–91.

Marmot M 2007. For the Commission on Social Determinants of Health. Achieving health equity: from root causes to fair outcomes. Lancet 370:1153–63.

Marmot M & Bell R 2011. Social determinants and dental health. Adv Dent Res 23:201–6.

Moynihan PJ & Kelly SAM 2014. 'Effect on caries of restricting sugars intake: systematic review to Inform WHO guidelines.' Journal of Dental Research 93(1):8–18.

National Advisory Council on Dental Health 2012. Report of the National Advisory Council on Dental Health. Canberra: Commonwealth of Australia.

OECD Stat 2016. Health status: dental health. DMFT at age 12. Accessed 2 November 2016 at: http://stats.oecd.org/Index.aspx?DataSetCode=HEALTH_STAT.

Ophaug RH, Singer L & Harland BF 1980. Estimated fluoride intakes of average two year old children in four dietary regions of the United States, J Dent Res 59(5):777–81.

Pendrys DG 2000. Risk of enamel fluorosis in nonfluoridated and optimally fluoridated populations: considerations for the dental professional. J Am Dent Assoc 131:746–55.

Riordan PJ 2002. Dental fluorosis decline after changes to supplement and toothpaste regimens. Community Dent Oral Epidemiol 30(3):233–40.

Roberts-Thomson KF & Spencer AJ 1999. Public knowledge of the prevention of dental decay and gum diseases. Aust Dent J 44:253–8.

Russell Al 1961. The differential diagnosis of fluoride and non-fluoride enamel opacities, J Pub Health Dent 21(4):143–6.

Sanders AE, Spencer AJ & Slade GD 2006. Evaluating the role of dental behaviour in oral health inequalities. Community Dent Health 34(1):71–9.

Slade G, Sanders A, Bill C & Do LG 2006. Risk factors for dental caries in the five-year-old South Australian Child Population. Aust Dent J 51:130–9.

Spencer AJ, Allister JH & Brennan DS 1995. Predictors of fixed orthodontic treatment in 15 year old adolescents in South Australia. Community Dent Oral Epidemiol 23:350–5.

Spencer AJ & Do LG 2008. Changing risk factors for fluorosis among South Australian children. Community Dent Oral Epidemiol 36(3): 210–18.

World Health Organization 2015. Guideline: sugars intake for adults and children. Geneva: World Health Organization.

Zohoori FV, Duckworth RM, Omid N, O'Hare WT & Maguire A 2012. Fluoridated toothpaste: usage and ingestion of fluoride by 4 to 6 year old children in England. Eur J Oral Sci 120(5):415-21.

13 Appendix

Appendix 1: Sociodemographic variables used in the raking ratio estimation procedure

Australian Capital Territory (ACT)
Child's age
1 = ACT& 5 years old (4,665)
2 = ACT& 6 years old (4,365)
3 = ACT& 7 years old (4,235)
4 = ACT& 8 years old (4,175)
5 = ACT& 9 years old (4,007)
6 = ACT& 10 years old (4,128)
7 = ACT& 11 years old (4,197)
8 = ACT& 12 years old (4,248)
9 = ACT& 13 years old (4,172)
10 = ACT& 14 years old (4,236)
Child's sex
1 = ACT& male (21,714)
2 = ACT& female (20,714)
Child's Indigenous status
1 = ACT& child non-Indigenous (41,276)
2 = ACT& child Indigenous (1,152)
Parents'/guardians' country of birth
1 = ACT& neither parent born overseas (27,124)
2 = ACT& either parent born overseas (15,304)
Parents'/guardians' education level
1 = ACT& neither parent has Bachelor degree or higher (20,543)
2 = ACT& either parent has Bachelor degree or higher (21,885)
Parents'/guardians' labour force status
1 = ACT& neither parent/guardian employed (3,413)
2 = ACT& either parent/guardian employed (39,015)
Household income
1 = ACT& low income (7,516)
2 = ACT& medium income (12,527)
3 = ACT& high income (22,385)
Family composition of household
1 = ACT& one-parent family (7,769)
2 = ACT& couple family (34,659)

Notes:
- Statistical Area Level 4 (SA4) regions are equivalent to GCCSA regions and therefore regional location was not required in the raking procedure.
- Remoteness area was excluded from the raking procedure as 99.8% of the child population aged 5 to 14 years resided in the Major cities remoteness area.

Oral health of Australian children

New South Wales (NSW)

Child's age

1 = Greater Sydney & 5 years old (58,662)
2 = Greater Sydney & 6 years old (56,773)
3 = Greater Sydney & 7 years old (55,339)
4 = Greater Sydney & 8 years old (55,105)
5 = Greater Sydney & 9 years old (53,645)
6 = Greater Sydney & 10 years old (54,454)
7 = Greater Sydney & 11 years old (54,670)
8 = Greater Sydney & 12 years old (53,886)
9 = Greater Sydney & 13 years old (54,130)
10 = Greater Sydney & 14 years old (55,155)
11 = Rest of NSW & 5 years old (33,470)
12 = Rest of NSW & 6 years old (32,588)
13 = Rest of NSW & 7 years old (32,220)
14 = Rest of NSW & 8 years old (32,340)
15 = Rest of NSW & 9 years old (32,793)
16 = Rest of NSW & 10 years old (33,727)
17 = Rest of NSW & 11 years old (34,039)
18 = Rest of NSW & 12 years old (34,537)
19 = Rest of NSW & 13 years old (34,654)
20 = Rest of NSW & 14 years old (34,899)

Child's sex

1 = Greater Sydney & male (283,832)
2 = Greater Sydney & female (267,987)
3 = Rest of NSW & male (172,631)
4 = Rest of NSW & female (162,636)

Child's Indigenous status

1 = Greater Sydney & child non-Indigenous (538,595)
2 = Greater Sydney & child Indigenous (13,224)
3 = Rest of NSW & child non-Indigenous (304,615)
4 = Rest of NSW & child Indigenous (30,652)

Parents'/guardians' country of birth

1 = Greater Sydney & neither parent born overseas (260,385)
2 = Greater Sydney & either parent born overseas (291,434)
3 = Rest of NSW & neither parent born overseas (282,319)
4 = Rest of NSW & either parent born overseas (52,948)

Parents'/guardians' education level

1 = Greater Sydney & neither parent has Bachelor degree or higher (338,671)
2 = Greater Sydney & either parent has Bachelor degree or higher (213,148)
3 = Rest of NSW & neither parent has Bachelor degree or higher (255,139)
4 = Rest of NSW & either parent has Bachelor degree or higher (80,128)

Parents'/guardians' labour force status

1 = Greater Sydney & neither parent employed (81,578)
2 = Greater Sydney & either parent employed (470,241)
3 = Rest of NSW & neither parent employed (58,270)
4 = Rest of NSW & either parent employed (276,997)

Household income

1 = Greater Sydney & low income (170,709)
2 = Greater Sydney & medium income (188,867)
3 = Greater Sydney & high income (192,243)
4 = Rest of NSW & low income (126,741)
5 = Rest of NSW & medium income (134,874)
6 = Rest of NSW & high income (73,652)

Family composition of household
1 = Greater Sydney & one-parent family (103,273)
2 = Greater Sydney & couple family (448,546)
3 = Rest of NSW & one-parent family (84,038)
4 = Rest of NSW & couple family (251,229)
Child's regional location — Local Health District (LHD) regions
1 = Sydney (51,743)
2 = South Western Sydney (124,132)
3 = South Eastern Sydney (82,984)
4 = Illawarra Shoalhaven (47,310)
5 = Western Sydney (113,504)
6 = Nepean Blue Mountains (46,865)
7 = Northern Sydney (101,669)
8 = Central Coast (41,168)
9 = Hunter New England (110,771)
10 = Northern NSW (35,917)
11 = Mid North Coast (26,003)
12 = Southern NSW (24,783)
13 = Murrumbidgee (32,288)
14 = Western NSW (37,896)
15 = Far West (3,859)
16 = Network with Vic (6,194)
Remoteness area
1 = NSW Major cities (638,936)
2 = NSW Inner regional (183,550)
3 = NSW Outer regional (59,146)
4 = NSW Remote (5,454)

Northern Territory (NT)
Child's sex
1 = Greater Darwin & male (8,387)
2 = Greater Darwin & female (8,379)
3 = Rest of NT & male (6,843)
4 = Rest of NT & female (6,319)
Child's Indigenous status by age group
1 = Greater Darwin & child non-Indigenous & 5–6 years old (2,863)
2 = Greater Darwin & child non-Indigenous & 7–8 years old (2,766)
3 = Greater Darwin & child non-Indigenous & 9–10 years old (2,818)
4 = Greater Darwin & child non-Indigenous & 11–12 years old (2,721)
5 = Greater Darwin & child non-Indigenous & 13–14 years old (2,765)
6 = Greater Darwin & child Indigenous & 5–6 years old (560)
7 = Greater Darwin & child Indigenous & 7–8 years old (522)
8 = Greater Darwin & child Indigenous & 9–10 years old (560)
9 = Greater Darwin & child Indigenous & 11-12 years old (540)
10 = Greater Darwin & child Indigenous & 13–14 years old (651)
11 = Rest of NT & child non-Indigenous & 5–6 years old (993)
12 = Rest of NT & child non-Indigenous & 7–8 years old (1,013)
13 = Rest of NT & child non-Indigenous & 9–10 years old (966)
14 = Rest of NT & child non-Indigenous & 11–12 years old (931)
15 = Rest of NT & child non-Indigenous & 13–14 years old (907)
16 = Rest of NT & child Indigenous & 5–6 years old (1,819)
17 = Rest of NT & child Indigenous & 7–8 years old (1,744)
18 = Rest of NT & child Indigenous & 9–10 years old (1,732)
19 = Rest of NT & child Indigenous & 11–12 years old (1,573)
20 = Rest of NT & child Indigenous & 13–14 years old (1,484)

Oral health of Australian children

Parents'/guardians' country of birth
1 = Greater Darwin & neither parent born overseas (10,612)
2 = Greater Darwin & either parent born overseas (6,154)
3 = Rest of NT & neither parent born overseas (11,403)
4 = Rest of NT & either parent born overseas (1,759)
Parents'/guardians' education level
1 = Greater Darwin & neither parent has Bachelor degree or higher (12,011)
2 = Greater Darwin & either parent has Bachelor degree or higher (4,755)
3 = Rest of NT & neither parent has Bachelor degree or higher (11,212)
4 = Rest of NT & either parent has Bachelor degree or higher (1,950)
Parents'/guardians' labour force status
1 = Greater Darwin & neither parent employed (2,000)
2 = Greater Darwin & either parent employed (14,766)
3 = Rest of NT & neither parent employed (3,851)
4 = Rest of NT & either parent employed (9,311)
Household income
1 = Greater Darwin & low income (3,852)
2 = Greater Darwin & medium income (6,269)
3 = Greater Darwin & high income (6,645)
4 = Rest of NT & low income (6,304)
5 = Rest of NT & medium income (4,056)
6 = Rest of NT & high income (2,802)
Family composition of household
1 = Greater Darwin & one-parent family (3,643)
2 = Greater Darwin & couple family (13,123)
3 = Rest of NT & one-parent family (3,576)
4 = Rest of NT & couple family (9,586)

Notes:

- Due to the large Indigenous population in the Northern Territory, the variables Indigenous status and Age were combined to create raking categories defined by GCCSA region by Indigenous status by two-year age group.
- Statistical Area Level 4 (SA4) regions are equivalent to GCCSA regions and therefore regional location was not required in the raking procedure.
- Remoteness area was excluded from the raking procedure as the process failed to converge when this variable was included. Despite this, the weighted sample totals derived from the final weights were similar to the population totals for this variable.

Queensland (Qld)

Child's age
1 = Greater Brisbane & 5 years old (28,793)
2 = Greater Brisbane & 6 years old (28,209)
3 = Greater Brisbane & 7 years old (27,283)
4 = Greater Brisbane & 8 years old (26,270)
5 = Greater Brisbane & 9 years old (26,967)
6 = Greater Brisbane & 10 years old (27,174)
7 = Greater Brisbane & 11 years old (26,758)
8 = Greater Brisbane & 12 years old (26,934)
9 = Greater Brisbane & 13 years old (27,225)
10 = Greater Brisbane & 14 years old (27,489)
11 = Rest of Qld & 5 years old (31,710)
12 = Rest of Qld & 6 years old (30,727)
13 = Rest of Qld & 7 years old (30,137)
14 = Rest of Qld & 8 years old (30,021)
15 = Rest of Qld & 9 years old (30,499)
16 = Rest of Qld & 10 years old (31,355)
17 = Rest of Qld & 11 years old (31,201)
18 = Rest of Qld & 12 years old (31,181)
19 = Rest of Qld & 13 years old (31,655)
20 = Rest of Qld & 14 years old (31,681)

Child's sex
1 = Greater Brisbane & male (140,118)
2 = Greater Brisbane & female (132,984)
3 = Rest of Qld & male (158,842)
4 = Rest of Qld & female (151,325)

Child's Indigenous status
1 = Greater Brisbane & child non-Indigenous (262,403)
2 = Greater Brisbane & child Indigenous (10,699)
3 = Rest of Qld & child non-Indigenous (280,386)
4 = Rest of Qld & child Indigenous (29,781)

Parents'/guardians' country of birth
1 = Greater Brisbane & neither parent born overseas (165,958)
2 = Greater Brisbane & either parent born overseas (107,144)
3 = Rest of Qld & neither parent born overseas (231,761)
4 = Rest of Qld & either parent born overseas (78,406)

Parents'/guardians' education level
1 = Greater Brisbane & neither parent has Bachelor degree or higher (181,151)
2 = Greater Brisbane & either parent has Bachelor degree or higher (91,951)
3 = Rest of Qld & neither parent has Bachelor degree or higher (240,155)
4 = Rest of Qld & either parent has Bachelor degree or higher (70,012)

Parents'/guardians' labour force status
1 = Greater Brisbane & neither parent employed (38,500)
2 = Greater Brisbane & either parent employed (234,602)
3 = Rest of Qld & neither parent employed (51,597)
4 = Rest of Qld & either parent employed (258,570)

Household income
1 = Greater Brisbane & low income (79,041)
2 = Greater Brisbane & medium income (108,327)
3 = Greater Brisbane & high income (85,734)
4 = Rest of Qld & low income (110,972)
5 = Rest of Qld & medium income (126,559)
6 = Rest of Qld & high income (72,637)

Oral health of Australian children

Family composition of household
1 = Greater Brisbane & one-parent family (140,118)
2 = Greater Brisbane & couple family (132,984)
3 = Rest of Qld & one-parent family (158,842)
4 = Rest of Qld & couple family (151,325)
Child's regional location — Statistical Area Level 4 (SA4) regions
1 = Brisbane — East (29,550)
2 = Brisbane — North (22,175)
3 = Brisbane — South (36,940)
4 = Brisbane — West (21,920)
5 = Brisbane Inner City (20,062)
6 = Cairns (32,390)
7 = Darling Downs — Maranoa (18,309)
8 = Fitzroy (30,975)
9 = Gold Coast (63,023)
10 = Ipswich (42,473)
11 = Logan — Beaudesert (44,098)
12 = Mackay (23,228)
13 = Moreton Bay — North (30,174)
14 = Moreton Bay — South (25,710)
15 = Queensland — Outback (13,548)
16 = Sunshine Coast (40,491)
17 = Toowoomba (20,016)
18 = Townsville (30,660)
19 = Wide Bay (37,527)
Remoteness area
1 = Qld Major cities (345,957)
2 = Qld Inner regional (126,136)
3 = Qld Outer regional (91,535)
4 = Qld Remote (19,641)

South Australia (SA)
Child's age
1 = Greater Adelaide & 5 years old (14,623)
2 = Greater Adelaide & 6 years old (14,094)
3 = Greater Adelaide & 7 years old (14,106)
4 = Greater Adelaide & 8 years old (13,955)
5 = Greater Adelaide & 9 years old (14,025)
6 = Greater Adelaide & 10 years old (14,185)
7 = Greater Adelaide & 11 years old (14,473)
8 = Greater Adelaide & 12 years old (14,801)
9 = Greater Adelaide & 13 years old (14,786)
10 = Greater Adelaide & 14 years old (14,934)
11 = Rest of SA & 5 years old (4,601)
12 = Rest of SA & 6 years old (4,671)
13 = Rest of SA & 7 years old (4,612)
14 = Rest of SA & 8 years old (4,580)
15 = Rest of SA & 9 years old (4,662)
16 = Rest of SA & 10 years old (4,700)
17 = Rest of SA & 11 years old (4,969)
18 = Rest of SA & 12 years old (4,965)
19 = Rest of SA & 13 years old (4,937)
20 = Rest of SA & 14 years old (5,083)

Childs sex
1 = Greater Adelaide & male (73,630)
2 = Greater Adelaide & female (70,352)
3 = Rest of SA & male (24,444)
4 = Rest of SA & female (23,336)
Child's Indigenous status
1 = Greater Adelaide & child non-Indigenous (140,181)
2 = Greater Adelaide & child Indigenous (3,801)
3 = Rest of SA & child non-Indigenous (44,289)
4 = Rest of SA & child Indigenous (3,491)
Parents'/guardians' country of birth
1 = Greater Adelaide & neither parent born overseas (93,955)
2 = Greater Adelaide & either parent born overseas (50,027)
3 = Rest of SA & neither parent born overseas (41,108)
4 = Rest of SA & either parent born overseas (6,672)
Parents'/guardians' education level
1 = Greater Adelaide & neither parent has Bachelor degree or higher (98,283)
2 = Greater Adelaide & either parent has Bachelor degree or higher (45,699)
3 = Rest of SA & neither parent has Bachelor degree or higher (39,994)
4 = Rest of SA & either parent has Bachelor degree or higher (7,786)
Parents'/guardians' labour force status
1 = Greater Adelaide & neither parent employed (22,336)
2 = Greater Adelaide & either parent employed (121,646)
3 = Rest of SA & neither parent employed (8,227)
4 = Rest of SA & either parent employed (39,553)
Household income
1 = Greater Adelaide & low income (49,083)
2 = Greater Adelaide & medium income (59,458)
3 = Greater Adelaide & high income (35,441)
4 = Rest of SA & low income (19,786)
5 = Rest of SA & medium income (20,791)
6 = Rest of SA & high income (7,203)
Family composition of household
1 = Greater Adelaide & one-parent family (32,477)
2 = Greater Adelaide & couple family (111,505)
3 = Rest of SA & one-parent family (11,066)
4 = Rest of SA & couple family (36,714)
Child's regional location — Statistical Area Level 4 (SA4) regions
1 = Adelaide Central and Hills (31,010)
2 = Adelaide North (50,357)
3 = Adelaide South (39,932)
4 = Adelaide West (22,683)
5 = Barossa — Yorke — Mid North (13,664)
6 = SA Outback (11,719)
7 = SA South East (22,397)
Remoteness area
1 = SA Major cities (134,682)
2 = SA Inner regional (22,907)
3 = SA Outer regional (26,304)
4 = SA Remote (7,869)

Oral health of Australian children

Tasmania (Tas)

Child's age
1 = Greater Hobart & 5 years old (2,710)
2 = Greater Hobart & 6 years old (2,624)
3 = Greater Hobart & 7 years old (2,489)
4 = Greater Hobart & 8 years old (2,565)
5 = Greater Hobart & 9 years old (2,544)
6 = Greater Hobart & 10 years old (2,676)
7 = Greater Hobart & 11 years old (2,601)
8 = Greater Hobart & 12 years old (2,674)
9 = Greater Hobart & 13 years old (2,672)
10 = Greater Hobart & 14 years old (2,689)
11 = Rest of Tas & 5 years old (3,662)
12 = Rest of Tas & 6 years old (3,554)
13 = Rest of Tas & 7 years old (3,484)
14 = Rest of Tas & 8 years old (3,448)
15 = Rest of Tas & 9 years old (3,673)
16 = Rest of Tas & 10 years old (3,693)
17 = Rest of Tas & 11 years old (3,912)
18 = Rest of Tas & 12 years old (4,008)
19 = Rest of Tas & 13 years old (3,847)
20 = Rest of Tas & 14 years old (4,091)

Child's sex
1 = Greater Hobart & male (13,662)
2 = Greater Hobart & female (12,582)
3 = Rest of Tas & male (19,243)
4 = Rest of Tas & female (18,129)

Child's Indigenous status
1 = Greater Hobart & child non-Indigenous (24,595)
2 = Greater Hobart & child Indigenous (1,649)
3 = Rest of Tas & child non-Indigenous (34,232)
4 = Rest of Tas & child Indigenous (3,140)

Parents'/guardians' country of birth
1 = Greater Hobart & neither parent born overseas (21,338)
2 = Greater Hobart & either parent born overseas (4,906)
3 = Rest of Tas & neither parent born overseas (32,266)
4 = Rest of Tas & either parent born overseas (5,106)

Parents'/guardians' education level
1 = Greater Hobart & neither parent has Bachelor degree or higher (18,773)
2 = Greater Hobart & either parent has Bachelor degree or higher (7,471)
3 = Rest of Tas & neither parent has Bachelor degree or higher (30,171)
4 = Rest of Tas & either parent has Bachelor degree or higher (7,201)

Parents'/guardians' labour force status
1 = Greater Hobart & neither parent employed (4,490)
2 = Greater Hobart & either parent employed (21,754)
3 = Rest of Tas & neither parent employed (7,314)
4 = Rest of Tas & either parent employed (30,058)

Household income
1 = Greater Hobart & low income (9,717)
2 = Greater Hobart & medium income (10,728)
3 = Greater Hobart & high income (5,799)
4 = Rest of Tas & low income (16,079)
5 = Rest of Tas & medium income (16,274)
6 = Rest of Tas & high income (5,019)

Family composition of household
1 = Greater Hobart & one-parent family (6,785)
2 = Greater Hobart & couple family (19,459)
3 = Rest of Tas & one-parent family (9,016)
4 = Rest of Tas & couple family (28,356)
Childs regional location — Statistical Area Level 4 (SA4) regions
1 = Hobart (26,244)
2 = Launceston and North East (17,801)
3 = South East (4,830)
4 = West and North West (14,741)
Remoteness area
1 = Tas Inner regional (41,227)
2 = Tas Outer regional/Remote (22,389)
Notes:
- Due to very few children being examined in remote areas of Tasmania the Remote category (1.8% of the child population) was combined with the Outer regional category (33.4% of the child population).

Victoria (Vic)
Child's age
1 = Greater Melbourne & 5 years old (51,632)
2 = Greater Melbourne & 6 years old (49,477)
3 = Greater Melbourne & 7 years old (48,903)
4 = Greater Melbourne & 8 years old (47,845)
5 = Greater Melbourne & 9 years old (47,323)
6 = Greater Melbourne & 10 years old (47,564)
7 = Greater Melbourne & 11 years old (47,813)
8 = Greater Melbourne & 12 years old (47,727)
9 = Greater Melbourne & 13 years old (47,754)
10 = Greater Melbourne & 14 years old (48,526)
11 = Rest of Vic & 5 years old (17,142)
12 = Rest of Vic & 6 years old (16,635)
13 = Rest of Vic & 7 years old (16,650)
14 = Rest of Vic & 8 years old (16,591)
15 = Rest of Vic & 9 years old (16,863)
16 = Rest of Vic & 10 years old (17,124)
17 = Rest of Vic & 11 years old (17,471)
18 = Rest of Vic & 12 years old (17,995)
19 = Rest of Vic & 13 years old (18,123)
20 = Rest of Vic & 14 years old (18,779)
Child's sex
1 = Greater Melbourne & male (248,024)
2 = Greater Melbourne & female (236,540)
3 = Rest of Vic & male (89,392)
4 = Rest of Vic & female (83,981)
Child's Indigenous status
1 = Greater Melbourne & child non-Indigenous (480,483)
2 = Greater Melbourne & child Indigenous (4,081)
3 = Rest of Vic & child non-Indigenous (168,357)
4 = Rest of Vic & child Indigenous (5,016)
Parents'/guardians' country of birth
1 = Greater Melbourne & neither parent born overseas (262,913)
2 = Greater Melbourne & either parent born overseas (221,651)
3 = Rest of Vic & neither parent born overseas (147,891)
4 = Rest of Vic & either parent born overseas (25,482)

Parents'/guardians' education level
1 = Greater Melbourne & neither parent has Bachelor degree or higher (296,819)
2 = Greater Melbourne & either parent has Bachelor degree or higher (187,745)
3 = Rest of Vic & neither parent has Bachelor degree or higher (130,711)
4 = Rest of Vic & either parent has Bachelor degree or higher (42,662)
Parents'/guardians' labour force status
1 = Greater Melbourne & neither parent employed (63,023)
2 = Greater Melbourne & either parent employed (421,541)
3 = Rest of Vic & neither parent employed (26,634)
4 = Rest of Vic & either parent employed (146,739)
Household income
1 = Greater Melbourne & low income (149,612)
2 = Greater Melbourne & medium income (185,932)
3 = Greater Melbourne & high income (149,020)
4 = Rest of Vic & low income (66,319)
5 = Rest of Vic & medium income (76,376)
6 = Rest of Vic & high income (30,678)
Family composition of household
1 = Greater Melbourne & one-parent family (88,004)
2 = Greater Melbourne & couple family (396,560)
3 = Rest of Vic & one-parent family (39,894)
4 = Rest of Vic & couple family (133,479)
Childs regional location – Dental Health Service (DHS) regions
1 = Barwon South West (46,439)
2 = Grampians (28,897)
3 = Loddon Mallee (40,974)
4 = Hume (35,693)
5 = Gippsland (32,306)
6 = Western Metro (95,098)
7 = Northern Metro (101,906)
8 = Eastern Metro (119,021)
9 = Southern Metro (157,603)
Remoteness area
1 = Vic Major cities (485,375)
2 = Vic Inner regional (140,379)
3 = Vic Outer regional (31,667)
4 = Vic Remote (516)

Western Australia (WA)

Child's age
1 = Greater Perth & 5 years old (23,081)
2 = Greater Perth & 6 years old (22,146)
3 = Greater Perth & 7 years old (21,925)
4 = Greater Perth & 8 years old (21,650)
5 = Greater Perth & 9 years old (21,300)
6 = Greater Perth & 10 years old (21,813)
7 = Greater Perth & 11 years old (22,031)
8 = Greater Perth & 12 years old (22,856)
9 = Greater Perth & 13 years old (22,850)
10 = Greater Perth & 14 years old (23,078)
11 = Rest of WA & 5 years old (7,509)
12 = Rest of WA & 6 years old (7,217)
13 = Rest of WA & 7 years old (7,049)
14 = Rest of WA & 8 years old (6,998)
15 = Rest of WA & 9 years old (7,190)
16 = Rest of WA & 10 years old (7,395)
17 = Rest of WA & 11 years old (7,393)
18 = Rest of WA & 12 years old (7,336)
19 = Rest of WA & 13 years old (6,889)
20 = Rest of WA & 14 years old (6,855)
Child's sex
1 = Greater Perth & male (113,897)
2 = Greater Perth & female (108,833)
3 = Rest of WA & male (36,221)
4 = Rest of WA & female (35,610)
Child's Indigenous status
1 = Greater Perth & child non-Indigenous (215,808)
2 = Greater Perth & child Indigenous (6,922)
3 = Rest of WA & child non-Indigenous (61,113)
4 = Rest of WA & child Indigenous (10,718)
Parents'/guardians' country of birth
1 = Greater Perth & neither parent born overseas (107,122)
2 = Greater Perth & either parent born overseas (115,608)
3 = Rest of WA & neither parent born overseas (53,547)
4 = Rest of WA & either parent born overseas (18,284)
Parents'/guardians' education level
1 = Greater Perth & neither parent has Bachelor degree or higher (146,848)
2 = Greater Perth & either parent has Bachelor degree or higher (75,882)
3 = Rest of WA & neither parent has Bachelor degree or higher (57,520)
4 = Rest of WA & either parent has Bachelor degree or higher (14,311)
Parents'/guardians' labour force status
1 = Greater Perth & neither parent employed (29,947)
2 = Greater Perth & either parent employed (192,783)
3 = Rest of WA & neither parent employed (11,710)
4 = Rest of WA & either parent employed (60,121)
Household income
1 = Greater Perth & low income (57,803)
2 = Greater Perth & medium income (80,149)
3 = Greater Perth & high income (84,778)
4 = Rest of WA & low income (23,921)
5 = Rest of WA & medium income (26,697)
6 = Rest of WA & high income (21,213)

Oral health of Australian children

Family composition of household
1 = Greater Perth & one-parent family (42,437)
2 = Greater Perth & couple family (180,293)
3 = Rest of WA & one-parent family (15,385)
4 = Rest of WA & couple family (56,446)
Childs regional location — Statistical Area Level 4 (SA4) regions
1 = Bunbury (22,655)
2 = Mandurah (10,811)
3 = Perth Inner (16,376)
4 = Perth North East (29,514)
5 = Perth North West (64,907)
6 = Perth South East (53,873)
7 = Perth South West (47,249)
8 = WA Outback (30,887)
9 = WA Wheat Belt (18,289)
Remoteness area
1 = WA Major cities (217,370)
2 = WA Inner regional (29,808)
3 = WA Outer regional (26,063)
4 = WA Remote (21,320)

Appendix 2: State and territory survey personnel

ACT

Survey manager	Amanda Blyton-Patterson
Co-ordinator	Amanda Blyton-Patterson
Dental examiners	Ruth Vosseler, Elizabeth Doyle, Patricia Mason, Heather Pinder
Dental recorders	Karen Harmsworth, Jenny Wardrobe, Brooke Morris, Kristin Alsemgeest, Danielle Pearce

NSW

Survey manager	Tanya Schinkewitsch
Co-ordinator	Tanya Schinkewitsch
Dental examiners	Leonie Green, Lynne Brissett, Katherine Price, Debbie McGibbon, Brianne Bartos, Julie Kelpsa, Angela Rankin, Jenny Lang, Sharyn James, Joanne Johnson, Hollie Day, Karen Kennedy, Helen Lee, Sharon Stuhl
Dental recorders	Michele Tait – Kerr, Beth Rieger, Leeona Harrison, Annette Dix, Elizabeth Di Meco, Sung Yang, Katherine Price, Natalie Jaksic, Cheryl Bedford, Lia Pagdanganan, Karen O'Grady.

NT

Survey manager	Patricia Slocum
Co-ordinator	Maria Ciarla
Dental examiners	Sally Finlay, Debbie Beldham, Lorrae Beckett, Imogen Hoppmann, Joanne Nelson, Melody Foh, Shavaya Huskinson
Dental recorders	Leanne Rigby, Pollyanna Walker, Tiffany Ammenhauser, Sarah Jones, Karen MacGregor, Khayla De Aussen

Qld

Survey manager	Ben Stute, Rhys Thomas
Co-ordinator	Zoe Johnson
Dental team members	Sue Batterham, Kym Baxter, Lauren Bonar, Susan Brain, Jo-Anne Bunyan, Kathy Burns, Michelle Campbell, Jillian Clyde, Amanda Corbett, Tonia Danes, Kathyrn Davis, Elizabeth De Silva, Wendy Doyle, Sue Douglass, Catherine Draney, Diana Hill, Colleen Hull, Maria Jones, Kerry Keene, Donna Knowles, Amanda Liddell, Gail Masters, Louise McGlinchey, Terri McIntosh, Cheryl McMahon, Margaret Moore, Kerrie O'Shea, Rebecca Osmond, Amanda Philp, Judith Plahn, Melissa Plath, Rhonda Roan, Jennifer Roberts, Terri Roser, Jenny Romagnolo, Lisa Rush, Tracy Sharp, Shelley Sinclair, Allison Smallwood, Kirrilea Smyth, Casey Soper, Christine Southall, Lauren Stockham, Deb Tector, Louise, Thompson, Lesley Toomey, Maria Turpie, Cathy Vaughan, Donna Weaver, Jane Yorkston

SA

Survey manager	Geoff Franklin
Co-ordinator	Anne Saunders
Dental examiners	Kerryn Aslin, Julie Brown, Marilyn Hutchison, Elizabeth Maddigan, Sue Neil, Rosie Winter, Brooke Breath
Dental recorders	Kristy Boord, Jacqueline Clark, Robyn Fanning, Marie Georgiou, Merridee Korner, Leanne Leicester, Lorraine Symons, Karen Miller, Erin Daniell

Vic

Survey manager	Andrea de Silva
Co-ordinator	Panagiota Gkolia
Dental examiners	Jane Abagia, Ashley Hew, Lina Koubar, Kristin Abdel-Nour, Cherie Borwick, Tracy Nguyen, Alison Avery, Mariam Botros
Dental recorders	Emilie Azzopardi, Ann Tudor, Ivanka Lazaneo, Yvette Hayward, Merala Lesevic, Catherine Kruljac, Marita Sorensen, Jiya Paul, Chris O'Dowd

Tas

Survey manager	Angie Byrom, Robyn Nikolai
Co-ordinator	Rosie Collier
Dental examiners	Jade Phillips, Lynn Cripps, Leigh Gorringe, Sally Page, Gail White, Rose Abbott, Sandra Martin, Sharon Smith
Dental recorders	Laura Rainbird, Mel Daniels, Julie Rush, Serena Summers, Kerrin Sykes, Ebony Skeggs, Tameika Cummings, Robyn Smith, Brooke Murfet

WA

Survey manager	Peter Arrow
Co-ordinator	Vicki Gatsos
Dental examiners	Jane King, Ms Sue Piggott, Ms Maree Waddell, Ms Anne-Marie Hayes
Dental recorders	Trina Donald, Ms Kerry Law, Ms Diana Reymond, Ms Dianne Winston

Note: Some examination team members in Qld acted as both examiners and recorders.

Symbols

$	Australian dollars
. .	not applicable
%	per cent
—	nil
n.p.	not published because estimate is statistically imprecise
>	greater than
<	less than
≥	greater than or equal to
≤	less than or equal to

Abbreviations

ABS	Australian Bureau of Statistics
AHMAC	Australian Health Ministers' Advisory Council
AIHW	Australian Institute of Health and Welfare
ARCPOH	Australian Research Centre for Population Oral Health
CD	Census collectors' district
dmfs/DMFS	Number of decayed, missing and filled permanent surfaces
ds/DS	Decayed surfaces
dmft/DMFT	Number of decayed, missing and filled permanent teeth
dt/DT	Decayed teeth
ERP	Estimated resident population
fs/FS	Filled surfaces
ft/FT	Filled teeth
ICC	Intra-class correlation coefficient
ICSEA	Index of Community Socio-Educational Advantage
IQR	Interquartile range
IRSAD	Index of Relative Socioeconomic Advantage/Disadvantage
mt/MT	Missing teeth
NACOH	National Advisory Committee on Oral Health
NCHS	US National Center for Health Statistics
NHANES	US National Health and Nutrition Examination Survey
NHMRC	National Health and Medical Research Council
NOHSA	National Oral Health Survey of Australia 1987–88
SEIFA	Socio-Economic Indexes for Areas
WHO	World Health Organization

Place names

ACT   Australian Capital Territory
NSW   New South Wales
NT   Northern Territory
Qld   Queensland
SA   South Australia
Tas   Tasmania
UK   United Kingdom
US   United States
Vic   Victoria
WA   Western Australia

Glossary

95% confidence interval Defines the uncertainty around an estimated value. There is a 95% probability that the true value falls within the range of the upper and lower limits.

Absolute difference The difference between two values calculated by subtracting one value from the other.

Birth cohort A group of people born during a particular period or year (also referred to as a generation).

Birth cohort analysis Analysis that evaluates changes within cohorts over time and between cohorts.

Calibration A procedure to promote standardisation between examiners performing the oral examinations.

Canine One of four 'eye teeth' positioned next to the incisors and used for tearing food.

Capital city The administrative seat of government of each of Australia's six states and two territories. Each capital city also represents the most populous location of its respective state or territory.

Census The Census of Population and Housing conducted every five years by the Australian Bureau of Statistics.

Coronal Pertaining to the crown of a tooth.

Crown The portion of tooth covered by white enamel that usually is visible in the mouth.

Dental attendance Behaviour related to the use of dental services.

Dental caries The process in which tooth structure is destroyed by acid produced by bacteria in the mouth. See Dental decay.

Dental caries experience The cumulative effect of the caries process through a person's lifetime, manifesting as teeth that are decayed, missing or filled.

Dental decay Cavity resulting from dental caries.

Dentition The set of teeth. A complete primary dentition comprises of 20 primary/deciduous teeth. A complete permanent dentition comprises 32 adult teeth.

dmfs/DMFS An index of dental caries experience measured by counting the number of decayed (d/D), missing (m/M), and filled (f/F) surfaces (s/S).

dmft/DMFT An index of dental caries experience measured by counting the number of decayed (d/D), missing (m/M), and filled (f/F) teeth (t/T).

Enamel Hard, white mineralised tissue covering the crown of a tooth.

Epidemiology The study of the distribution and causes of health and disease in populations.

Erupted tooth A tooth that has emerged through the gums into the mouth.

Examination protocol Methods and guidelines for conducting standardised oral examinations conducted in a survey.

Extraction Removal of a natural tooth.

Fluoride A naturally occurring trace mineral that helps to prevent tooth decay.

Fluorosis Discolouration or pitting of the dental enamel caused by exposure to excessive amounts of fluoride during enamel formation.

Gingiva Gum tissue.

Gingivitis Redness, swelling or bleeding of the gums caused by inflammation.

Incisor One of eight front teeth used during eating for cutting food.

Index of Relative Socioeconomic Advantage/Disadvantage (IRSAD) One of four indices measuring area-level disadvantage derived by the Australian Bureau of Statistics. The IRSAD is derived from attributes such as low income, low educational attainment, high unemployment and jobs in relatively unskilled occupations.

Index of Community Socio-Educational Advantage (ICSEA) an indication of the socio-educational backgrounds of students at a certain school.

Indigenous identity A person who states that they are of Aboriginal and/or Torres Strait Islander descent is an Indigenous Australian.

Interproximal Between the teeth.

Intra-class correlation coefficient A statistical term referring to a measure of agreement between two or more examiners.

Mandible Lower jaw.

Maxilla Upper jaw.

Mean The arithmetic average of a set of values.

Molar One of 8 primary or 12 permanent back teeth used in grinding food.

Natural teeth Refers to a person's own teeth as opposed to artificial teeth.

Participation rate The proportion of people from whom survey information is collected from among the total number of people selected as intended study participants.

Permanent teeth Adult teeth (secondary teeth).

Plaque A film composed of bacteria and food debris that adheres to the tooth surface.

Prevalence The proportion of people with a defined disease within a defined population.

Primary teeth Deciduous/baby teeth.

Public dental care state- or territory-funded dental care.

Recorder A person, usually a dental assistant, who recorded the results of an oral examination onto a laptop computer.

Relative difference The difference between two values calculated as a ratio of one value divided by another.

Restoration A filling to repair a tooth damaged by decay or injury.

Oral health of Australian children

Sampling bias A flaw in either the study design or selection of participants that leads to an erroneous interpretation.

Socio-Economic Indexes for Areas (SEIFA) A set of four indices derived by the Australian Bureau of Statistics from population census data to measure aspects of socioeconomic position for geographic areas.

Socioeconomic position Descriptive term for a position in society and usually measured by attributes such as income, education, occupation or characteristics of residential area.

State/territory Geographic regions of Australia. The nation has six states and two territories.

Statistical significance An indication from a statistical test that an observed association is unlikely (usually less than 5% probability) to be due to chance created when a random sample of people is selected from a population.

Trend The general direction in which change over time is observed.

Unerupted tooth A tooth that has failed to emerge through the gums into the mouth.

Weights Numbers applied to groups of study participants to correct for differences in probability of selection and in participation.

List of tables

Oral health of Australian children

List of figures

Electronic Index

This book is available as a free fully-searchable ebook from
www.adelaide.edu.au/press